Orbital Reconstruction

Editors
LEANDER DUBOIS
ALFRED G. BECKING

ATLAS OF THE ORAL AND MAXILLOFACIAL SURGERY CLINICS OF NORTH AMERICA

www.oralmaxsurgeryatlas.theclinics.com

Consulting Editor
RUI P. FERNANDES

March 2021 • Volume 29 • Number 1

ELSEVIER

1600 John F. Kennedy Boulevard • Suite 1800 • Philadelphia, Pennsylvania, 19103-2899
http://www.oralmaxsurgeryatlas.theclinics.com

ATLAS OF THE ORAL AND MAXILLOFACIAL SURGERY CLINICS OF NORTH AMERICA Volume 29, Number 1 March 2021 ISSN 1061-3315 ISBN-13: 978-0-323-79073-4

Editor: John Vassallo; j.vassallo@elsevier.com
Developmental Editor: Laura Fisher

Reprints. For copies of 100 or more of articles in this publication, please contact the Commercial Reprints Department, Elsevier Inc., 360 Park Avenue South, New York, NY 10010-1710. Tel.: 212-633-3874; Fax: 212-633-3820; E-mail: reprints@elsevier.com.

Atlas of the Oral and Maxillofacial Surgery Clinics of North America (ISSN 1061-3315) is published biannually by Elsevier, 360 Park Avenue South, New York, NY 10010-1710. Months of issue are March and September. Periodicals postage paid at New York, NY and additional mailing offices. Subscription prices are $474.00 for international individual, $396.00 for US individual, $416.00 for Canadian individual; $220.00 for international student, $100.00 for US student and Canadian student; $615.00 for international institution, $615.00 for Canadian institution, $600.00 for US institution. Foreign air speed delivery is included in all *Clinics* subscription prices. All prices are subject to change without notice. POSTMASTER: Send address changes to *Atlas of the Oral and Maxillofacial Surgery Clinics of North America*, Health Sciences Division, Subscription Customer Service, 3251 Riverport Lane, Maryland Heights, MO 63043. Tel: 1-800-654-2452 (U.S. and Canada); 314-447-8871 (outside U.S. and Canada). Fax: 314-417-8029. E-mail: journalscustomerservice-usa@elsevier.com (for print support); journalsonline support-usa@elsevier.com (for online support).

Atlas of the Oral and Maxillofacial Surgery Clinics of North America is covered in *MEDLINE/PubMed (Index Medicus)*.

Printed in the United States of America.

Contributors

CONSULTING EDITOR

RUI P. FERNANDES, MD, DMD, FACS, FRCS(Ed)
Clinical Professor and Chief, Division of Head and Neck Surgery, Program Director, Head and Neck Oncologic Surgery and Microvascular Reconstruction Fellowship, Departments of Oral and Maxillofacial Surgery, Neurosurgery, and Orthopaedic Surgery and Rehabilitation, University of Florida Health Science Center, University of Florida College of Medicine-Jacksonville, Jacksonville, Florida, USA

EDITORS

LEANDER DUBOIS, DDS, MD, DMD, PhD
Department of Oral and Maxillofacial Surgery, Amsterdam University Medical Centers, University of Amsterdam, Academic Center of Dentistry Amsterdam (ACTA), Amsterdam, the Netherlands; Department of Oral and Maxillofacial Surgery, St Antonius Hospital Utrecht/Nieuwegein/Woerden, the Netherlands

ALFRED G. BECKING, DDS, MD, DMD, PhD, FEBOMS
Department of Oral and Maxillofacial Surgery, Amsterdam University Medical Centers, University of Amsterdam, Academic Center of Dentistry Amsterdam (ACTA), Amsterdam, the Netherlands; Department of Oral and Maxillofacial Surgery, MKA Kennemer & Meer, Haarlem, the Netherlands

AUTHORS

ALFRED G. BECKING, DDS, MD, DMD, PhD, FEBOMS
Department of Oral and Maxillofacial Surgery, Amsterdam University Medical Centers, University of Amsterdam, Academic Center of Dentistry Amsterdam (ACTA), Amsterdam, the Netherlands; Department of Oral and Maxillofacial Surgery, MKA Kennemer & Meer, Haarlem, the Netherlands

RICHARD BRYAN BELL, MD, DDS, FACS, FRCS (Ed)
Attending, Earle A. Chiles Research Institute at Robert W. Franz Cancer Center, Providence Head and Neck Cancer Program and Clinic, Providence Cancer Institute, Portland, Oregon, USA

J. EELCO BERGSMA, MD, DMD, PhD
Department of Oral and Maxillofacial Surgery, Amphia Hospital Breda, Breda, the Netherlands

MICHAEL BLUMER, Dr med, Dr med dent
Klinik für Mund-, Kiefer- und Gesichtschirurgie, UniversitätsSpital Zürich, Zürich, Switzerland

YVETTE BRAAKSMA-BESSELINK, CO, MMedSci
Department of Ophthalmology, Amsterdam University Medical Centers, University of Amsterdam, Amsterdam, the Netherlands

JONATHAN CHODROFF, DDS, MD, MEd
Resident, Department of Oral and Maxillofacial Surgery, Oregon Health & Science University, Portland, Oregon, USA

CARL PETER CORNELIUS, MD, DDS
Associate Professor, Klinik und Poliklinik für Mund-, Kiefer- und Gesichtschirurgie der der Ludwig-Maximilians-Universität München, Innenstadtcampus, München, Bavaria, Germany

RONALD O.B. DE KEIZER, MD
Department of Oculoplastic, Orbital and Lacrimal Surgery, The Rotterdam Eye Hospital, Rotterdam, the Netherlands

JASJIT DILLON, MD, DMD, PhD
Clinical Associate Professor, Chief of Service and Program Director, Department of Oral and Maxillofacial Surgery, University of Washington, Harborview Medical Center, Seattle, Washington, USA

LEANDER DUBOIS, DDS, MD, DMD, PhD
Department of Oral and Maxillofacial Surgery, Amsterdam University Medical Centers, University of Amsterdam, Academic Center of Dentistry Amsterdam (ACTA), Amsterdam, the Netherlands; Department of Oral and Maxillofacial Surgery, St Antonius Hospital Utrecht/Nieuwegein/Woerden, the Netherlands

NADIR ELIAS, DMD, MSc
Fellow, Advanced Craniomaxillofacial Surgery and Trauma (2020-2021), Legacy Emanuel Medical Center, Head and Neck Institute, Portland, Oregon, USA

HARALD ESSIG, PD, Dr med, Dr med dent
Klinik für Mund-, Kiefer- und Gesichtschirurgie, UniversitätsSpital Zürich, Zürich, Switzerland

NILS-CLAUDIUS GELLRICH, MD, DDS
Department of Oral and Maxillofacial Surgery, Hannover Medical School, Hannover, Germany

PETER J.J. GOORIS, MD, DMD, PhD, FEBOMFS
Affiliate Professor, Department of Oral and Maxillofacial Surgery, University of Washington, Washington, USA; Staff Member, Department of Oral and Maxillofacial Surgery, University Medical Centre Amsterdam, the Netherlands; Department of Oral and Maxillofacial Surgery, Amphia Hospital Breda, Breda, the Netherlands

GIJSBERT J. HÖTTE, MD
Department of Oculoplastic, Orbital and Lacrimal Surgery, The Rotterdam Eye Hospital, Rotterdam, the Netherlands

SIMON HOLMES, FDS, RCS, FRCS
Professor of Craniofacial Traumatology, Consultant, Maxillofacial Surgeon, Department of Oral and Maxillofacial Surgery, Royal London Hospital and Queen Mary University of London, London, United Kingdom

JESPER JANSEN, MD, DMD, PhD
Orbital Research Group (ACOR), Resident, Department of Oral and Maxillofacial Surgery, University Medical Center Amsterdam, University of Amsterdam, Academic Center of Dentistry Amsterdam, Amsterdam, the Netherlands

HINKE MARIJKE JELLEMA, CO, MMedSci, PhD
Department of Ophthalmology, Amsterdam University Medical Centers, University of Amsterdam, Amsterdam, the Netherlands

CORNELIS KLOP, MSc
Department of Oral and Maxillofacial Surgery, Amsterdam UMC Location AMC and Academic Center for Dentistry Amsterdam (ACTA), University of Amsterdam, Amsterdam, the Netherlands

THOMAS J.J. MAAL, MSc, PhD
Department of Oral and Maxillofacial Surgery, Amsterdam UMC Location AMC and Academic Center for Dentistry Amsterdam (ACTA), University of Amsterdam, Amsterdam, the Netherlands; Department of Oral and Maxillofacial Surgery, Radboud University Medical Centre Nijmegen, Nijmegen, the Netherlands

MARC CHRISTIAN METZGER, MD, DMD
Professor, Klinik für Mund-, Kiefer- und Gesichtschirurgie der, Albert-Ludwigs Universität Freiburg, Freiburg, Baden-Württemberg, Germany

FLORIAN PROBST, MD, DMD, PhD
Klinik und Poliklinik für Mund-, Kiefer- und Gesichtschirurgie der Ludwig-Maximilians-Universität München, Innenstadtcampus, München, Bavaria, Germany

ALEXANDER SCHRAMM, MD, DDS
Department of Oral, Maxillofacial and Plastic Surgery, German Armed Forces Hospital of Ulm, Department of Oral and Maxillofacial Surgery, University Hospital, Ulm University, Ulm, Germany

RUUD SCHREURS, MSc
Orbital Research Group (ACOR), 3D Laboratory, Department of Oral and Maxillofacial Surgery, Amsterdam UMC Location AMC and Academic Center for Dentistry Amsterdam (ACTA), University of Amsterdam, Amsterdam, the Netherlands; Department of Oral and Maxillofacial Surgery, Radboud University Medical Centre Nijmegen, Nijmegen, the Netherlands

CONG VO, DDS, MD
Resident, Department of Oral and Maxillofacial Surgery, Oregon Health & Science University, Portland, Oregon, USA

MAXIMILIAN EBERHARD HERMANN WAGNER, Dr med univ, Dr med dent
Klinik für Mund-, Kiefer- und Gesichtschirurgie, UniversitätsSpital Zürich, Zürich, Switzerland

MICHAEL WHITCOMB, DMD, MD
Resident, Department of Oral and Maxillofacial Surgery, Oregon Health & Science University, Portland, Oregon, USA

FRANK WILDE, MD, DDS
Department of Oral, Maxillofacial and Plastic Surgery, German Armed Forces Hospital of Ulm, Department of Oral and Maxillofacial Surgery, University Hospital, Ulm University, Ulm, Germany

Contents

ATLAS OF THE ORAL AND MAXILLOFACIAL SURGERY CLINICS OF NORTH AMERICA

FORTHCOMING ISSUES

September 2021

Zygomatic Implants
Salam Salman and Anastasiya Quimby, Editors

March 2022

Common Procedures in Craniofacial Surgery
Mark A. Miller and David M. Yates, *Editors*

PREVIOUS ISSUES

September 2020

Computer-Guided Oral and Maxillofacial Surgery
Kevin Arce, *Editor*

March 2020

Reconstruction of Facial Skin Defects
Anthony M. Bunnell, *Editor*

Preface

Up-to-Date on Orbital Trauma and Reconstruction

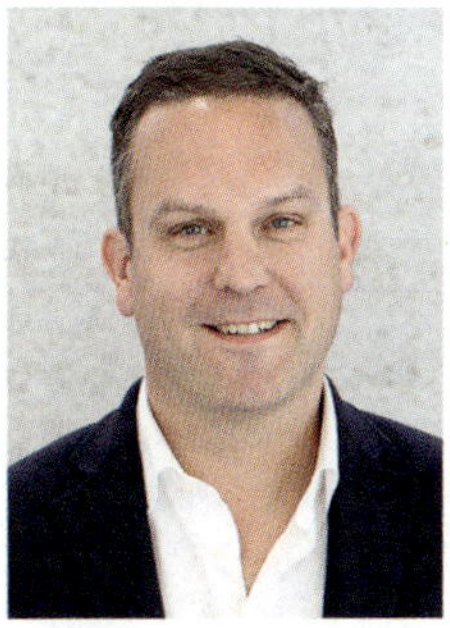

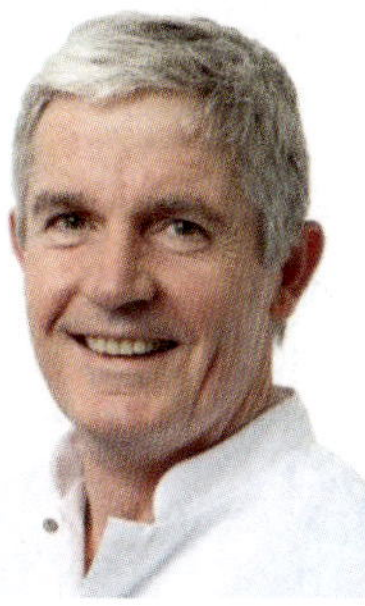

Leander Dubois, DDS, MD, DMD, PhD   Alfred G. Becking, DDS, MD, DMD, PhD, FEBOMS

Editors

The orbit is a complex area with crucial anatomic structures packed into a small space. In orbital fractures not only the bone is involved but also the periorbit with vulnerable soft tissues. Orbital reconstruction is a delicate procedure with the protruding orbital soft tissues limiting the surgical overview. Technological developments like preoperative planning, navigation, additive manufacturing techniques, and intraoperative imaging have increased the predictability of the bony reconstruction in the recent years and are thought to have a favorable effect on the clinical outcome. So, anatomic knowledge and proper indications, combined with a good implemented clinical protocol can help to improve the quality of life for our patients. Above all, orbital fracture management has become a multidisciplinary matter.

This *Atlas of the Oral and Maxillofacial Surgery Clinics of North America* focuses on orbital fracture management for both primary and secondary trauma care. This issue begins with the anatomy of the orbit (Cornelius, Probst, Metzger, and Gooris), ocular injury and emergencies around the globe (Hötte and De Keizer), and the main controversies in orbital reconstructions regarding indications, timing, and biomaterials (Dubois, Dillon, Jansen, and Becking). In order to understand diplopia, the importance of orthoptic evaluation (Braaksma and Jellema) is underlined and how this can be implemented in an evidence-based clinical protocol (Gooris, Jansen, Bergsma, and Dubois). The primary fracture care (Holmes) and best implant for the right are further discussed. The fundamentals of 3D virtual planning

Atlas Oral Maxillofacial Surg Clin N Am 29 (2021) xi–xii
1061-3315/21/© 2020 Published by Elsevier Inc.
https://doi.org/10.1016/j.cxom.2020.11.001

(Schreurs, Klop, and Maal) are explained and how this could be used for intraoperative feedback (Schreurs, Wilde, Schramm, and Gellrich). The complexity of secondary reconstructions is illustrated in solitary orbital fractures (Essig, Wagner, and Blumer) and in combination with NOE, ZMC, or panfacial fractures (Bell). The final article gives a scientific overview of which advanced technology could be used to improve the predictability of the reconstruction (Schreurs, Becking, Jansen, and Dubois).

We want to thank all the authors for their important contributions to this issue of *Atlas of the Oral and Maxillofacial Surgery Clinics of North America*. We especially wish to thank Nils Gellrich, Majeed Rana, and Harald Essig for introducing us to the field of navigation and Peerooz Saeed, Hinke Marijke Jellema, and Maarten Mourits for sharing their valuable insights in ophthalmology and orbital surgery.

Leander Dubois, DDS, MD, DMD, PhD
Department of Oral and Maxillofacial Surgery
Amsterdam University Medical Centers
University of Amsterdam
Academic Center of Dentistry Amsterdam
Amsterdam, The Netherlands

Department of Oral and Maxillofacial Surgery
St Antonius Hospital
Utrecht/Nieuwegein/Woerden, The Netherlands

Alfred G. (Eddy) Becking, DDS, MD, DMD, PhD, FEBOMS
Department of Oral and Maxillofacial Surgery
Amsterdam University Medical Centers
University of Amsterdam
Academic Center of Dentistry Amsterdam
Amsterdam, The Netherlands

Department of Oral and Maxillofacial Surgery
MKA Kennemerland, The Netherlands

E-mail addresses:
l.dubois@amsterdamumc.nl (L. Dubois)
ag.becking@amsterdamumc.nl (A.G. (Eddy) Becking)

Anatomy of the Orbits

Skeletal Features and Some Notes on the Periorbital Lining

Carl Peter Cornelius, MD, DDS [a,*], Florian Probst, MD, DMD, PhD [a],
Marc Christian Metzger, MD, DMD [b], Peter J.J. Gooris, MD, DMD, PhD, FEBOMFS [c,d]

KEYWORDS

• Orbits • Skeletal framework • Periorbital lining • Neural • Vascular pathways

KEY POINTS

- The skeletal framework around the anterior aperture of each orbit and the 4 walls of the orbital cavity can be conceived as a pyramid with a quadrangular base. This pyramid transforms into to a 3-sided posterior apex, because the orbital floor ends at the posterior basin of the inferior orbital fissure.
- Bony openings (canals, grooves, fissures, foramina, notches) provide the pathways for the neurovascular structures linking the intraorbital structures inside the periorbital sac to the cranial cavity, ethmoid and skull base, infratemporal fossa, and face.
- A system of 3 sagittal buttresses along the inferomedial orbital walls contributes to the stability (biomechanical resistance) of the internal orbit.
- Besides the overall dimension of the orbital cavity, the contours and sloping of the inferomedial wall orbital surfaces, with the posteromedial bulge as predominantly, are the key determinants for globe height and globe projection.

Introduction

The orbits are two inversely corresponding bony housings at the transition between the skull base and the midface. They contain the visual organ, consisting of the eyeballs with the refractive apparatus, retinal receptors and the auxilliary adnexa, in particular the lacrimal system and the extraocular muscles (EOM) and moreover the adipose body including innervation [optomotor, special (CN II) and general (CN V) somatosensory, parasympathetic and sympathetic] and vascular supply.

Orbital cavity—bony skeleton

Systematic skeletal description

Each orbit is assembled of 7 bones: zygoma, maxilla, palatine, ethmoid, lacrimal, sphenoid, and frontal. In highly simplified terms, the skeletal components outline a cone-shaped or pear-shaped cavity with a thick marginal rim framing the aperture at its base in contrast to the thin-walled internal orbit (Fig. 1A–D). Various bony openings (canals, grooves, fissures, foramina, and notches) are pathways for neural and vascular linkages to the cranial cavity, infratemporal fossa, paranasal sinuses, inner nose, and the face (see Fig. 1A, B).

Geometric concept

In geometric abstraction, the orbit can be described as a pyramid with a quadrangular base, which converts into a 3-sided tip or apex (Fig. 2A).

The open base, or *aditus ad orbitam*, projects frontolaterally and the apex posteromedially toward the optic foramen.

The junctions of the walls in the superomedial, superolateral, inferolateral, and inferomedial quadrants, or "pyramidal corners", are curved as a matter of fact (Fig. 2B, C).

Orbital walls

The superior orbital wall (roof) to its largest extent consists of the orbital part of the frontal bone (see Fig. 2B; Fig. 3A, B).

The most posterior minor portion at the apex is formed by the lesser wing of the sphenoid (LWS). The orbital roof takes a triangle shape bent up into a concavity. The lacrimal fossa is a shallow depression anterolaterally for the lacrimal gland. The trochlear fovea conforms to the anteromedial adherence zone of the trochlear fiber condensations.

The inferior orbital wall (floor) incorporates the orbital plate of the maxilla as the major area, the orbital plate of the zygoma as anterolateral contribution, and the upper surface (plate) of the orbital process of the palatine bone at the posteromedial end position (see Fig. 1B, C). Analogous to the

[a] Klinik und Poliklinik für Mund-, Kiefer- und Gesichtschirurgie der der Ludwig-Maximilians-Universität München, Innenstadtcampus, Lindwurmstr. 2a, 80337 München, Bavaria, Germany
[b] Klinik für Mund-Kiefer- und Gesichtschirurgie der, Albert-Ludwigs Universität Freiburg, Hugstetter Str. 55, 79106 Freiburg, Baden Württemberg, Germany
[c] Department of Oral and Maxillofacial Surgery, Amphia Hospital Breda, Molengracht 1, 4818 CK Breda, The Netherlands
[d] University Medical Centre Amsterdam, The Netherlands
* Corresponding author.
E-mail address: Peter.Cornelius@med.uni-muenchen.de

Atlas Oral Maxillofacial Surg Clin N Am 29 (2021) 1-18

https://doi.org/10.1016/j.cxom.2020.10.001

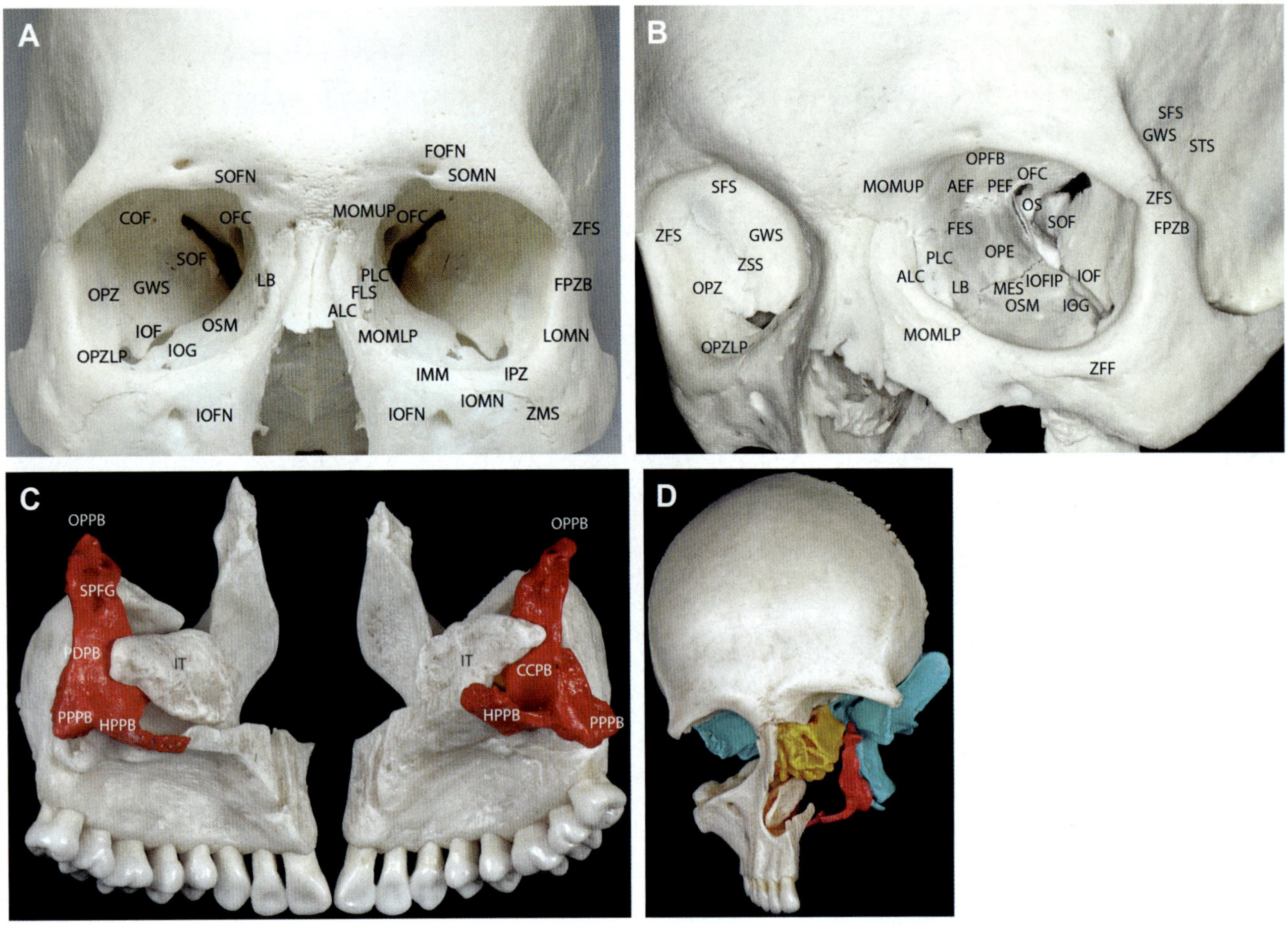

Fig. 1 (*A*) Orbits—anterior view—rim circumference. The broad blending of the anterior and posterior lacrimal crest results in discontinuity and ambiguity at the medial orbital rim. The anterior view limits the visibility over the internal orbital surfaces. (*B*) Orbits—left antero-oblique view to get insight into the inferomedial and anterolateral orbital walls concurrently. (*C*) Posterior view of the maxillae (swung out) to appreciate the orbital process of palatine bones (*red*) as robust constituent of the posterior orbital floor. (*D*) Osseous model set up demonstrating the origin of the posterior ledge—the orbital process of the palatine bone (*red*) reaches to the rearmost portion of the orbital floor with its orbital plate (facies orbitalis) (corresponding to "posterior ledge"); it is contiguous to the perpendicular and horizontal plate. Ethmoid bone (*yellow*), sphenoid (*turquoise*) with GWS, LWS, and pterygoid process—outer plate and hamulus. ALC, Anterior Lacrimal Crest; CCPB, Conchal Crest of Palatine Bone; COF, Cranioorbital Foramen; FES, Frontoethmoidal Suture; FLS, Fossa for Lacrimal Sac; FOFN, Frontal Foramen / Notch; FPZB, Frontal Process of Zygoma Bone; GWS, Greater Wing of Sphenoid; HPPB, Horizontal Process of Palatine Bone; IMM, Infraorbital Margin of Maxilla; IOF, Inferior Orbital Fisssure; IOFIP, IOF Isthmus Promontory; IOG, Infraorbital Groove; IOMN, Infraorbital Margin; IPZ, Infraorbital Process of Zygoma; IT, Inferior Turbinate; LB, Lacrimal Bone; LOMN, Lateral Orbital Margin; LWS, Lesser Wing of Sphenoid; MES, Maxilloethmoidal Suture Line; MOMLP, Medial Orbital Margin - Lower Part; MOMUP, Medial Orbital Margin - Upper Part; OFC, Optic Foramen/Canal; OPE, Orbital Plate of Ethmoid; OPFB, Orbital Plate of Frontal Bone; OPPB, Orbital Process and Plate of Palatine Bone; OPZ, Orbital Plate of Zygoma, OPZLP, Orbital Plate of Zygoma Lower Part; OSM, Orbital Surface of Maxilla; OS, Optic Strut; PDPB, Perpendicular plate of palatine bone (nasal surface); PPPB, Pyramidal Process of Palatine Bone; PLC, Posterior Lacrimal Crest; SFS, Sphenofrontal Suture; SOF, Superior Orbital Fissure; SOFN, Supraorbital Foramen/Notch; SOMN, Supraorbital Margin; SPFG, Sphenopalatine foramen/groove; STS, Sphenotemporal Suture; ZFF, Zygomaticofacial Foramen; ZFS, Zygomaticofrontal Suture, ZMS, Zygomaticomaxillary Suture; ZSS, Zygomaticosphenoid Suture (*Courtesy of* C. P. Cornelius, F. Probst, M. C. Metzger, and P. J. J. Gooris.)

orbital roof, it takes a triangular shape, however, with a limitation through the inferior orbital fissure (IOF). The orbital floor is shorter in anteroposterior extent than the 3 other orbitals walls and thus is missing in the orbital apex.

The medial wall is part of the centrofacial or naso-orbito-ethmoid unit and begins at the anterior lacrimal crest of the frontonasal process of the maxilla, followed by the lacrimal bone, the rectangular lamina papyracea of the ethmoid as the largest component, and the lateral sphenoid body posteriorly (Fig. 4A, B).

The frontoethmoidal suture line (FES) marks the level of the ethmoidal roof. The cribriform plate, however, may lie up to 10 mm caudal to the FES. A firm bony thickening results from support of the underlying basal (ground) lamina of the middle turbinate and reinforces the track of the maxilloethmoidal suture line. Therefore, it is referred to as inferomedial orbital strut (IOS).

The lateral orbital wall consists of the orbital plate (facies) of the zygoma anteriorly and the greater wing of the sphenoid (GWS) posteriorly (see Fig. 5A,B and Fig. 6), forming a flat

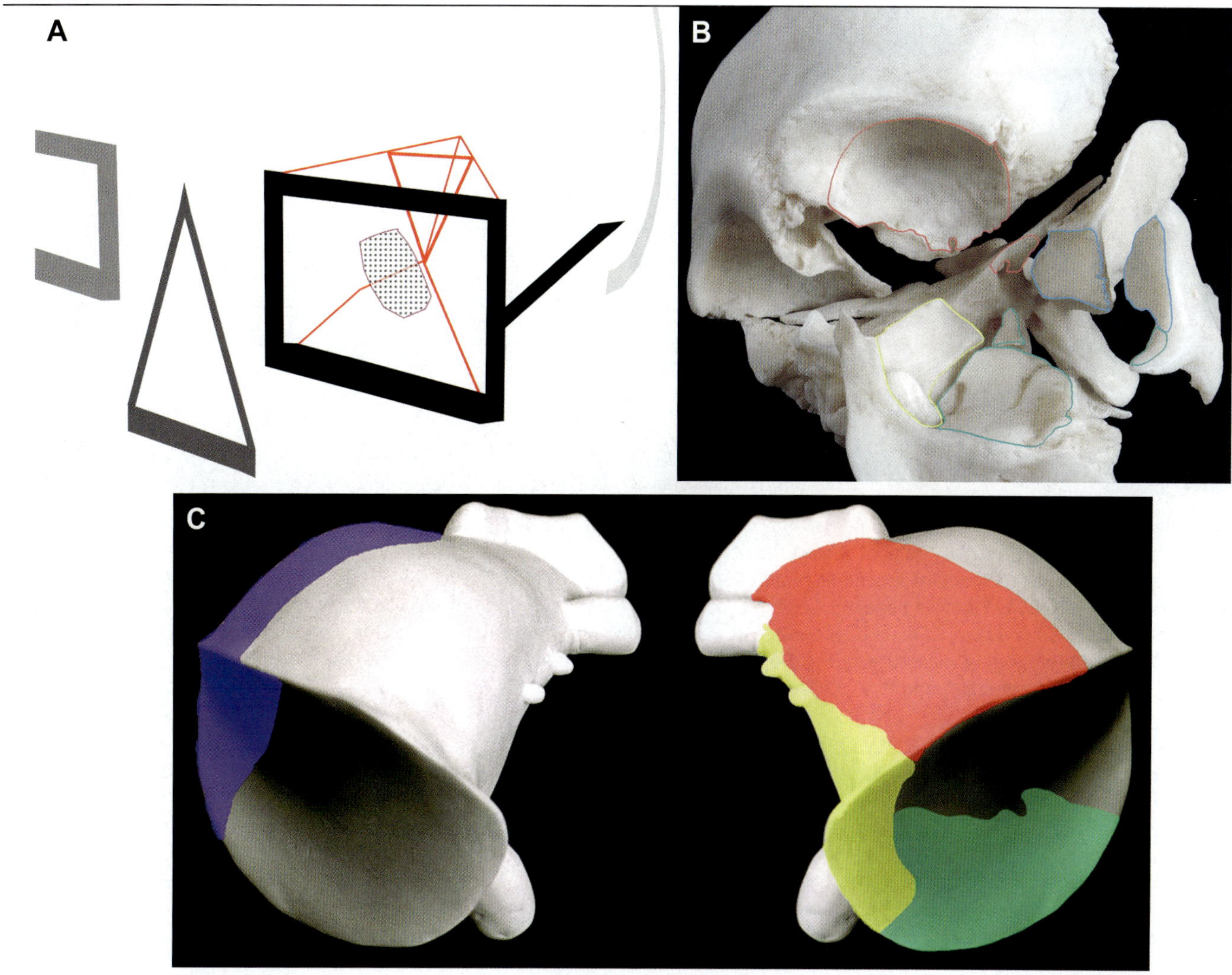

Fig. 2 (*A*) Geometric scheme of the orbit—a quadrangular pyramid converts into a tetrahedron posteriorly. Accordingly, there is a triangular frontal cross-section in the apex. Dot matrix designates posteromedial bulge. (*B*) Exploded skull model of left orbit—walls of the orbital cavity and their bone components. Color code: floor—green, medial wall—yellow, roof—red, and lateral wall—blue/purple (matching Fig. 2C). (*C*) Color-marked cast specimens of the internal orbits (color coding of the walls [see Fig. 2B]). ([*A*] Used by permission from *Orbital Fractures* by Beat Hammer, ISBN 0-88937-139-3 and ISBN 3-8017-0785-2 ©1995 by Hogrefe & Huber Publishers (now Hogrefe Publishing), www.hogrefe.com; and [*B*, *C*] *Courtesy of* C. P. Cornelius, F. Probst, M. C. Metzger, and P. J. J. Gooris.)

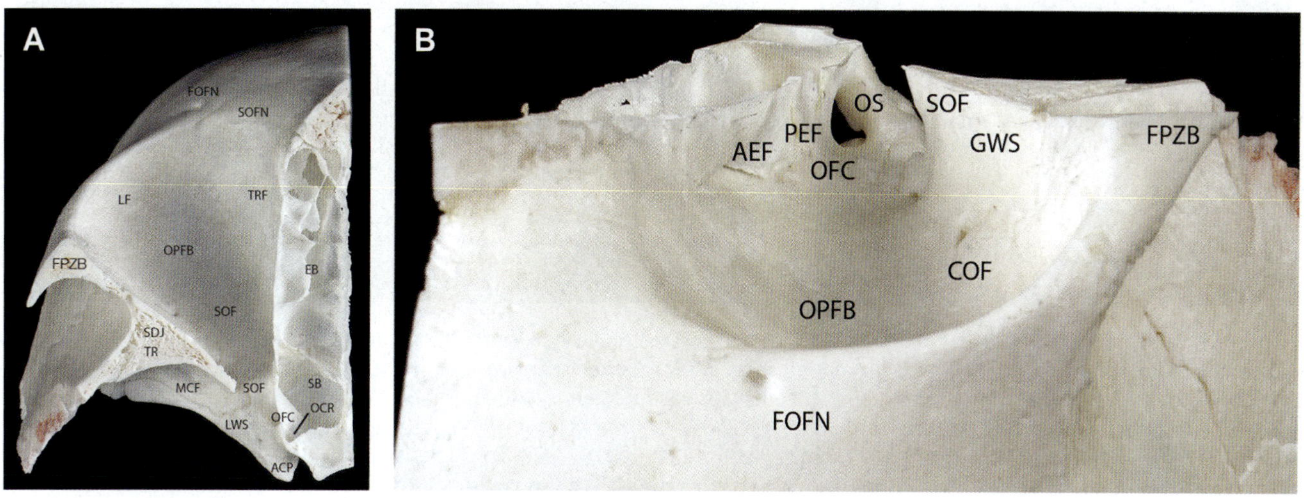

Fig. 3 (*A*) Orbital roof (*right side of anatomic specimen*) from below (*B*) Orbital roof—upside down/inferodorsal view revealing a look into the superomedial corner of the orbital apex with the optic foramen/canal (OFC) turned medially as upward just like the optic strut and the narrow superior lateral SOF sector. The optic strut and the narrow superior lateral SOF sector. ACP, Anterior Clinoid Process; AEF, Anterior Ethmoidal Foramen; EB, Ethmoid Bone; FPZB, Frontal Process of Zygoma Bone; LF, Lacrimal Fossa; MCF, Middle Cranial Fossa; OCR, Opticocarotid Recess; OS, Optic Strut; PEF, Posterior Ethmoidal Foramen; SB, Sphenoid Bone; SDJ, Sphenoid Door Jamp; TR, Trigone (GWS); TRF, Trochlear Fovea (*Courtesy of* C. P. Cornelius, F. Probst, M. C. Metzger, and P. J. J. Gooris.)

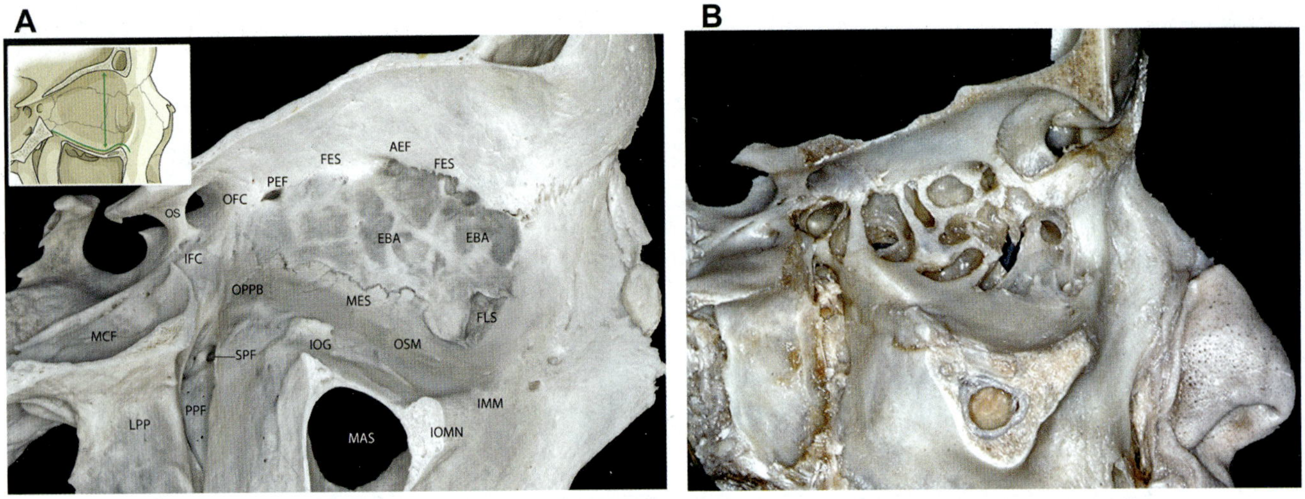

Fig. 4 (*A*) Medial orbital wall—lateral to medial view offering a look into the optic foramen/canal (OFC) and the PPF along the medial IOF margin and retrotuber maxillary region. (*Inset*) Vertical extent of the postentry zone behind the infraorbital and supraorbital rim (*vertical green arrow*). Lazy S shape of ascending orbital floor (*green line*). (*B*) Medial orbital wall—lateral view, ethmoid, sphenoid, and frontal air cells opened. EBA, Ethmoid Bone/Air Cells; IFC, Infraoptic Canal; LPP, Lateral Pterygoid Plate; MAS, Maxillary Antrum/ Sinus; MES, Maxilloethmoidal Suture Line; OSM, Orbital Surface of Maxilla; PPF, Pterygopalatine Fossa; SPF, Sphenopalatine Foramen. (inset [*A*] *Source:* AO Surgery Reference, www.aosurgery.org. Copyright by AO Foundation, Switzerland; and [Fig. 4A and Fig. 4B] *Courtesy of* C. P. Cornelius, F. Probst, M. C. Metzger, and P. J. J. Gooris.)

plane surface angulated approximately 45° toward the sagittal plane. The GWS separates the orbit from the middle cranial fossa and is part of the vertical pterygomaxillary buttress. Axial cross-sections unveil the posterior GWS as a central trigone, with a spongious bone space between the orbital, temporal, and cranial cortical surfaces (Fig. 5B). This potential space for surgical decompression is termed, the sphenoid door jamb (SDJ). More anteriorly, the lateral orbital wall turns into a monocortical layer with the zygomaticosphenoid suture (ZSS) line located in the thinnest portion. The ZSS is a reliable reference for the reduction of zygoma fractures from inside the orbit.

The marginal orbital tubercle (Whitnall tubercle) on the frontal zygomatic process (Fig. 6) binds the attachments of the

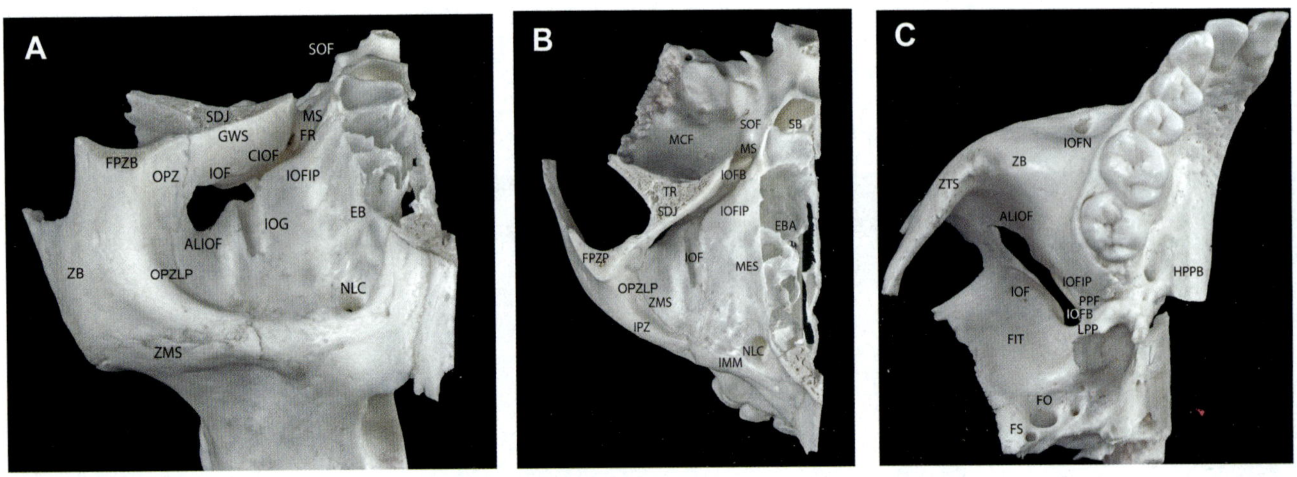

Fig. 5 (*A*) Orbital floor (*right side of anatomic specimen*)—anterocranial view (infraorbital margin tilted downward). The IOF communicates with the infratemporal and pterygopalatine fossa (PPF). Rather than a simple punched perforation in a shelf, the IOF is configured as a ravine with steep sides, basins, and affluents, such as foramen rotundum, pterygoid canal, and inferior orbital groove. (*B*) Orbital floor (*right*) from above. The posterior end of the IOF ends in a basin in front of the maxillary strut. Thus, the orbital floor does not contribute to the apex (ie, posterior orbit). (*C*) Assembly of maxilla, zygoma, and sphenoid bone (right)—inferolateral aspect showing retrotuber and infratemporal region. The ravine-like character of the IOF with a robust posterior bony border (sphenoidal trigone and medial IOF margin) is confirmed. ALIOF, Anterior Loop of Inferior Orbital Fissure; CIOF, Confluence/IOF Isthmus; FIT, Fossa Infratemporalis; FO, Foramen Ovale; FS, Foramen Spinosum; FR, Foramen Rotundum; IOFB, Inferior Orbital Fissure/Basin; IOFIP, Isthmus Promontory; LPP, Lateral Pterygoid Plate; MES, Maxilloethmoidal Suture Line; MS, Maxillary Strut; NLC, Nasolacrimal Canal/Groove; OPZLP, Orbital Plate of Zygoma Lower Part; ZB, Zygomatic Bone; ZTS, Zygomaticotemporal Suture (*Courtesy of* C. P. Cornelius, F. Probst, M. C. Metzger, and P. J. J. Gooris.)

lateral retinacular suspension complex. It is a rounded blunt eminence of 2 mm or 3 mm diameter arising 2 mm to 4 mm behind the orbital rim and approximately 1 mm below the zygomaticofrontal suture (ZFS).

Bony openings—fissures, canals, grooves, foramina, and connections encountered during periorbital dissection

Optic canal

The optic canal opens into the superomedial corner of the orbital apex, where the posterior medial wall extension meets with the roof. It has an elliptical cross-section (approximate diameter 4–9.5 mm) a length of over 5.5 mm up to 11.5 mm and passes upward (15°) and inward (45°) until it ends medial to the anterior clinoid process in the middle cranial fossa. The canal is formed by the sphenoid body inferomedially, by the anterior root of the LWS superiorly, and by the optic strut laterally (Fig. 7A–C). The optic strut is a bony abutment linking the sphenoid body and the anterior clinoid process that separates the optic canal from the superior orbital fissure (SOF).

Superior orbital fissure

The SOF frequently is a club-shaped or L-shaped gap interposed between the LWS and the GWS or the orbital roof and the lateral wall, respectively (Fig. 7A–D). It slopes from the lateral apex inferomedially, where it levels along the sphenoid body and at the top of the maxillary strut, which is a transverse bony confluence above the foramen rotundum. The ring of Zinn (common tendinous ring/annular tendon), which is the origin of the 4 extraocular rectus muscles, subdivides the SOF into 3 individual hubs. The lateral half of the tendon ring (lateral and inferior rectus muscles) encircles a large outlet at the central or midlevel SOF sector, the superolateral annular foramen. The upper and lower divisions of the oculomotor nerve (CN III), the abducens nerve (CN VI), the nasocliary nerve (branch of CN V2), sympathetic nerve fibers, and the superior ophthalmic vein pass through this foramen and thereupon into the intraconal space of the orbit. The upper and innermost half of the annular ring (superior and medial rectus muscles) girdles the superomedial foramen, which funnels the optic nerve at its entrance into the optic foramen. The narrow superior lateral SOF sector outside and above the annulus transmits the frontal and lacrimal nerves (branches of CN V2) as well as the trochlear nerve (CN IV) into the extraconal space.

The inferior SOF sector underneath the annulus gives passage to the inferior ophthalmic vein and the sympathetic root as well as the long root of the ciliary ganglion (CG). A posterior extension of Müller's orbital smooth muscle recedes into the lower boundary of this sector and stretches over the posterior IOF basin.

Cranio-orbital foramen

The cranio-orbital foramen (COF) (orbitomeningeal foramen) (see Fig. 1A) is the exit point of the recurrent meningeal artery, which is an inconstant vessel (occuring in approximately in 40%-50% only) with a rather varying branching pattern. The COF is located either separately in the GWS next to the superolateral end of the SOF or it is even merging with the latter. The COF may be joining the orbit to the anterior (A-type) or middle (M-type) cranial fossa.

Inferior orbital fissure

Prototypically, the IOF outlines display a silhouette resembling a cat-tongue chocolate inside the orbit, although overall it is a complex 3-dimensional (3-D) opening of varying shapes (Fig. 5A–C). The long axis runs a posteromedial to anterolateral route, starting at the maxillary strut, to a loop in-between the lateral and the medial surfaces of the zygoma. The IOF separates the orbital floor from the lateral orbital wall. The infraorbital neurovascular bundle and the zygomatic nerve ascend from the pterygopalatine fossa (PPF) through the posterior IOF basin to reach either the infraorbital groove or the lateral orbital wall. The narrowing in the center of the IOF (isthmus promontory) originates from a crescent-shaped overhang of the orbital floor next to the surface of the palatine bone.

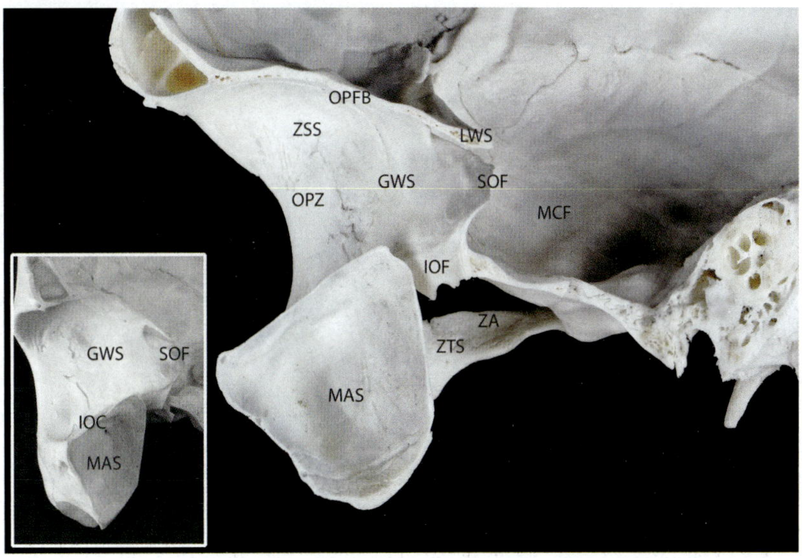

Fig. 6 Lateral orbital wall—medial view. (*Inset*) Oblique medial view. ZA, Zygomatic Arch. (*Courtesy of* C. P. Cornelius, F. Probst, M. C. Metzger, and P. J. J. Gooris.)

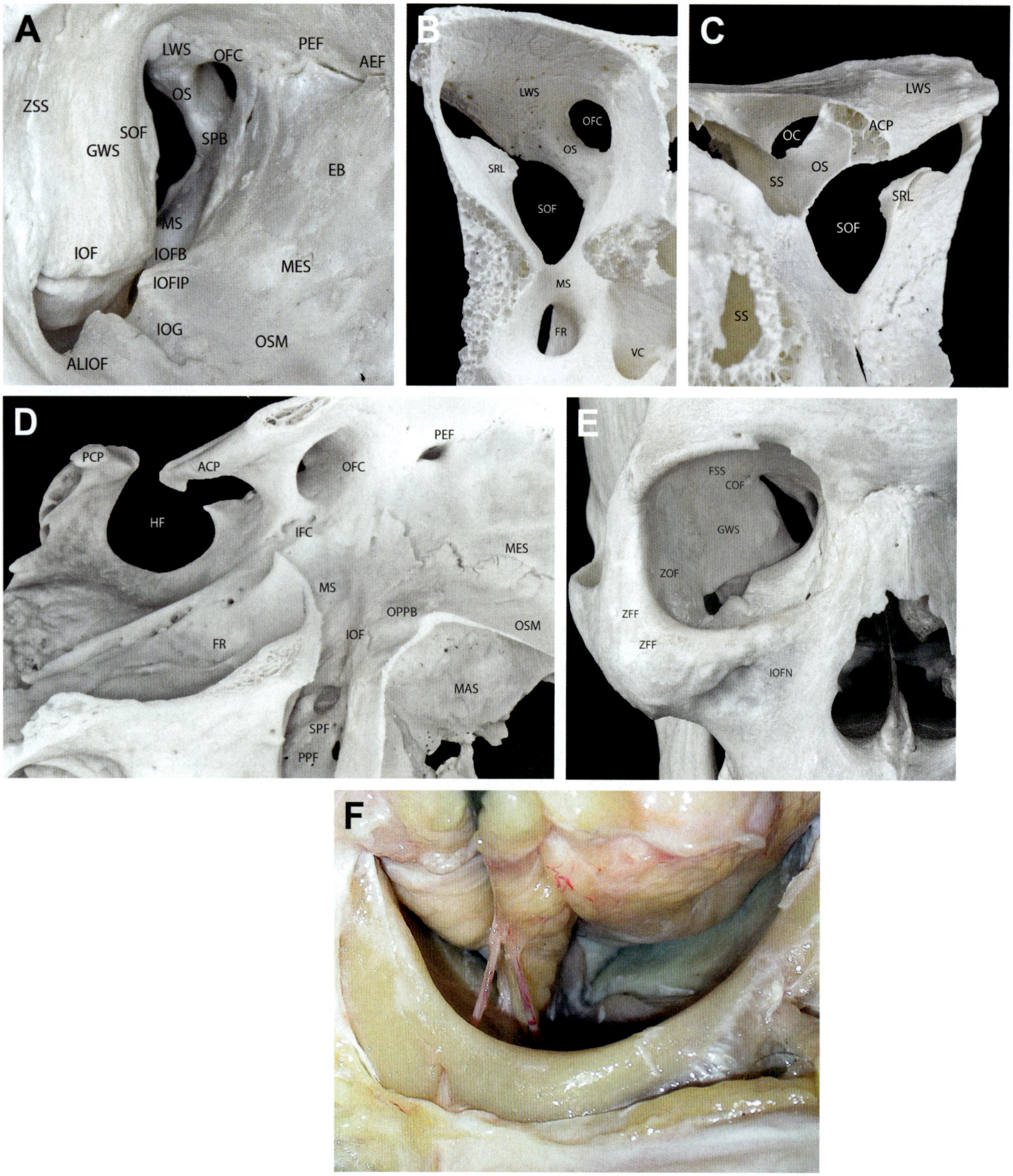

Fig. 7 (*A*) Architecture of the orbital fissure system (on right side of specimen taking the form of an uppercase L, seen as mirrored image as shown here; on left hand side in form of an uppercase L, unmirrored (not shown)) extending into the apex and optic canal—anterior close up view of the major bony pathways in and out of the orbit. Besides the optic nerve (CN II), the optic canal transmits the ophthalmic artery and accompanying autonomous nerve fibers. (*B*) Orbital apex (*right side of specimen*)—frontal bone slice—the triangular cross-section is defined by the lateral, medial, and superior orbital wall. The central and inferior SOF sectors lie below the OFC and are widened compared with the lateral superior sector. The lateral rectus spine (SRL) indicates the attachment of Zinn annular ring at GWS and the borderline between the upper and the central SOF sectors. (*C*) Intracranial view of apical tip (flip side of Fig. 7A). Anterior clinoid process (ACP) partially removed and lateral sphenoid sinus wall partially drilled away to show pneumatization of the optic struct, which is the equivalent to the optico-carotid recess. (*D*) Junction of orbital apex and lateral sellar region/middle cranial fossa (*right*)—lateral view. The infraoptic groove (sulcus), tubercle or canal is the origin of the common annular tendon (Zinn ring). (*E*) Foramina in inferolateral orbital quadrant and surface of zygomatic body. (*F*) Inferolateral orbital quadrant—zygomaticofacial neurovascular bundles. FSS, Frontosphenoid Suture; FR, Foramen Rotundum; HF, Hypophyseal Fossa; OC, Optic canal, Intracranial End; PCP, Posterior Clinoid Process; SPF, Sphenopalatine Foramen; SRL, Spina Rectus Lateralis; SS, Sinus Sphenoidalis; VC, Vidian Canal / Pterygoid Canal; ZOF, Zygomaticoorbital Foramen; ZTF, Zygomaticotemporal Foramen. (*Courtesy of* C. P. Cornelius, F. Probst, M. C. Metzger, and P. J. J. Gooris.)

In contrast to the SOF, densely packed with nerves and vessels (Table 1), the IOF encloses a continuation of the buccal fad pad into the orbital cavity (see Fig. 17A). The fatty IOF backfill tissue intermingles with smooth muscle fibers (musculus orbitalis Müller), vessels (infraorbital vein/plexus pterygoideus, minor arterial branches), and parasympathetic nerve endings.

Foramen rotundum—maxillary strut—pterygoid (Vidian) canal

The foramen rotundum penetrates the base of the pterygoid process (see Figs. 2B, 5A, and 7B) and is the path of communication for the maxillary nerve (CN V2) between the middle cranial fossa and the PPF. The maxillary strut relates to the bony bridge across the foramen rotundum. The opening of the pterygoid (Vidian) canal lies inferomedially to the foramen rotundum. It traverses the base of the medial pterygoid plate and exits into the PPF.

Ethmoidal foramina

The ethmoidal foramina (EF) are laid out in an anterior-posterior row along the FES line (see Figs. 4A, B and 13A, B). Most of the time, there are 2 foramina —an anterior EF (AEF) and posterior EF (PEF). They may be supernumerary up to a maximum of 6. The topography of the holes (discussed later) varies not only in the sagittal direction but also vertically, with an intrasutural (frequency 85%) or extrasutural position, below or above the FES.

Awareness of the proximity of the posterior-most foramen to the optic canal is regarded as critically important in the prevention of optic neuropathy and amaurosis. Injuries of the ethmoid arteries may result in massive hemorrhage or retro-orbital hematomas. Predictably, deroofing the ethmoidal canals above the FES level carries increased risk for bleeding and accidental entry into the anterior cranial fossa.

Infraorbital foramen

The infraorbital canal opens with an identically named foramen at the anterior facial wall (see Fig. 1A, B, D). The canal begins as a conduit suspended on a bony beam underneath the anterior orbital floor and turns into the infraorbital groove (sulcus) as it runs backwards to the floor surface and its end at the IOF rear sink (posterior basin). Typically, the foramen is located 7 mm to 10 mm below the infraorbital margin on a plumb line passing through the midpupil.

Supraorbital and frontal foramina/notches

The supraorbital margin can embody supraorbital foramina and frontal foramina and/or passages formed as incisurae (notches) (see Figs. 1A, B and 3A). Their vertical heights differ—notches are contiguous with the margin; foramina are located superior to the rim. Although supraorbital foramina/notches (SOFNs) are a constant finding, frontal foramina/notches (FOFNs) are facultative, with varying frequency. The sizes and shapes of the apertures are rather diverse. Supraorbital emerging points are located on an imaginary borderline between the medial third and the lateral two-thirds of the bony rim, while frontal exits lie in the superolateral quadrant within a short range (0.5 cm) of SOFNs.

Zygomatico-orbital, zygomaticofacial, and zygomaticotemporal foramina

The openings and subsequent intrabony courses of the zygomatico-orbital foramen (ZOF), zygomaticofacial foramen (ZFF), and zygomaticotemporal foramen (ZTF) follow various patterns. As the name indicates, ZOF refers to single or multiple openings in the inner surface of the anterior inferolateral orbital quadrant (Fig. 7E, F). Each ZOF represents the entrance to a separate or an interconnected canal, which exits at the facial (ZFF) and/or temporal (ZTF) zygomatic surface. Hence, there can be an array of independent canals (ie, ZOF—ZFF and ZOF—ZTF) exclusively as well as a principal interconnected canal system with a Y-type division/subdivision standing either alone or with additional independent connections.

Nasolacrimal groove/canal

The frontonasal maxillary process, the lacrimal bone, and the lacrimal process of the inferior turbinate configure the nasolacrimal groove/canal (NLC) with the anterior and posterior lacrimal crests encompassing the fossa for the lacrimal sac at the medial orbital wall (see Fig. 5A, B and 4A, B). The amphora-like inlet of the membranous sac converges into the lacrimal duct (diameter 4—5 mm), which continues over a distance of at least 12 mm to the lower outlet, that is, the lacrimal plica underneath the anterior lower nasal concha.

Internal orbital buttresses

A set of 3 buttresses running in parallel stabilizes the orbital floor in the sagittal direction (Fig. 8A, B), the IOS along the maxillo-ethmoidal suture line, the intermediary bony underpinning of the infraorbital groove/canal, and the reinforcement along the medial IOF margin laterally. The involvement and fragmentation of the buttresses are indicators of the severity of the trauma.

Orbital dimensions, volume, surface contours, and 3-dimensional globe position—interrelationship

Numerous factors determine the 3-D position of the ocular globe inside the orbit, its anterior projection, and radial relationships to the orbital rims; these are the overall dimension and volume as well as the geometry and surface contours of the internal orbit, such as slopes, angles, planes, concavities, and convexities—in particular, the so-called posteromedial bulge within the inferomedial wall transition.

The overall dimensions (Fig. 9A) and volumes of the orbit show great variations owing to age, gender, and ethnicity—4-cm horizontal × 3.5-cm vertical are typical average values for the adult aditus, the anteroposterior depth is 4.5 cm to 5 cm approximately, and the overall volume of the orbital cavity measures up to 30 mL, including the ocular globe, a sphere of 22 mm to 27 mm in diameter, up to 7 mL in volume and 69 mm to 85 mm in equatorial circumference.

The sagittal projection of the globe (corneal apex plane and/or equator) is referenced relative to the sagittal projection of the orbital rims, traditionally to the retruded lateral orbital rim only (exophthalmometry) and more recently using 360° polar plots (CT morphometry) to measure distances to

Table 1 Bony openings related to nerval and vascular orbital pathways

	Acronym	Location	Nerve(s)	Artery(ies)	Vein(s)	Further Structure(s)
Supraorbital Notch/ Foramen	SONF	supraorbital margin	sensory branch of CN V1 (– frontal nerve): supraorbital nerve	supraorbital artery	supraorbital vein	
Frontal Notch/Foramen	FONF	supraorbital margin	sensory branch of CN V1 (frontal nerve): supratrochlear nerve	supratrochlear artery	supratrochlear vein	
Infraorbital Groove/ Canal	IOG	orbital plate of maxilla/orbital floor	sensory branch of CN V2 (maxillary nerve): infraorbital nerve	infraorbital artery (+ perforators)	infraorbital vein	periorbital lining
Infraorbital Foramen	IOFN	facial antral wall	sensory branch of CN V2 (maxillary nerve): infraorbital nerve	infraorbital artery	infraorbital vein	periorbital lining
Inferior Orbital Fissure	IOF	GWS, ZB, MB, PB	- sensory branches of CN V2: - zygomatic nerve [infraorbital nerve] - parasympathetic branches from pterygopalatine ganglion	infraorbital artery	inferior ophthalmic vein/ communication with pterygoid plexus	periorbital lining orbital muscle - Müller; extension of buccal fat pad
Inferior Orbital Fissure – Posterior Basin/ Pterygopalatine Fossa		GWS, MB, PB	via foramen rotundum: CN V2 – maxillary nerve pterygoid canal (Vidian): nerve of pterygoid canalie, (= deep and greater petrosal nerve)			
Anterior Ethmoidal Foramen/Canal	AEF	anterior fronto-ethmoidal junction	anterior ethmoidal nerve	anterior ethmoidal artery	anterior ethmoidal vein	periorbital lining
Posterior Ethmoidal Foramen/Canal	PEF	posterior fronto-ethmoidal junction	posterior ethmoidal nerve	posterior ethmoidal artery	posterior ethmoidal vein	periorbital lining
Nasolacrimal Groove/ Fossa/Canal	NLC	frontal corner of inferomedial orbita quadrant				nasolacrimal sac and duct
Zygomaticoorbital Foramen-ina/Canals	ZOF	OPZ	sensory branch of CN V2 (– maxillary nerve): zygomatic nerve	collateral arterioles	collateral venules	periorbital lining
Zygomaticofacial Foramen/Canal	ZFF	facial surface of zygomatic body	branch of zygomatic nerve (z) zygomatico facial nerve	collateral arterioles	collateral venules	periorbital lining
Zygomaticotemporal Foramen/Canal	ZTF	internal/posterior surface of zygomatic body and /or OPZ	branch of zygomatic nerve (z) zygomatico temporal nerve	collateral arterioles	collateral venules	periorbital lining
Superior Orbital Fissure – Above Zinn's Ring Lateral Superior SOF Sector	SOF	LWS and GWS	CN V1 branch: lacrimal nerve CN V1 branch: frontal nerve CN IV: trochlear nerve	[recurrent meningo-lacrimal artery; – facultative occurrence middle meningeal artery]	superior ophthalmic vein	periorbital lining
Superior Orbital Fissure – Through Zinn's Ring Central SOF Sector			CN V1 branch: nasociliary nerve CN III: superior and inferior division of oculomotor nerve CN VI: abducens nerve Sympathetic root of ciliary ganglion			
Superior Orbital Fissure – Below Zinn's Ring Inferior Medial SOF Sector					inferior ophthalmic vein	periorbital lining
[Cranio-orbital Foramen] facultative occurrence	COF			[recurrent meningo-lacrimal artery; – facultative occurrence middle menigeal artery]		
Optic Foramen/Canal	OFC	between sphenoid body and anterior LWS root and OS	CN II: optic nerve sympathetic fibers from internal carotid plexus	ophthalmic artery		periorbital lining meningeal sheaths

Abbreviations; ICP, Internal Carotid Plexus; MB, Maxillary Bone; PB; Palatine Bone; ZB, Zygomatic Bone.

preassigned points all over the outer rim periphery (Eckstein and colleagues 2011).

The globe projection in the coronal plane or the vertical/horizontal globe position is correlated to the delineation, shape, and curvatures of the orbital aditus (square, rectangle, trapezoid, polygon, or circular rim aperture) and the interorbital distance.

The inclination of the medial part of the inferior rim is parallel to the angle of the orbital floor (Fig. 9B). The lateral parts of the rim and the floor both run in a horizontal plane. The lowest lateral point of the orbital floor is located next to the anterior IOF loop. With aging, both the lower rim and the floor shift posteriorly and inferiorly, so that the anteroposterior rim angle flattens, but the height and width of the aditus to the orbit do not change significantly.

The lowest portion of the orbital floor coincides with a short-pathed, circumferentially running concavity just behind the orbital rims. Originating from the periorbital dissection sequence, this widening is named, *the postentry zone* (see Fig. 4A). The orbital floor steadily ascends from the bottom of the postentry zone until it reaches the convex top site of the orbital process of the palatine bone (posterior ledge). Because this process curves down abruptly backward into the posterior IOF basin, the paramedian portion of the orbital floor assumes an undulating shape in the sagittal direction, which is termed, *the lazy S configuration*. The bony surface relief in the posterior transition of the orbital floor into the medial orbital wall is upraised by the focal convexity, as aforementioned, the posterior medial bulge (Fig. 10A–C). This spot in the surface profile is referred to as *Beat Hammer's key area*, because this

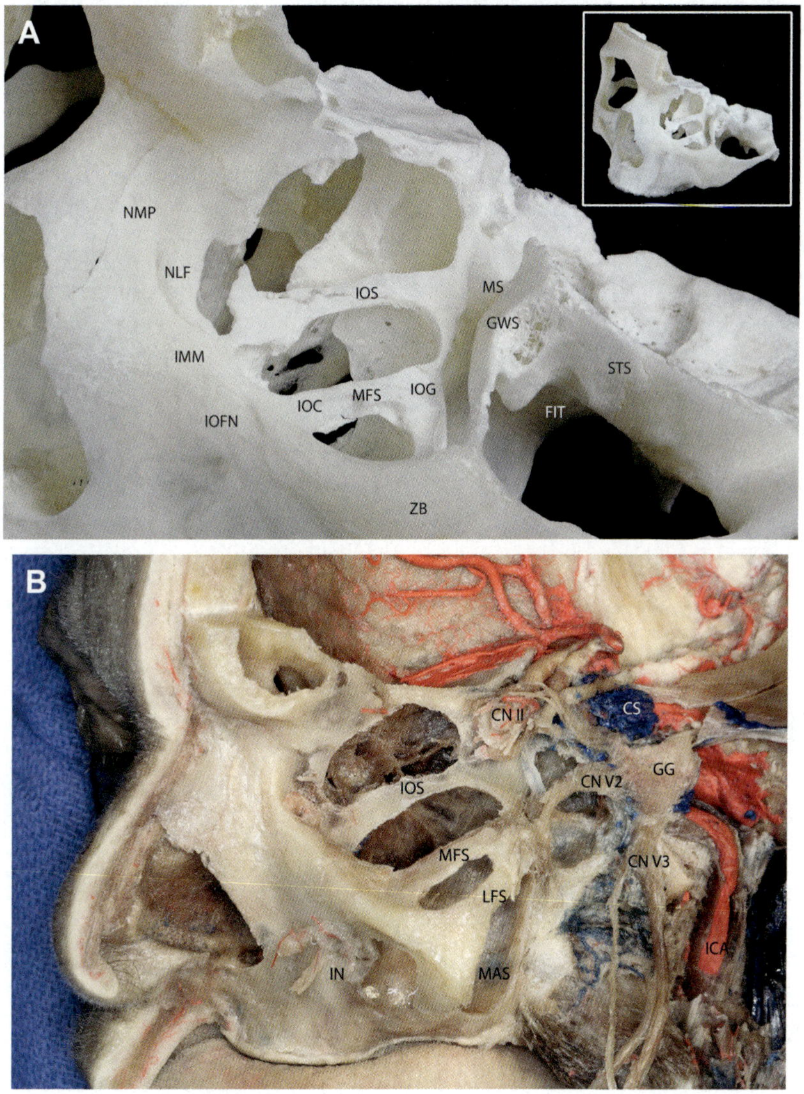

Fig. 8 (*A*) Sagittal internal orbital buttresses in parallel after removal of thin interjacent bony plates: IOS along the articulation of orbital floor and medial orbital wall with a strong anterior portion around the nasolacrimal duct, weaker midportion because of lamina papyracea as well as aeration by ethmoidal bulla and solid wide posterior palatine bone portion; midway floor strut surrounding the infraorbital groove and canal; lateral floor strut along anterior/lateral IOF edge. (*Inset*) Overview midface skeleton. (*B*) Sagittal internal orbital buttresses and soft tissue relations (left zygoma, anterior and middle skull base removed to expose LFS). CN II, Optic Nerve; CN V2, Trigeminal Nerve - Maxillary Nerve Division; CN V3, Trigeminal Nerve - Mandibular Nerve Division; CS, Cavernous Sinus; FIT, Fossa Infratemporalis; GG, Ganglion Gasseri / Trigeminal Ganglion; ICA, Internal Carotid Artery; IN, Infraorbital Nerve; IOC, Infraorbital Canal; IOS, Inferomedial Orbital Strut; LFS, Lateral Floor Strut; MFS, Midway Floor Strut; MS, Maxillary Strut; NLF, Nasolacrimal Fossa; NMP, Nasomaxillary Process; STS, Sphenotemporal Suture. (*Courtesy of* C. P. Cornelius, F. Probst, M. C. Metzger, and P. J. J. Gooris.)

author [Hammer, 1995] has stressed its tremendous importance for the appropriate surgical reconstruction of the internal orbit (Fig. 11A, B). The difficulty of procuring accurate and reproducible anatomic boundaries of the posterior medial bulge long has been recognized in statistical shape analysis. In consequence, still no mapping technique exists that displays increasing contour lines to estimate the steepness gradient of the all-important sloping hillside and select an appropriate implant immediately.

Traumatic orbital wall defects involving the key area most of the time pass by the orbital process of the palatine bone, so that this intact bony ledge can serve as support in reconstruction.

The internal surface of lateral orbital wall equates to a straight and even plane between the lateral rim and the SOF entrance (see Figs. 9A and 10A).

Anterior orbit—midorbit—posterior orbit (apex)

Often, the length (anteroposterior extension) of the orbit is divided into thirds. This division is intuitive and not based on anatomical references or numerical distances between measuring points, and the shorter orbital floor length is not taken into consideration. A more pragmatic approach is a partitioning into an anterior orbit, a midorbit, and a posterior orbit using the IOF (Fig. 12). The extent of the IOF between the anterior loop and the maxillary strut designates the boundaries of the midorbit, whereas the anterior orbit lies in front and the posterior orbit in the rear of the IOF.

Deep orbit versus rule of halves: 24 to 12 to 6

The anterior IOF loop has been proposed as an anatomic landmark to define the point of entrance into the deep orbit in posttraumatic surgical dissection and repair, with the 2 arguments that the frontal orbital cross-section begins to taper backward continuously from there on, making a subperiosteal (periorbital) dissection progressively difficult and with the high frequency at which it is involved by relevant traumatic defects. The concept of the deep orbit (Evans and Webb, 2007) suggests using the following 4 hard and soft tissue structures for orientation and pathfinding during dissection of the inferior and lateral wall:

- Infraorbital nerve (canal—groove/sulcus)
- IOF
- GWS (central trigone part/sphenotemporal buttress)
- Upper plate of the orbital process of the palatine bone

These structures concenter at the confluence of the orbit, which corresponds to the area in direct proximity of IOF isthmus (see Figs. 5A, B, 10A, and 15).

Often, orbital depth gauging data derived from anthropometric studies cannot provide appropriate guidelines for safe distance dissection because of variation, particularly in trauma due to severe multifragmentation, displacement, soft tissue disruption, and fat herniation. So, the preferences is to dissection in a subperiosteal (subperiorbital) plane to identify the lead structures. Apart from the EF, the medial orbit does not feature any orientation aid to prevent interference with the optic foramen and nerve.

Despite the well-known uncertainties in terms of number and zonal location of the EF, their potential distances in relation to the lacrimal crest, among each other, and to the optic foramen (Fig. 13A) are referred to by a well-known mnemonic—the rule of halves: 24 mm to 12 mm to 6 mm (Rontal and colleagues, 1979) brings one to remind the distances (Fig. 13B).

Orbital soft tissue contents

Orbital septum

The aditus to the orbit is closed off by the septum, a fibroelastic multilayered diaphragm separating the eyelids

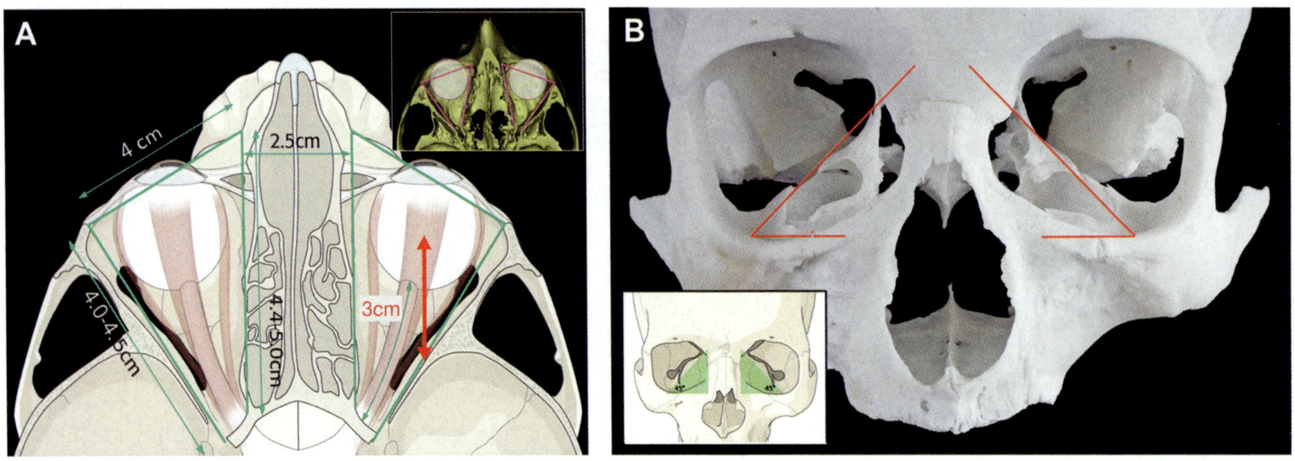

Fig. 9 (*A*) Average dimensions and angular relationships of the orbits and interorbital space. (*Inset*) Routine 3-D reformatted CT scan showing that individual angulation and measurements can vary widely with the diploic space (SDJ) within GWS yielding a major contribution. (*B*) Frontal view of both orbits. Lateral orbital walls removed allowing a look into the diploic space (SDJ) within the GWS, and the infratemporal and temporal spaces. Inferomedial walls and ethmoidal cells partially removed showing maxillary sinuses and posterior ledges. Line sketch of so-called orbital angle (*red*), that is, the inclination of the orbital floor to horizontal plane. (*Inset*) Orbital angles (45°) along intact orbital floor surfaces. ([Fig. 9A and Fig. 9B *inset*] *Source:* AO Surgery Reference, www.aosurgery.org. Copyright by AO Foundation, Switzerland; and [Fig. 9A *inset* and Fig. 9B] *Courtesy of* C. P. Cornelius, F. Probst, M. C. Metzger, and P. J. J. Gooris.)

(preseptal) from the orbital contents (postseptal/retroseptal). The septum lies deep to the orbicularis oculi muscle (suborbicular). It is one of the components building up the middle lamellae of the upper and lower eyelids. In the upper eyelid, it fuses with the anterior layer of the levator aponeurosis and in the lower eyelid to the capsulopalprebral fascia below the tarsal plate. The thickness of the orbital septum is not homogenous. The lateral portion is thicker than the medial portion.

Periorbita—periosteal lining—periorbitum

The periosteal lining of the internal orbit is denoted as periorbita, or by some investigators as periorbitum, taking the final syllable of periosteum into linguistic consideration.

The periosteal/periorbital sac is a thin but resistant fibrous envelope that provides protection to the orbital soft tissue contents (Fig. 14). It sends sleeves and prolongations into the canals, foramina, and fissures (see Figs. 13A and 14) to blend with the dura or the adjacent periosteum. The fusion zone over the orbital rims is thickened and sets up the arcus marginalis, which is the origin of the orbital septum. The infraorbital neurovascular bundle is completely wrapped in kind of a mesoperiosteum to keep it in direct contact with the orbital floor lining along the infraorbital groove. Tiny branches arising from the infraorbital artery penetrate the sheath to anastomose with muscular branches of the ophthalmic artery near the inferior rectus and oblique muscles (Fig. 15A, B).

A distinction has to be drawn between the extraperiosteal space or bony side and the intraperiosteal space or visceral side of the periorbita.

As a whole, the periorbita is only loosely adherent to the bony surfaces. It is fixed more firmly to the trochlea, Whitnall tubercle, and the deep limb of the medial canthus/lacrimal sac and the infraorbital groove.

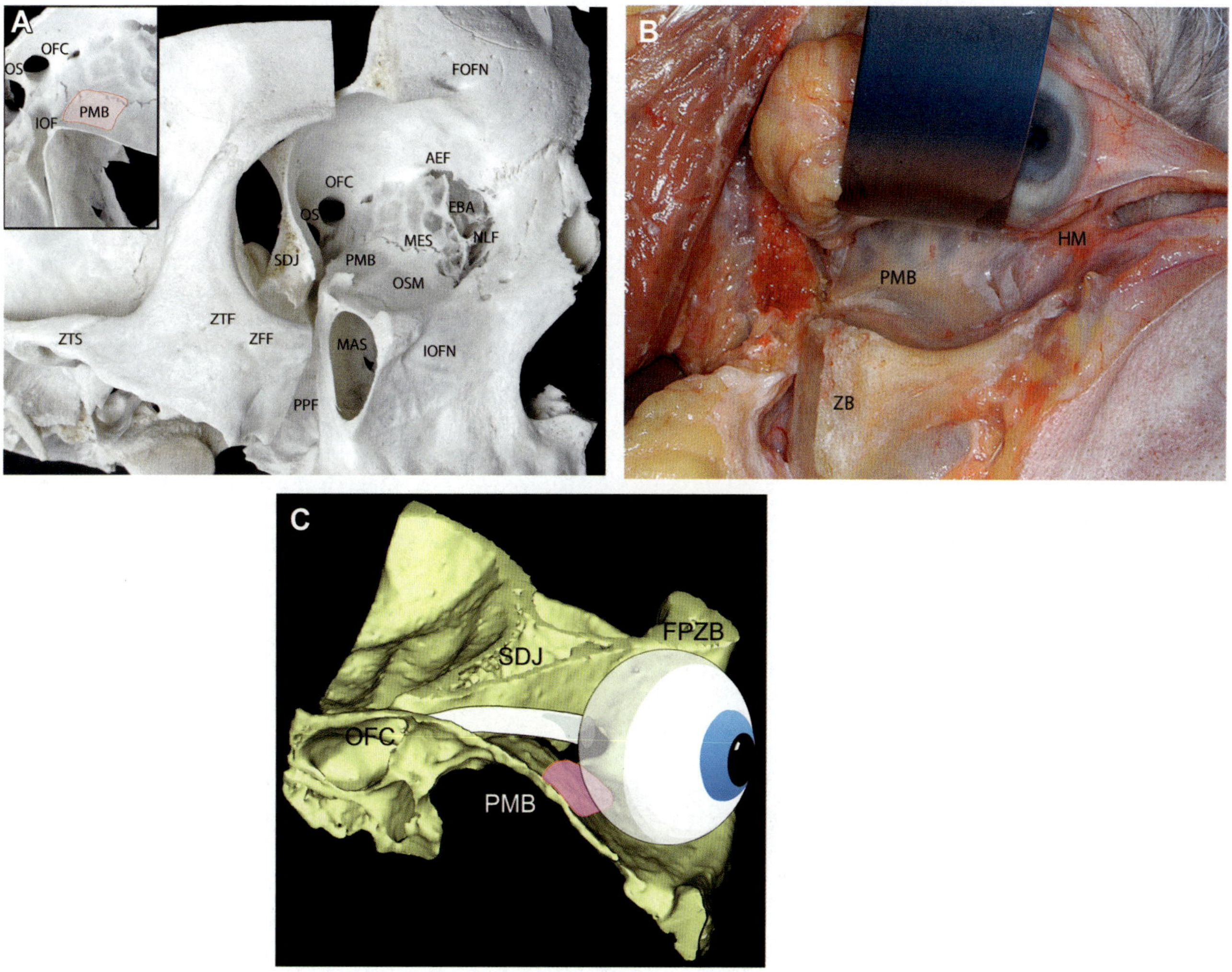

Fig. 10 (*A*) Orbit (right)—staggered partitions after midline sagittal plane section. Lazy S becomes obvious along the medial orbital floor. The lateral orbital wall reveals as a flat plane. (*Inset*) Convexity of the posterior inferomedial wall with key area outlined provisorily (*red rectangle*). (*B*) Exposure of lazy S and key area—by superior retraction of the orbital soft tissue contents and swinging of the eyelids anteriorly (zygoma and GWS/SDJ removed). (*C*) Globe height and globe projection—graphic illustration based on 3-D reformatted CT scan of left orbit. The bulge configuration of the posterior inferomedial orbital walls (key area) in conjunction with the angulated plane of the lateral orbital wall are the primary determinants for the vertical and sagittal globe position. HM, Horner's Muscle; PMB, Posterior Medial Bulge. (*Courtesy of* C. P. Cornelius, F. Probst, M. C. Metzger, and P. J. J. Gooris.)

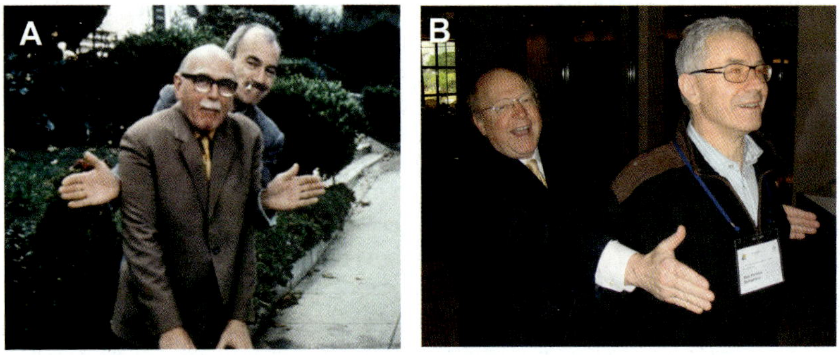

Fig. 11 (*A*) Globe height and globe projection—the fanlike divergence of the orbital walls is comparable to a pair of hands holding the globe in its forward position. Demonstrated by Paul Tessier and John Clark (Jack) Mustardé—on the occasion of a University of California Los Angeles meeting about orbital and eyelid surgery in the late 1970s: "Jack Mustardé said that posttraumatic enophthalmos was not correctable, which was the dogma at that time. Tessier said, No Jack, you are wrong, and he got behind him and pushed him forward by bringing his arms together. He said my arms are the walls of the orbit." (*B*) Globe height and globe projection—in line with history the orbital wall—globe relationship replayed by Paul Manson and Beat Hammer—on the occasion of 3rd European Advanced Symposium in Orbital Reconstruction, Chalkididi/Greece, April 2008. ([*A*] *Courtesy of* Dr S. Anthony Wolfe, Miami, FL; and [*B*] *Courtesy of* C. P. Cornelius, F. Probst, M. C. Metzger, and P. J. J. Gooris.)

An intimately linked framework of diversified connective tissue components extends from the inner or visceral side of the periorbita to support the ocular globe and the entirety of muscular and neural and vascular elements (ie, Koornneef system of radial and interlocking septa [Koornneef 1976, 1977, Demer 2002, Miller 2019], extraocular muscle pulleys, and many more other concepts).

To avoid confusion, the term, *periorbita*, generally is used to refer to the area around the orbit and the globes (forehead, hairy eyebrows, brow eyelids continuum, eye spacing, palpebral fissures, lacrimal puncta, eyelids, midcheek, and temples) in the widest sense of a periocular or periorbital region instead of the periosteal covering inside the orbit.

Dissection of the periorbital lining

A systematic dissection, separating the periorbital lining from the underlying bony surface relief into the deep orbit, comes across landmark structures of particular note, some of them associated with potential risk for injury (Fig. 16). Unlike classic anatomy, which typically describes the soft contents of the orbit in craniocaudal layers after removal of the floor of the anterior cranial fossa, namely, the orbital roof, a periorbital dissection proceeds in anteroposterior direction without osteotomies of the bony rims or walls starting at the aditus over the midorbit toward the entrance into the apex along the lower and/or upper bony circumference. The extent of bone that can be exposed depends on the placement and size of the skin incision and subsequent surgical access. As a consequence, any look into the orbital cavity is restricted to a limited segment, and a 360° visualization of the whole internal orbit is achievable only by piecing together the perspectives from all sides to a panorama in one's mental imagination.

Successive transection of the periorbital invaginations and through the contents of the IOF starting at its anterior loop widens the view within the inferolateral orbital quadrant.

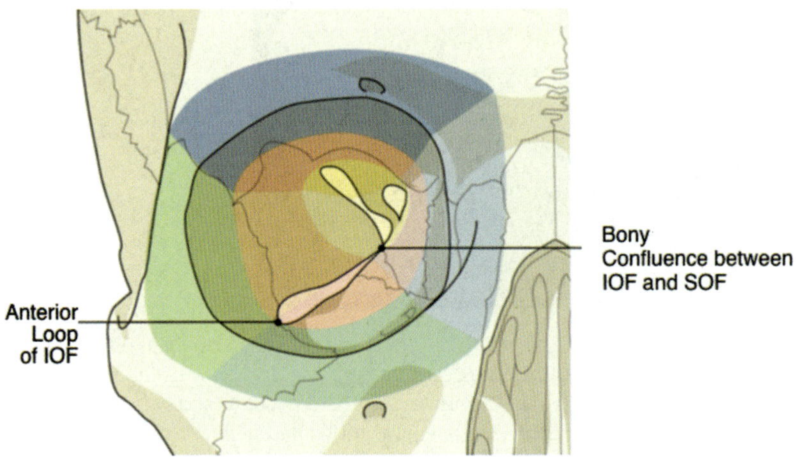

Fig. 12 Start and ending of IOF correspond to the spatial boundaries of the concentric circles of the anterior, mid, and posterior orbit. (*Source:* AO Surgery Reference, www.aosurgery.org. Copyright by AO Foundation, Switzerland.)

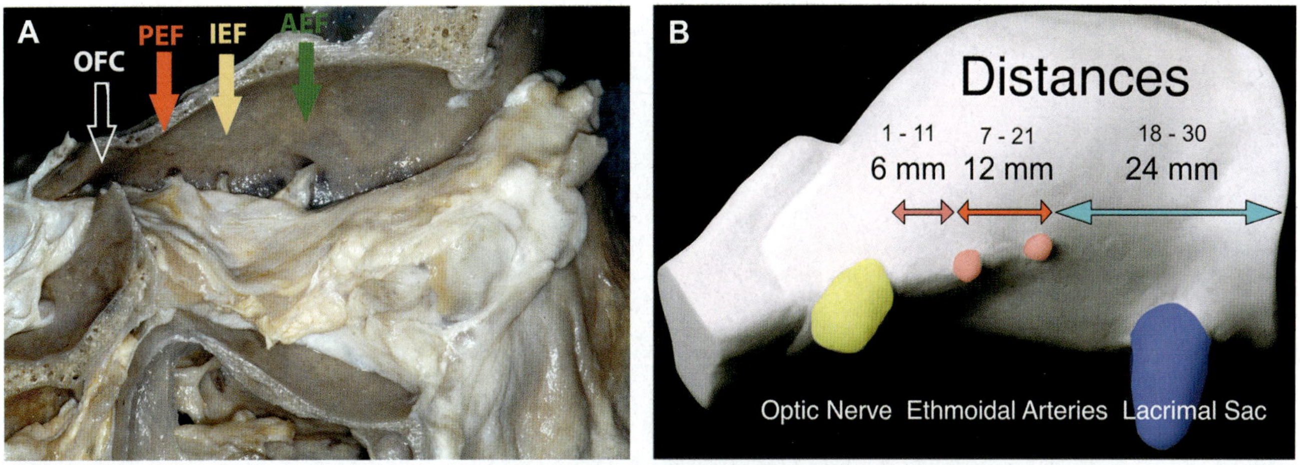

Fig. 13 (*A*) Variation of EF—periorbital sac emptied to show the sleevelike extensions to AEF, IEF, PEF, and optic foramen/canal (OFC). (*B*) Rule of halves—24 mm to 12 mm to 6 mm—average distance of 24 mm from anterior lacrimal crest to AEF, 12 mm between AEF and PEF, and another 6-mm span from PEF to OFC. AEF, Anterior Ethmoidal Foramen; IEF, Intermediate Ethmoidal Foramen; OFC, Optic Foramen / Canal; PEF, Posterior Ethmoidal Foramen. (*Courtesy of* C. P. Cornelius, F. Probst, M. C. Metzger, and P. J. J. Gooris.)

There is no harm to the posterior portion of the infraorbital nerve, because this is settled low in the IOF basin/PPF and does not reach up to the level of the orbital floor (Fig. 17A–C).

The landmarks and structures at risk along the 4 orbital walls appear in a prototypical sequence, with the periorbital dissection going posteriorly (Fig. 18).

Further thought should be given to the fact that all attempts to push the limits of the periorbital dissection far back through the concentrically aligned walls of the midorbit toward the tight apex using instrumentation and spatulas build up soft tissue pressure. The compressing effects may be as detrimental to the optic nerve or the SOF contents as direct mechanical impingement at the optic foramen (Fig. 19).

Ipsilateral pupillary mydriasis and anisocoria encountered during deep periorbital dissection and fracture repair are well-known but still distressing phenomena. Manipulation and interference with the long inferior oblique muscle (IOM) branch of the inferior oculomotor division (see Fig. 15A) and/or the CG represent possible causes of intraoperative pupillary dilatation.

Ciliary ganglion

The CG is the pre–postganglionic relay center of the CN III parasympathetic pathway. It lies embedded in fat between the lateral

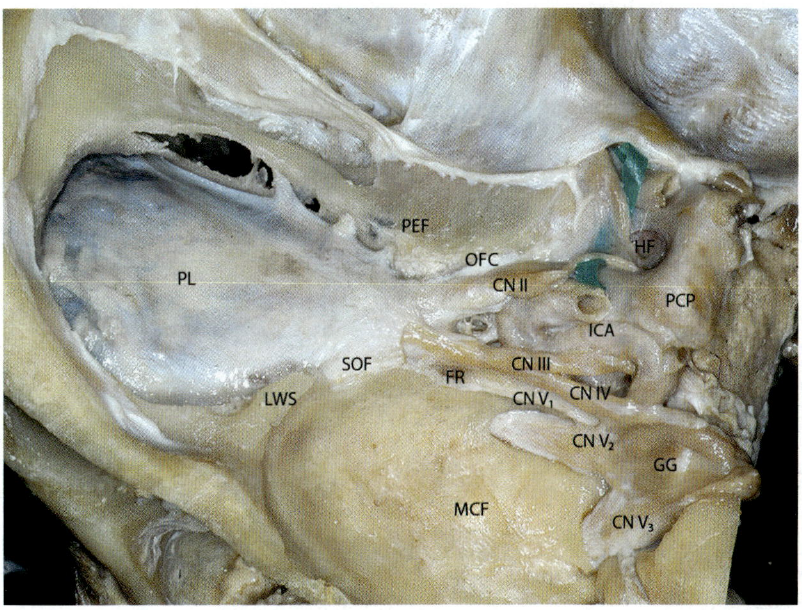

Fig. 14 Periorbital sac—intracranial view after removal of lateral orbital wall and roof (*left*). Medial cranial fossa with exposed ganglion Gasseri and trigeminal nerve divisions. CN III, Oculomotor Nerve; CN IV, Trochlear Nerve; CN V1, Trigeminal Nerve - Ophthalmic Nerve Division; HF, Hypophyseal Fossa; ICA, Internal Carotid Artery; PL, Periorbital Lining. (*Courtesy of* C. P. Cornelius, F. Probst, M. C. Metzger, and P. J. J. Gooris.)

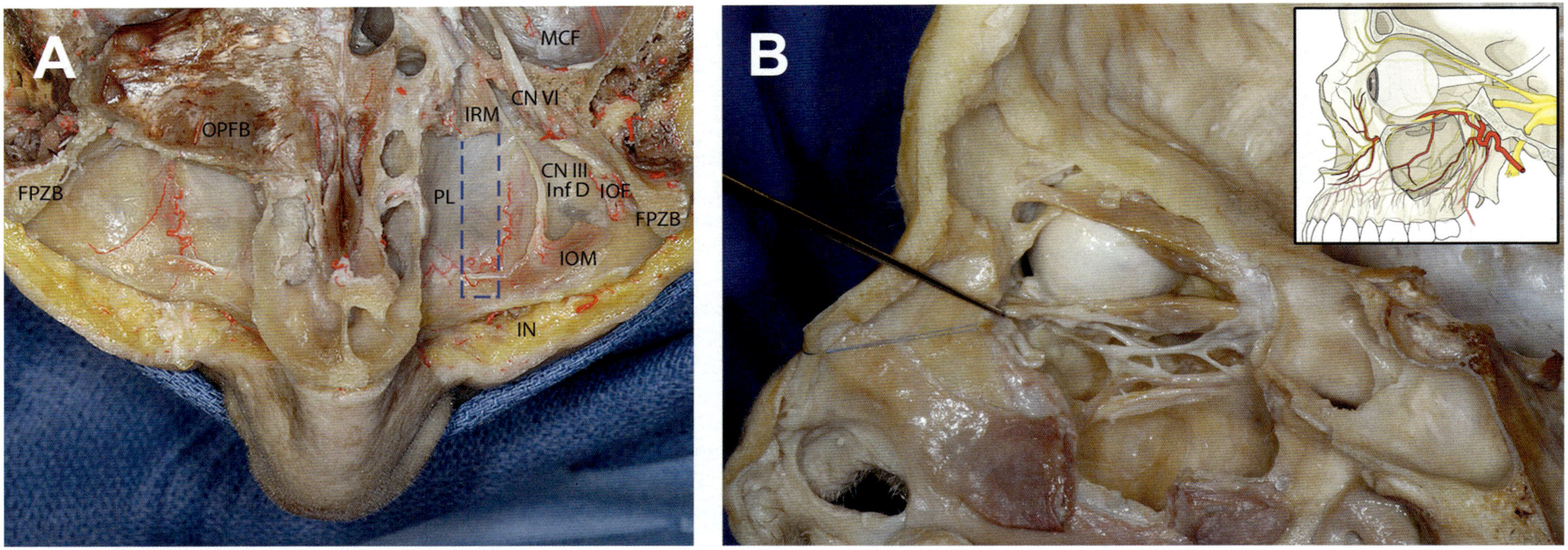

Fig. 15 (*A*) Both orbital floors viewed from above with periorbital coverage intact. Perforators run along the course of the infraorbital neurovascular bundle on its visceral side (this means in effect within the intraperiorbital space). Left orbit: IOM originating immediately lateral to NLC, the long branch of the inferior division of CN III to IOM runs in parallel to the IOG, IOC and the lateral border of the IRM (*striped lines*). (*B*) Orbital contents and infraorbital neurovascular bundle perforators—medial approach. IOM and attached CN III motor branch hook retracted. The arterial strand divides into numerous smaller branches (perforators) which connect to the periorbita and IRM along the top side of the infraorbital groove. These vessels must be meticulously bipolar cauterized during deep subperiorbital dissection of the orbital floor. (*Inset*) Distribution of infraorbital neurovascular bundle and vessel entrance into the periorbital sac. CN III Inf D, Oculomotor Nerve Inferior Division; CN VI, Cranial Nerve VI - Abducens Nerve; IOM, Inferior Oblique Muscle; IRM, Inferior Rectus Muscle. ([*A, B*] *Courtesy of* C. P. Cornelius, F. Probst, M. C. Metzger, and P. J. J. Gooris; and [*B inset*] *Source:* AO Surgery Reference, www.aosurgery.org. Copyright by AO Foundation, Switzerland.)

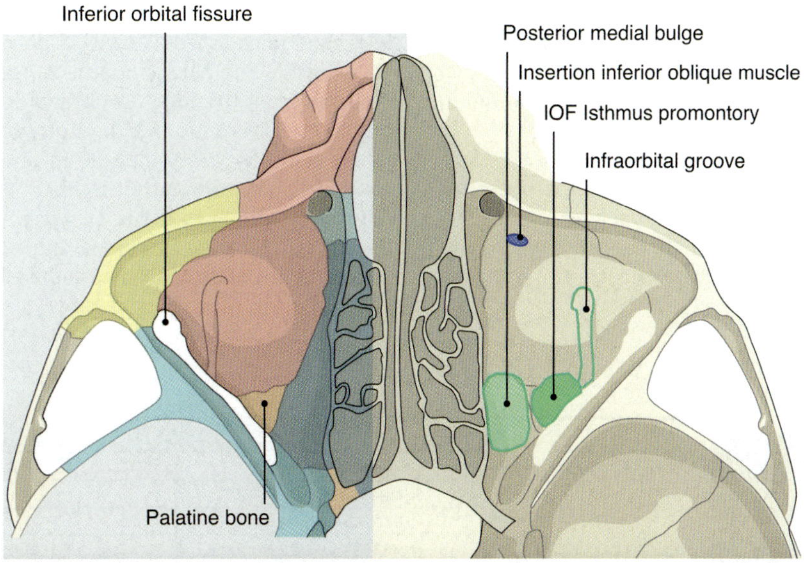

Fig. 16 Axial plane after transverse head section at intermediate height level of the orbits—view from above. Left lower circumference displays bone components making up the orbital floor and bordering the IOF. Right lower circumference with markings of relevant landmarks/structures at risk along the periorbital dissection route on the floor surface. (*Source:* AO Surgery Reference, www.aosurgery.org. Copyright by AO Foundation, Switzerland.)

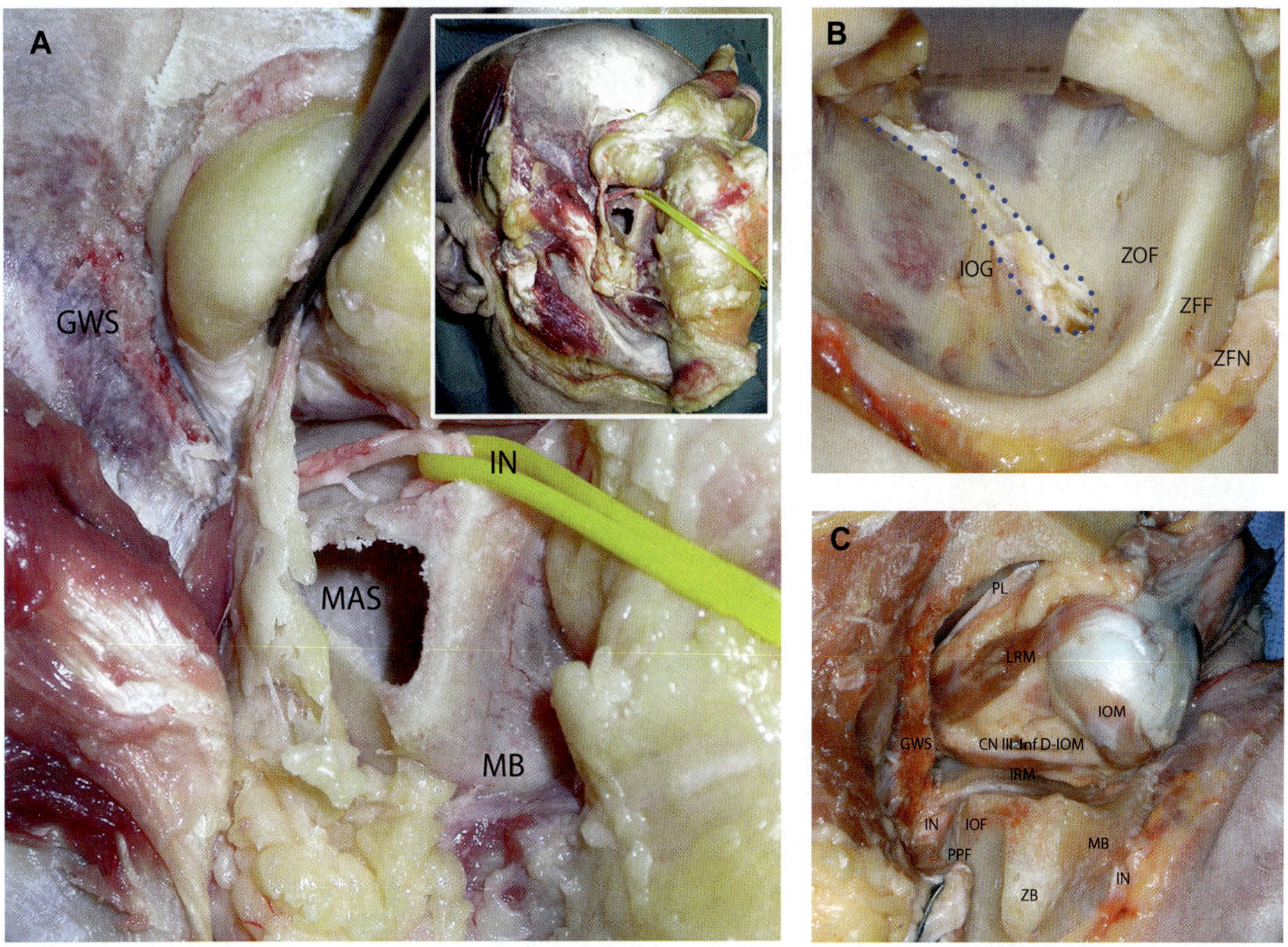

Fig. 17 (*A*) Content of the IOF—periorbital invagination and fat filling the IOF for the whole length—retracted upwards. Orbital fat and buccal fat pad communicate. The infraorbital neurovascular bundle pulled out and upward of the IOG. (*Inset*) Topographic overview. (*B*) Augmented exposure of inferolateral orbital quadrant after transsection of the IOF contents (*dotted outline*). (*C*) Posterior portion of infraorbital nerve residing in the posterior IOF basin/PPF below the level of the IOF and orbital floor. IN, Infraorbital Nerve; LRM, Lateral Rectus Muscle; ZFF, Zygomaticofacial Foramen; ZFN, Zygomaticofacial Nerve. (*Courtesy of* C. P. Cornelius, F. Probst, M. C. Metzger, and P. J. J. Gooris.)

aspect of CN II and the lateral rectus muscle, most often in the midhalf between Zinn ring and the back of the eyeball (Fig. 20). It can have a round, ovoid, or an starlike flat-end shape. The mean size approximates to 2.5 mm in horizontal diameter, 1.5 mm in vertical height, and 0.5 mm to 1 mm in thickness.

CG has inputs by sensory, sympathetic, and parasympathetic fiber projections, which join it from the posterior aspect and is why they are named roots.

The sensory root runs through a single branch diverting of the nasociliary nerve proximal to Zinn ring. The sympathetic root corresponds to a thin filament containing fibers from the intracavernous internal carotid plexus (ICP) reaching the CG via the SOF. The parasympathetic root commonly is single and emerges from the long IOM branch of the inferior oculomotor division (ie, ramus n. oculomotorii ad ganglion ciliare). The CG is traversed by the sympathetic and sensory fibers. The preganglionic parasympathetic fibers with their origin in the Edinger-Westphal nucleus synapse within the ganglion. The postganglionic neurons leave the CG and combine with the main bundles of up to 8 to 10 short ciliary nerves and innervate

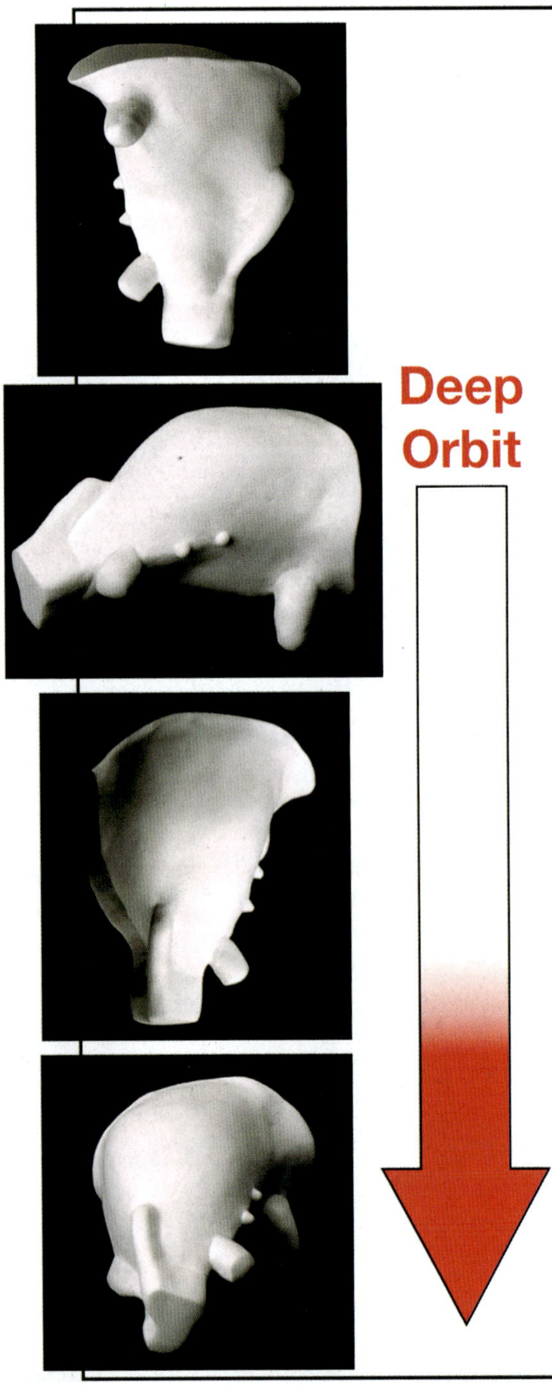

Anterior Orbit	
Landmarks	**Structures at Risk**
Septum Orbitale	
Arcus Marginalis	
Postentry Expansion	Insertion of IOM
Nasolacrimal Fossa /Canal	Lacimal Sac /Duct
	Medial Retinaculum
Zygomatico Orbital Foramen/-ina	Zygomatic Nerve
Trochlear Fovea	Trochlea
Whitnall's Tubercle	Lateral Retinaculum
Midorbit	
Landmarks	**Structures at Risk**
Anterior Loop of IOF	
Greater wing of Sphenoid	Zygomatic Nerve Lacrimal Nerve
Zygomaticosphenoid Suture	
Infraorbital Groove	Perforators from Infroarbital Neurovascular Bundle
Internal Orbital Buttress (MES)	
Posterior Medial Bulge	
Anterior Ethmoidal Foramen	Anterior Ethmoidal Neurovascular Bundle
Intermediate Ethmoidal Foramina	Supernumery Ethmoidal Neurovascular Bundles
IOF Isthmus / IOFIP	Infraorbital nerve Zygomatic nerve
	Ciliary Ganglion (CG)
IOF Basin	Inraorbital Nerve Parasympathetic Branches for Lacrimal
Posterior Orbit (Apex)	
Landmarks	**Structures at Risk**
Posterior Ethmoidal Foramen	Posterior Ethmoidal Neurovascular Bundle
Optic Foramen	Optic Nerve Ophthalmic Artery
Maxillary Strut / (Foramen Rotundum)	Maxillary Nerve
Lower medial SOF Sector	Inferior Ophthalmic Vein
COF	Recurrent Meningo-Lacrimal Artery / ? Ophthalmic Artery originating from Middle Meningeal Artery ?
Lateral Superior SOF Sector	LS SOF S Contents: CN IV, CN V1- branches - Lacrimal Nerve Frontal Nerve. Superior Ophthalmic Vein
Central SOF Sector	C SOF S Contents: Nasociliary Nerve CN III, CN VI Sympathetic CG Roots
Optic Strut	

Fig. 18 Periorbital dissection sequence—silhouettes of right periorbital sac (inferior–medial–superior–posterior) to indicate approximate position of landmarks and related structures at risk. (*Courtesy of* C. P. Cornelius, F. Probst, M. C. Metzger, and P. J. J. Gooris.)

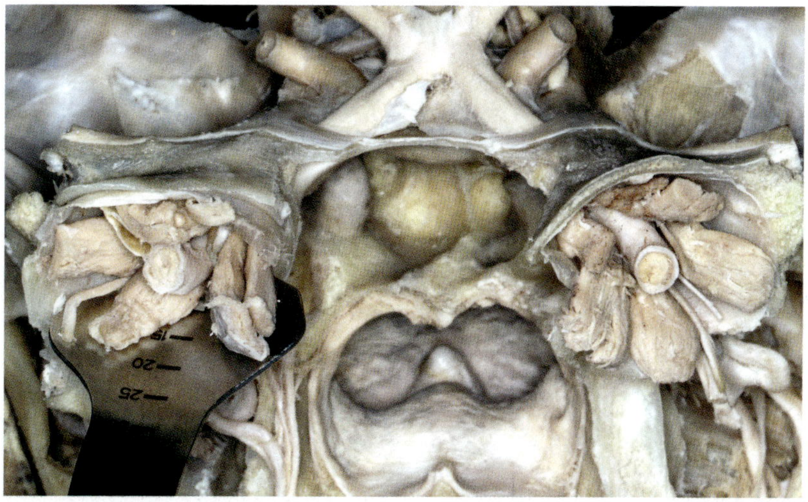

Fig. 19 Frontal section at the transition of midorbit into posterior orbit—view of both apical cross-sections and their contents (fat removed). The tip of the spatula elevating the periorbita might exert indirect compressional effects on CN II, the SOF fillings and extraocular muscles. (*Courtesy of* C. P. Cornelius, F. Probst, M. C. Metzger, and P. J. J. Gooris.)

the sphincter pupillae of the iris and the ciliary muscle to control pupil constriction and regulate ocular accommodation. The short ciliary nerve bundles are of a tiny (0.2-mm) diameter. In their initial course, they stay in a lateral position to CN II. Then they undergo further divisions, which revolve around the whole CN II circumference to pierce the sclera at the posterior globe. The sensory fibers contained in the short ciliary nerve bundles convey sensation from the eyeball and the cornea; the sympathetic fibers are in charge of vasoconstriction.

The long ciliary nerves, side branches of the nasociliary nerve, mingle with the short ciliary nerve bundles and carry sympathetic fibers. These fibers supply the pupillary dilator muscle.

Clinics care points

- Dissection of the periorbital lining away from the bony surfaces of the internal orbit must proceed with forethought and precaution, while watching out for neurovascular structures and suspension (eg, trochlea and retinacula) or insertion (eg, inferior oblique muscle) sites. Topographic orientation in reference to anatomic landmarks is the preferable safeguard as opposed to average depth-gauge measurements.
- The approach into the tight spatial confines of the deep orbit using spatulas generates compressive forces to the intraorbital portion of the optic nerve beyond the risk of direct mechanical nerve injuries next to the optic foramen and superior orbital fissure.

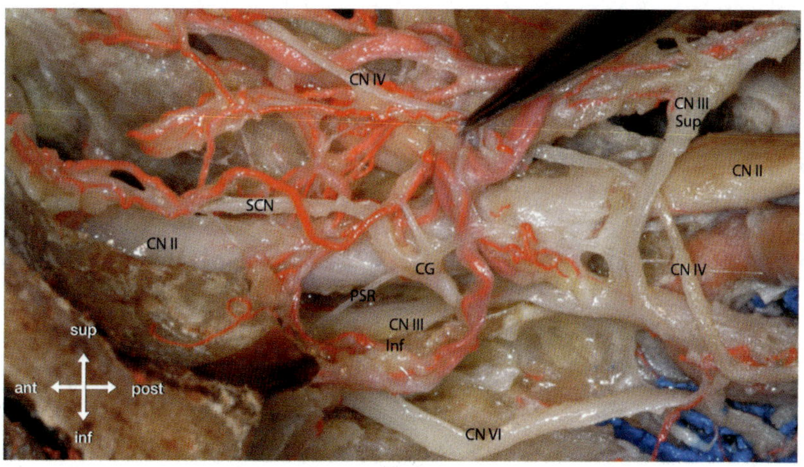

Fig. 20 CG—lateral view in posterior left orbit. Starlike appearance with multiple nerval inlets and outlets, including the parasympathetic radix (PSR). ant, anterior; post, posterior; sup, superior; inf, inferior; CG, Ciliary ganglion; CN III Inf D, Oculomotor Nerve Inferior Division; CN III Sup D, Oculomotor Nerve Superior Division; PSR, Parasympathetic Radix; SCN, Short Ciliary Nerve. (*Courtesy of* C. P. Cornelius, F. Probst, M. C. Metzger, and P. J. J. Gooris.)

Acknowledgments

A big kudos and many thanks go to the photographers Gerhard Poetzel and Rudolf Herzig, OMFS/FPS Departement Ludwig-Maximilians-University, Munich, for their enormous help!

Disclosure

The authors have nothing to disclose. Dissections of anatomic specimens were conducted in compliance with state and local laws.

Further readings

Cornelius CP, Mayer P, Ehrenfeld M, et al. The orbits-anatomical features in view of innovative surgical methods. Facial Plast Surg 2014; 30(5):487–508.

Demer JL. The orbital pulley system: a revolution in concepts of orbital anatomy. Ann N Y Acad Sci 2002;956:17–32.

Dutton JJ. Atlas of clinical and surgical orbital anatomy. 2nd Edition. Philadelphia (PA): Saunders; 2011.

Eckstein LA, Shadpour JM, Menghani R, et al. The relationship of the globe to the orbital rim. Arch Facial Plast Surg 2011;13(1): 51–6.

Ellis E III, Zide MF. Surgical approaches to the facial skeleton. 2nd edition. Philadelphia: Lippincott Williams & Wilkins; 2006.

Evans BT, Webb AA. Post-traumatic orbital reconstruction: anatomical landmarks and the concept of the deep orbit. Br J Oral Maxillofac Surg 2007;45(3):183–218.

Gooris PJJ, Muller BS, Dubois L, et al. Finding the ledge: sagittal analysis of bony landmarks of the orbit. J Oral Maxillofac Surg 2017; 75(12):2613–27.

Gregory GL. Eye and brain: the psychology of seeing. 5th Edition. Oxford: Oxford University Press; 1998.

Hammer B. Orbital fractures. Diagnosis, operative treatment, secondary corrections. Seattle Toronto Bern: Hofgrefe & Huber; 1995.

Holmes S, Blythe J. Orbit and orbital trauma,. In: Brennan PA, Standring SM, Wiseman SM, editors. Gray's surgical anatomy. 1st edition. Amsterdam: Elsevier; 2020.

Jansen J, Dubois L, TJJ Maal, et al. A nonsurgical approach with repeated orthoptic evaluation is justified for most blow-out fractures. J Craniomaxillofac Surg 2020;48(6):560–8.

Kim HS, Oh JH, Choi DY, et al. Three-dimensional courses of zygomaticofacial and zygomaticotemporal canals using micro-computed tomography in Korean. J Craniofac Surg 2013;24(5):1565–8.

Kawamoto HK Jr. Late posttraumatic enophthalmos: a correctable deformity? Plast Reconstr Surg 1982;69(3):423–32.

Kazak Z, Celik S, Ozer MA, et al. Three-dimensional evaluation of the danger zone of ethmoidal foramens on the frontoethmoidal suture line on the medial orbital wall. Surg Radiol Anat 2015;37(8): 935–40.

Koornneef L. Spatial aspects of orbital musculofibrous tissue in man [PhD thesis]. Amsterdam and Lisse: University of Amsterdam: Swets & Zeitlinger; 1976.

Koornneef L. The architecture of the musculo-fibrous apparatus in the human orbit. Acta Morphol Neerl Scand 1977;15(1):35–64.

Manson PN, Iliff N. Surgical anatomy of the orbit. In: Marsh JL, editor. Current therapy in plastic and reconstructive surgery Vol1 : head and Neck. Toronto: Decker; 1989. p. 117–22.

Miller JM. EOM pulleys and sequelae: a critical review. Invest Ophthalmol Vis Sci 2019;60(15):5052–8.

Peris-Celda M, Martinez-Soriana F, Rhoton AL Jr. Rhoton's Atlas of head, neck, and brain: 2d and 3d images. New York (NY): Thieme Medical Publishers, Inc.; 2018.

Regoli M, Bertelli E. The revised anatomy of the canals connecting the orbit with the cranial cavity. Orbit 2017;36(2):110–7.

Rhoton AL, Natori Y. The orbit and sellar region: microsurgical anatomy and operative approaches. New York (NY): Thieme Medical Publishers; 1996.

Rontal E, Rontal M, Guilford FT. Surgical anatomy of the orbit. Ann Otol Rhinol Laryngol 1979;88(3 Pt 1):382–6.

Rootman J. Orbital surgery - a conceptual approach. 2nd Edition. Philadelphia (PA): Lippincott Williams & Wilkins; 2014. Rootman 2nd.

Zide BM. Surgical anatomy around the orbit. The system of zones. Philadelphia (PA): Lippincott Williams and Wilkins; 2006.

Ocular Injury and Emergencies Around the Globe

Gijsbert J. Hötte, MD*, Ronald O.B. De Keizer, MD

KEYWORDS

• Ocular trauma • Eyelid laceration • Canalicular laceration • Orbital compartment syndrome

KEY POINTS

- Retrobulbar hemorrhage in the setting of orbital trauma can cause orbital compartment syndrome, which may result in irreversible vision loss. Immediate action through a lateral canthotomy and cantholysis is required.
- Ocular examination should be performed by an ophthalmologist in any case of periocular trauma. If globe laceration is suspected, any manipulation of the area should be avoided until integrity of the globe has been confirmed or sufficiently restored.
- Adequate knowledge of the anatomy and functional and dynamic behavior of the eyelids is paramount when performing repair of an eyelid laceration.
- Repair of canalicular lacerations should be attempted in all cases within 48 hours by a surgeon experienced in lacrimal surgery.

Introduction

The orbital soft tissues include various important structures such as the eyelids, lacrimal drainage system, extraocular muscles, the optic nerve, and the globe. Although protected by the bony orbit, these structures are prone to traumatic injuries which, as discussed in this chapter, include orbital compartment syndrome, globe laceration, eyelid laceration, and damage to the lacrimal drainage system. It is paramount that such injury is timely recognized and adequately dealt with, and a thorough examination should therefore be performed by an ophthalmologist in any case of orbital trauma. However, because of the multidisciplinary nature of the orbital region, it is important that other physicians also are familiar with these injuries.

Retrobulbar hemorrhage and orbital compartment syndrome

Etiology and clinical assessment

The intraorbital structures are confined within a closed and rigid compartment consisting of the bony orbital walls and the orbital septa and eyelids (Box 1). As such, there is little space to accommodate a sudden increase in orbital pressure. Orbital compartment syndrome (OCS) occurs when the intraorbital pressure exceeds the arterial perfusion pressure, resulting in ischemia and irreversible damage to the optic nerve and retina within 100 minutes.[1] The most common cause of such an increase in orbital pressure is retrobulbar hemorrhage, as may occur in the setting of periocular trauma.

Department of Oculoplastic, Orbital and Lacrimal Surgery, The Rotterdam Eye Hospital, PO Box 70030, Rotterdam 3000 LM, the Netherlands

* Corresponding author.

E-mail address: g.hotte@oogziekenhuis.nl

Treatment: lateral canthotomy and cantholysis

In line with the previously mentioned etiology, emergency treatment is directed at opening up the closed compartment. This is accomplished in the first place by performing a lateral canthotomy and cantholysis, a technique that any emergency physician or medical specialist involved in the orbital region should be familiar with. The canthal ligaments (sometimes referred to as tendons) are the structures that attach the eyelid tarsi to the bony orbit, with the lateral ligament being the most easily accessible. Releasing the eyelid from its attachment to the lateral orbital wall opens up the orbital compartment and allows for an anterior movement of the globe, thereby decreasing the intraorbital pressure. Sometimes the question is raised whether this anterior movement of the globe does not stretch the optic nerve, causing permanent damage as well. However, the length of the orbital part of the optic nerve is somewhat redundant, allowing for some degree of exophthalmos before the nerve fibers are put on stretch. Even more so, tensile forces on the optic nerve are far less harmful than ischemia.

Lateral canthotomy and cantholysis is performed as follows:

- Canthotomy (Fig. 1A): Use scissors to make a cut in the lateral canthal angle, directed away from the globe, up to the lateral orbital rim. The cut is made through all layers of the lateral canthal angle at once: skin, orbicularis muscle, lateral canthal ligament, palpebral conjunctiva. Make sure not to cut the bulbar conjunctiva, as this may cause symblepharon. This first cut effectively divides the lateral canthal ligament into an inferior and superior limb.

Atlas Oral Maxillofacial Surg Clin N Am 29 (2021) 19–28

https://doi.org/10.1016/j.cxom.2020.11.002

Box 1. Signs of orbital compartment syndrome

Progressive proptosis
Decreased visual acuity
Relative afferent pupillary defect (RAPD)
Concentric motility impairment
Pain
Increased intraocular pressure
Tight orbital tissues
Chemosis
Decreased retinal perfusion, as noted on fundoscopy

- Skin-muscle flap (Fig. 1B): By blunt dissection, you can now create a skin-muscle flap inferior to the lateral canthal angle.
- Inferior cantholysis (Fig. 1C): When you raise the skin-muscle flap, the underlying inferior limb of the lateral canthal ligament is exposed, but often not clearly distinguishable. With tooth forceps, grasp the eyelid margin of the lower eyelid near the lateral canthal angle and pull the eyelid medially and anteriorly. By doing so, the inferior limb of the lateral canthal ligament is put on stretch. With the tip of the closed scissors you can now feel the inferior limb of the canthal ligament as a tight string. Open up the scissors around this string and cut it with your scissors directed directly inferior. Again, feel with your scissors for residual attachments and cut them. Repeat this until the cantholysis is completed and the eyelid is freely mobile. Note that the lateral canthal ligament is continuous with fibers from the orbital septum. Therefore, the cut may need to be extended to include the septum to acquire adequate mobility.
- Superior cantholysis: If you feel that inferior cantholysis has yielded insufficient release of the compartment syndrome, superior cantholysis can be performed in a similar fashion. It is advisable to direct this cut superiorly as well as slightly laterally to avoid cutting into the lacrimal gland, which may cause brisk bleeding and can result in severe dry eye.
- Repair of the lateral canthal angle: After approximately 2 weeks, the canthal angle can be closed; however, in most cases, repair is not necessary, as spontaneous granulation usually provides adequate results.

It should be noted that in the setting of an orbital fracture (mostly the floor or medial wall), the compartment may have been opened up sufficiently by the fracture itself and cantholysis may not be necessary. However, OCS still can occur if the periorbita remains intact. Conversely, if inferior and superior cantholysis have been performed without the desired effect, emergency orbital decompression, including opening of the periorbita, must be considered.

Orbital compartment syndrome and imaging

The indication for imaging in the context of OCS, as well as the precise indications to perform cantholysis, are source of debate. We advise the following rules of thumb:

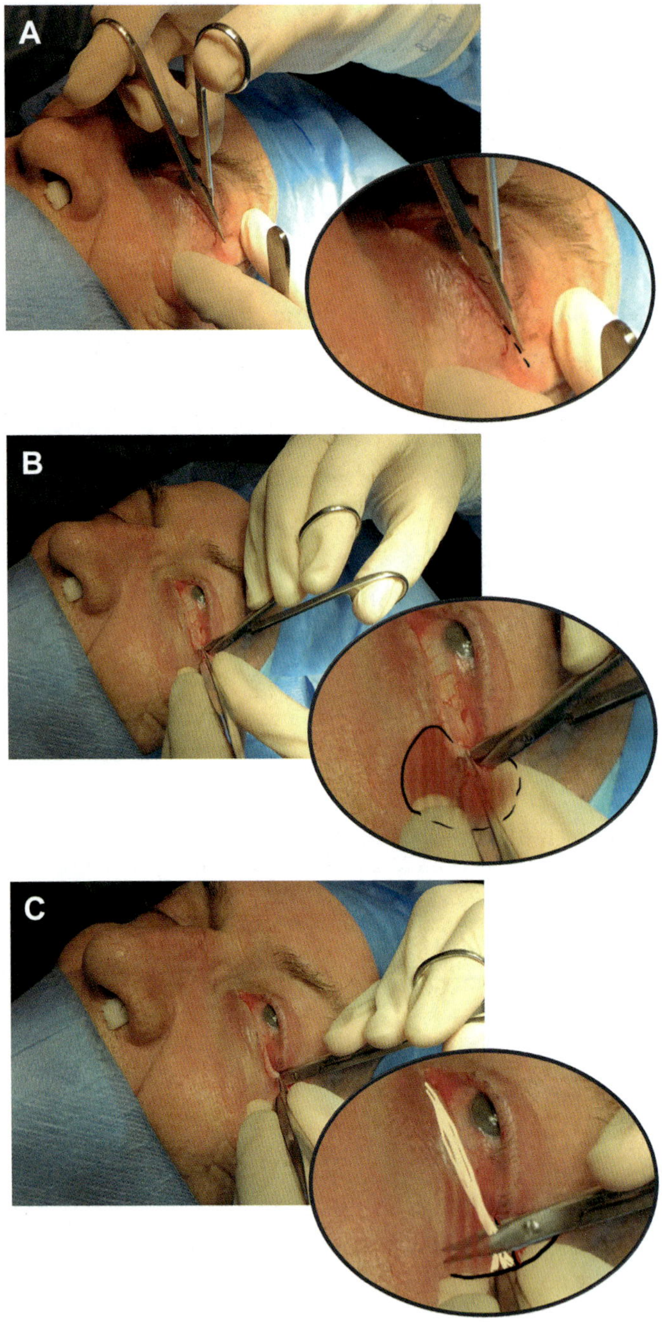

Fig. 1 Technique for lateral canthotomy and inferior cantholysis. (*A*) Lateral canthotomy. (*B*) Dissection of a skin-muscle flap. (*C*) Inferior cantholysis.

- Do not delay treatment awaiting radiological evaluation:The decision to perform inferior cantholysis should be made based on clinical signs, not solely on the findings of computed tomography (CT) imaging. Although a retrobulbar hemorrhage can be easily seen on CT imaging, the urgency of the situation dictates to act immediately when OCS is suspected, without delay for radiological evaluation. Conversely, a small retrobulbar hemorrhage that is noted on CT imaging without clinical manifestations of OCS may be left untreated.
- When in doubt, make the cut: Remember that not performing a cantholysis when you should have done so, may

Box 2. Ocular assessment by emergency physician

Confirm integrity of the globe
Visual acuity
Red cap test
Confrontational visual field
Ocular Motility
Pupillary test, including RAPD

result in permanent and profound loss of vision. On the other hand, an adequately executed, inferior cantholysis rarely causes permanent complaints after healing.

Trauma to the globe

Ocular examination

It is important to remember that damage to the intraocular structures can occur even in apparently mild cases of trauma, and thorough ocular examination should therefore be performed by an ophthalmologist in any case of periocular trauma. The first assessment, however, can be performed by the emergency physician (Box 2). We believe that the ophthalmologist should be involved directly in the emergency room in any of the circumstances, as listed in Box 3. In any other case, more detailed examination by an ophthalmologist can be performed within the next few days.

Globe laceration

Laceration of the globe can occur in penetrating or blunt periocular trauma and accordingly should be ruled out in all cases of periocular trauma. Signs of globe laceration are listed in Box 4.

If a globe laceration is indeed suspected, the following should be initiated:

- Place a protective shield (not a pressure bandage!)
- Ask the ophthalmologist for urgent consultation
- Make sure the patient is kept on a nil per os regimen
- Provide with adequate systemic analgesics
- Avoid any manipulation of the globe and eyelids:
  - Do not administer topical medication unless necessary
  - Provide with adequate sedatives in case of anxiety
  - Provide with adequate antiemetics, as vomiting may give increased pressure on the globe
  - If possible, postpone examination or treatment of other injuries until integrity of the globe has been confirmed or sufficiently restored by an ophthalmologist.

Box 3. Indications for ocular assessment by an ophthalmologist

Suspected intraorbital hemorrhage
Suspected globe laceration
Suspected extraocular muscle entrapment
Exophthalmos or tenting of the optic nerve
Eyelid and/or lacrimal lacerations
Decreased vision
Unconscious patients

Box 4. Signs of globe laceration

Prolapse of uvea, vitreous, or retina (Fig. 2)
Intraocular foreign body (as noted on biomicroscopy/fundoscopy or orbital imaging)
Orbital imaging suggestive of globe laceration
Leakage of intraocular fluids as demonstrated by a positive Seidel test
History of sharp periocular trauma
Eyelid laceration
Extensive subconjunctival hemorrhage
Peaked pupil (see Fig. 2)
Shallow anterior chamber
Hypotony

Other traumatic ocular injury

Although a detailed description is beyond the scope of this article, other complications of ocular trauma are listed in Box 5.

Eyelid lacerations

Eyelid lacerations not involving the eyelid margin

Although repair of eyelid lacerations that do not involve the eyelid margin may seem relatively straightforward, adequate knowledge of the anatomy and dynamic behavior of the eyelids is paramount to reduce the risk of complications. We recommend the following principles:

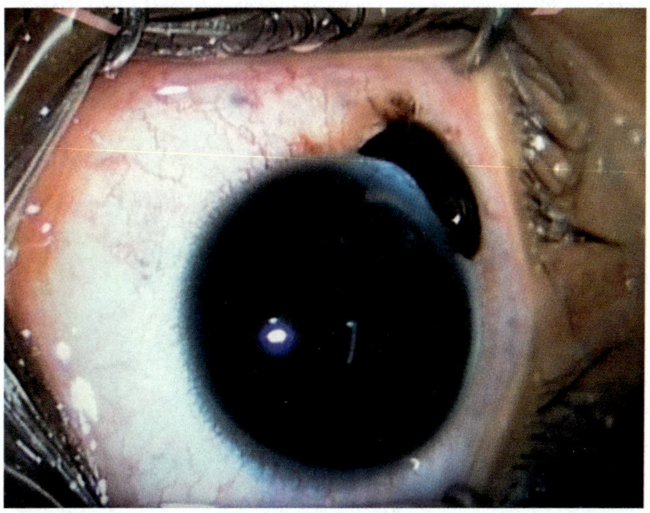

Fig. 2 Small globe laceration at the level of the limbus. Note the peaked pupil pointing toward the location of the uveal prolapse. (*Courtesy of* J. De Faber, MD, Rotterdam, The Netherlands.)

Box 5. Other complications of ocular injury

Corneal erosion
Hyphema (Fig. 3)
Iridodialysis (Fig. 4)
Cataract
Lens luxation (Fig. 5)
Vitreous hemorrhage
Commotio retinae
Choroidal rupture
Retinal breaks and detachment
Traumatic optic neuropathy
Optic nerve avulsion

- Always confirm integrity of the globe: The eyelids are only thin protection of the globe. Therefore, an eyelid laceration should always prompt assessment of the globe's integrity.
- Conservative wound debridement: Parts of the skin that are unviable can be removed by wound debridement; however, vascularization of the eyelids is excellent, so that debridement usually does not have to be performed aggressively. Moreover, remember that excessive debridement may lead to a relative skin deficiency, which may cause cicatricial ectropion or lagophthalmos. Free, relatively clean, avascularized flaps may be sutured back in their anatomic location.

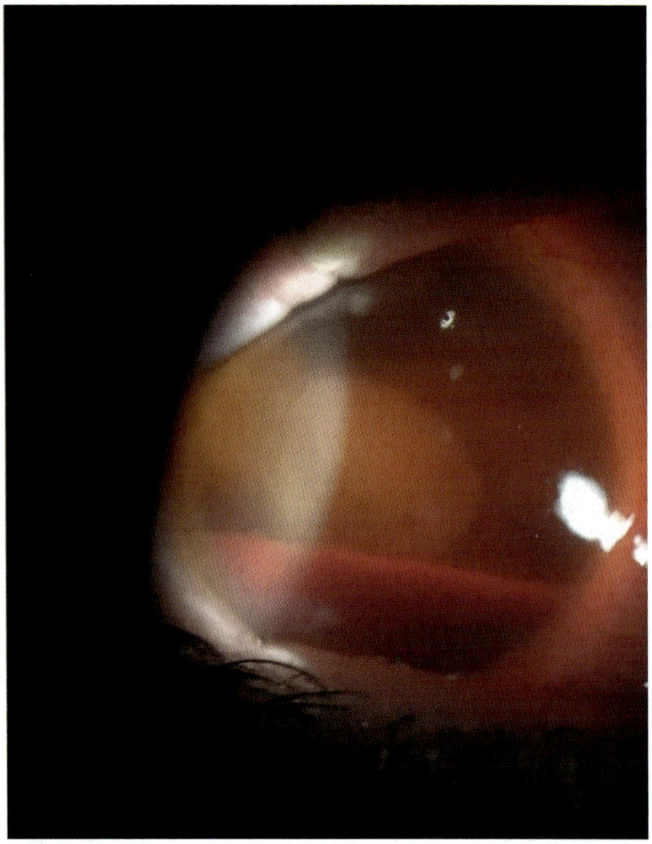

Fig. 3 Hyphema. (*Courtesy of* J. De Faber, MD, Rotterdam, The Netherlands.)

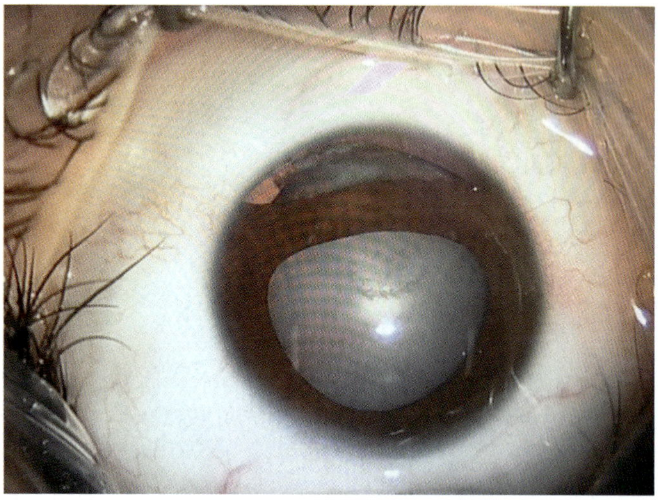

Fig. 4 Iridodialysis. (*Courtesy of* J. De Faber, MD, Rotterdam, The Netherlands.)

- Do not close the orbital septum: The orbital septum is a sheet of fibrous tissue that extends from the orbital rims to fuse with the eyelid retractors. If the orbital septum is violated in an eyelid laceration, closing of the septal defect is not advisable, as this may lead to shortening of the septum. As the septum is a rigid structure firmly attached to the orbital rim, shortening may lead to a hang up of the eyelid causing lagophthalmos and exposure of the globe.

Eyelid lacerations involving the eyelid margin

It is important to understand that the eyelid margin is crucial for both functional and esthetic aspects of the eyelid and adequate restoration of eyelid margin is paramount. Various suture techniques have been described. For all techniques, good functional and esthetic results are obtained only if the following rules are followed:

- Protect the globe: Working closely to the ocular surface, it is advisable to protect the globe with either a protective shield or Jäger plate.

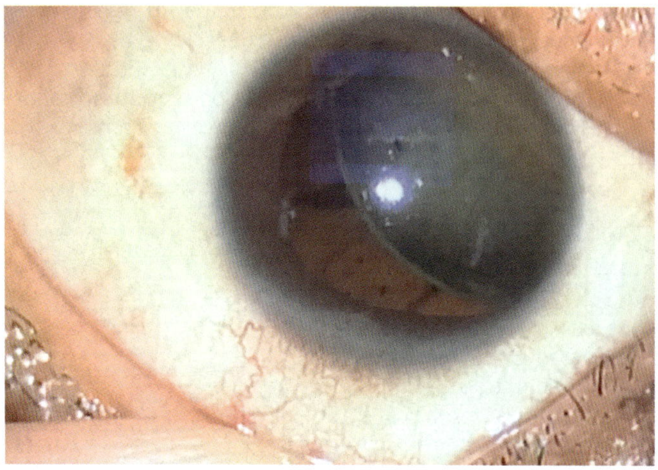

Fig. 5 Lens luxation. (*Courtesy of* J. De Faber, MD, Rotterdam, The Netherlands.)

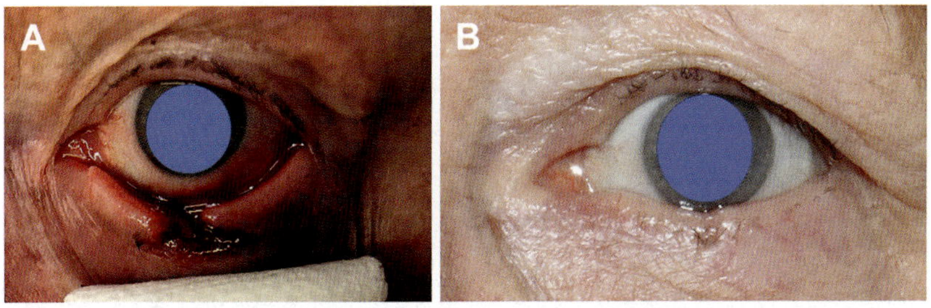

Fig. 6 Laceration of the eyelid margin. (*A*) Traumatic laceration of the central inferior eyelid involving the eyelid margin. (*B*) Small notch after repair.

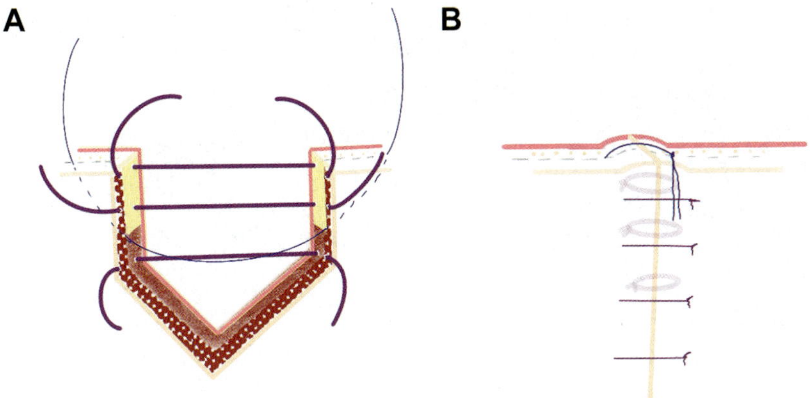

Fig. 7 Closure of an eyelid margin defect in 2 layers. (*A*) Placement of the deep tarsal sutures (*purple*) and eyelid margin suture (*blue*). (*B*) The eyelid margin suture is left long and tied down with the skin sutures. (*Courtesy of* W. Van den Bosch, MD, PhD, Rotterdam, The Netherlands.)

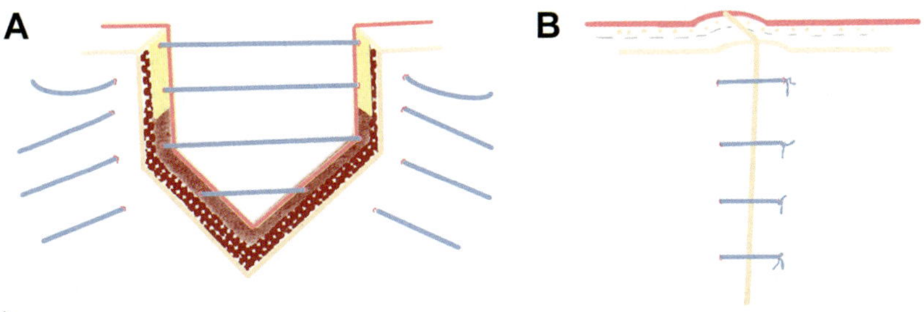

Fig. 8 Closure of an eyelid margin defect in one layer. (*A*) Single-layered suture for skin, orbicularis muscle, and tarsus. (*B*) An additional eyelid margin suture can be placed if needed, but is not shown here. (*Courtesy of* D. Paridaens, MD, PhD, Rotterdam, The Netherlands.)

- Do not pass through the conjunctiva: In any technique for eyelid closure, care is taken not to breach the conjunctiva because the suture may cause irritation to the ocular surface, resulting in corneal abrasion or even ulcers. Also, place the knot anteriorly so that it does not erode through the conjunctiva.
- Mirror the sutures: The sutures are "mirrored," both in an anterior-posterior and superior-inferior direction. This means that the height and depth of the suture should be exactly equal on both sides of the wound. If this is not done properly, a notch in the eyelid margin will result (Fig. 6).
- If unsatisfied, try again: It is easier to obtain adequate eyelid position during the primary repair than to do so at a later stage. Therefore, if you feel that the wound margins do not approximate nicely, remove the sutures and try again.
- Timing: Primary closure of eyelid laceration is preferably performed within 24 hours, although we believe that good results can be obtained up to 48 hours.[2]

Most surgeons use a double-layered suture technique, which consists of deep tarsal sutures together with superficial skin sutures. Although many techniques are described, we usually use the following:[3]

- Deep tarsal sutures (Fig. 7A): Just inferior to the eyelid margin, a Vicryl 6-0 or 5-0 suture is passed into the

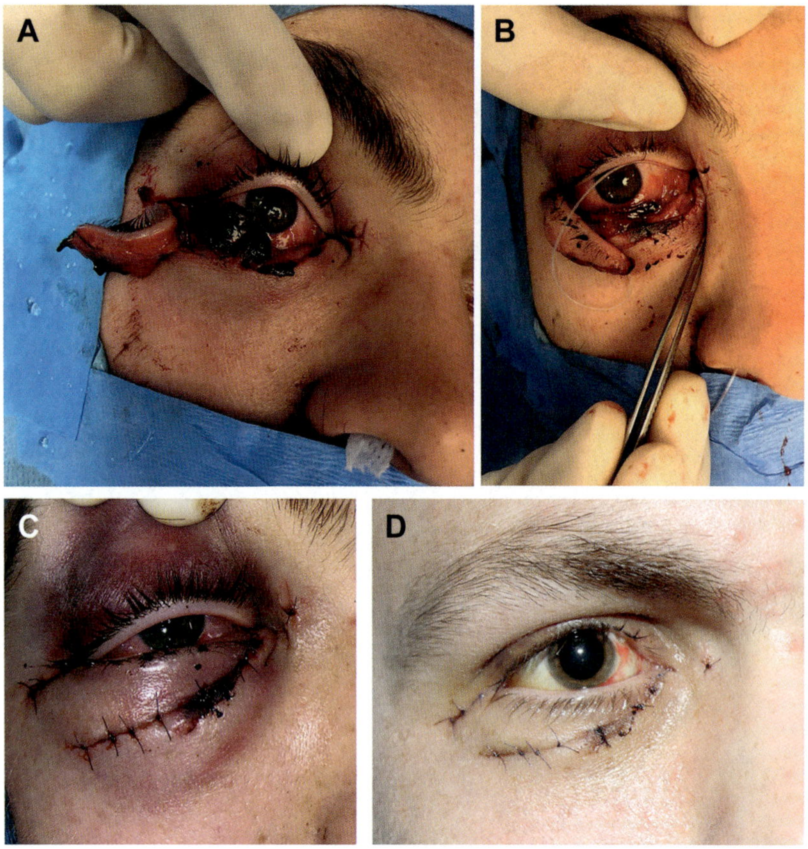

Fig. 9 Large eyelid laceration including the inferior canaliculus. (*A*) Eyelid laceration involving the lateral canthal ligament, medial canthal ligament, inferior canaliculus, and inferior fornix. The eyelid is now only vascularized through a small laterally based pedicle of skin and muscle. (*B*) Note the proximal end of the stent fixated inside the inferior punctum, whereas the distal end runs through the distal cut end and exits from the nose. (*C*) Note the triangle of darkened skin just inferior to the laceration, which is often wrongly chosen to be removed by excessive debridement. (*D*) One week after reconstruction. Note that the eyelid as a whole and the triangle of darkened tissue more specifically prove to be viable although it was vascularized only through the small laterally based pedicle.

orbicularis muscle and out through the underlying tarsus. In the opposite wound edge, the suture is then passed through the tarsus and back out through the overlying orbicularis muscle. As noted previously, the height and depth of these passes should be exactly mirrored so that the wound edges approximate correctly. By pulling each end to the opposing side, you can confirm that the position of the suture is adequate. Now, before tying the first suture, a second suture is placed in a similar fashion just 2 to 3 mm inferiorly. If necessary, another third suture can be placed, again 2 to 3 mm inferiorly. The first suture is now tied. This often results in an angled apposition of the wound edges, which is corrected by tying the second and possibly third suture. Note that only 2 or 3 of these sutures are needed in the lower eyelid, whereas usually 3 or 4 are needed for closure of the upper eyelid, as it has a much higher tarsal plate.

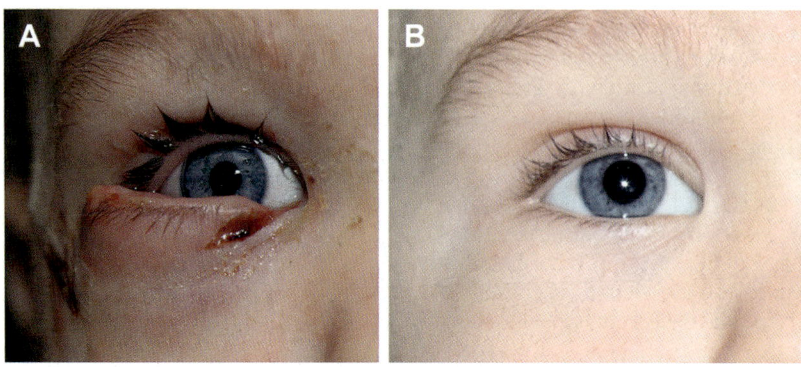

Fig. 10 Laceration of the medial and lateral canthal ligaments. (*A*) Eyelid laceration involving the medial and lateral canthal ligament in a child. (*B*) Three months after reconstruction of the lateral canthal ligament, medial canthal ligament, and inferior canaliculus.

- Eyelid margin suture (Fig. 7B): Although the deep tarsal sutures are the most important for reconstruction and integrity of the eyelid margin, a subtle indentation at the level of the gray line may remain. Therefore, some surgeons prefer to place an additional 6-0 or 7-0 fast-absorbing suture through the gray line. Because of its proximity to the ocular surface, this suture may cause irritation. To prevent this, the ends of the suture are usually left long and will be tied down with the skin sutures.
- Skin sutures (see Fig. 7B): Either nonabsorbable sutures such as Prolene 6-0 or fast-absorbing sutures such as Vicryl Rapide 6-0 are used to close the skin. As mentioned, these sutures can be used to tie down the ends of the eyelid margin suture.

Although variations of the previously mentioned double-layered suture technique have been used historically, a single-layered technique can give similar results[4]:

- Single-layered suture for skin, orbicularis muscle and tarsus (Fig. 8A): Just inferior to the eyelid margin, a Prolene or Vicryl 6-0 is passed through skin and orbicularis muscle and exits through the underlying tarsus. In the opposing wound edge, the suture is then passed through the tarsus and back out through the overlying orbicularis muscle and skin. Again, before tying this suture, a second suture is placed in a similar manner 2 to 3 mm inferiorly.
- Eyelid margin suture (Fig. 8B): If needed, an additional eyelid margin suture can be placed and tied down with the other sutures.

Traumatic injury to the lacrimal drainage system

Canalicular laceration

Periocular trauma often causes horizontal traction on the eyelid. When this happens, the eyelid may rupture at its weakest points: the medial and/or lateral canthal ligaments (Figs. 9 and 10). These ligaments connect the eyelid tarsi to the bony orbit.

The lateral canthal ligament attaches to the lateral orbital tubercle (Whitnall tubercle), and avulsion of this ligament is relatively easily repaired, although a frequently made mistake is to reattach the lateral canthal ligament too far inferiorly, causing unsightly down slant of the eyelid.

On the other hand, the medial canthal ligament has a more complex anatomy. It is composed of an anterior and a posterior limb that are attached to the anterior and posterior lacrimal crest, respectively. Although the posterior limb is more subtle, its patency is crucial for an adequate position of the eyelid, following the curvature of the globe posteriorly. More importantly, the medial canthal ligament has an intricate relationship with the lacrimal drainage system, which is why periocular trauma and eyelid lacerations are relatively often associated with canalicular laceration.

Literature shows that canalicular repair must be performed if both canaliculi are involved (Fig. 11); however, some investigators claim that in case of a single canalicular laceration, epiphora may not occur if one patent canaliculus remains.[5] Even so, it must be said that if epiphora does occur, secondary repair of the canaliculus can be extremely challenging.

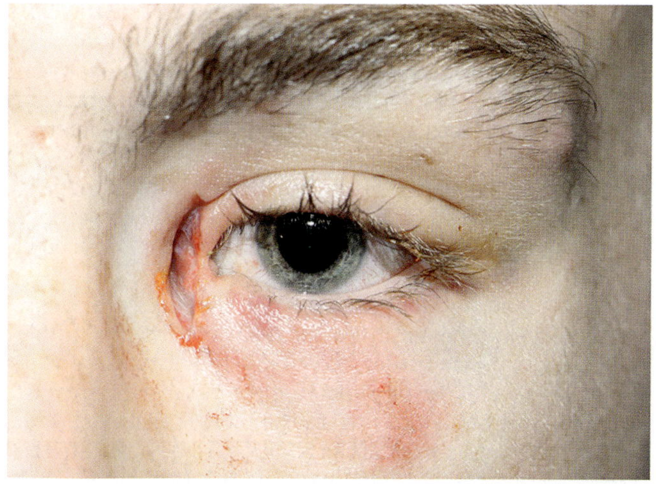

Fig. 11 Laceration after sharp trauma just medial to the medial canthal angle. Note the displacement and rounding of medial canthal angle, a sign that the medial canthal ligament has been cut. In this case, both inferior and superior canaliculi were lacerated and successfully reconstructed using 2 monocalicular stents.

Therefore, we advise to always attempt repair of the canaliculus as soon as possible but at least within 48 hours. Because of the complex anatomy and importance of primary repair, it is important that the canalicular reconstruction is performed only by surgeons experienced in lacrimal surgery.

Advice in canalicular repair

- General anesthesia: Although small superficial lacerations may be reconstructed under local anesthesia (Fig. 12), we advise general anesthesia for most cases. It provides a better controlled environment for the reconstruction, which at times can be challenging and frustrating. Moreover, local anesthesia results in additional tissue swelling,

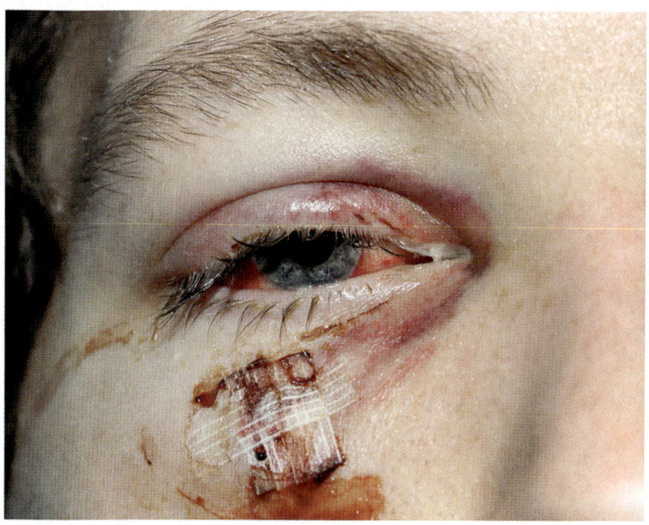

Fig. 12 Obscured canalicular laceration. In periocular trauma, small canalicular lacerations may be easily overlooked. In this case, it appears to be only a superficial laceration of the lower eyelid; however, below the plug of mucus a laceration through the upper canaliculus was found on closer examination.

which may obscure the distal end of the cut canaliculus, especially when the rupture is near the lacrimal sac.

- Inspection of the punctum: The first step is to perform inspection of the punctum to see if it is still intact. In most cases, the laceration occurs a few millimeters medially to the punctum.
- Confirming laceration of the canaliculus: After stretching the punctum with a punctal dilator, a Bowman probe is inserted. Visualization of the probe within the wound confirms canalicular laceration.
- Identification of the distal end of the cut canaliculus: Although at times easily visible as a white "mouth" within the red and pink tissues, identifying the distal cut end of the canaliculus can be difficult. If the distal end cannot be found, one can try to irrigate the intact canaliculus with fluorescein, saline, or air. In addition, some advocate the use of pigtailed probes through the intact canaliculus, although we advise to use them cautiously, as they may cause iatrogenic damage to the intact canaliculus and lacrimal sac.
- Use a monocanalicular stent: In canalicular repair, it is paramount to place a temporary silicone stent. Traditionally, a bicanalicular stent is used, with one end advanced through the upper canaliculus and the other end through the lower canaliculus. These stents are then fixated inside the nose. We, however, recommend the use of a monocanalicular stent, as they have certain advantages. For one, it omits the need to stent the remaining intact canaliculus, reducing the risk of iatrogenic damage. Moreover, monocanalicular stents come with a plug at the proximal end that fits securely in the lacrimal punctum (Fig. 13), reducing the risk of stretching the punctum and canaliculus (known as cheese wiring), as may be seen in the bicanalicular system. Monocanalicular stents come in 2 versions. One has a metal probe attached to the distal end of the stent, whereas the other has not. With this probe, it can be easier to engage the distal end of the lacerated canaliculus. The probe then has to be advanced through the nasolacrimal duct and retrieved from the nose, which may be difficult at times and may cause iatrogenic

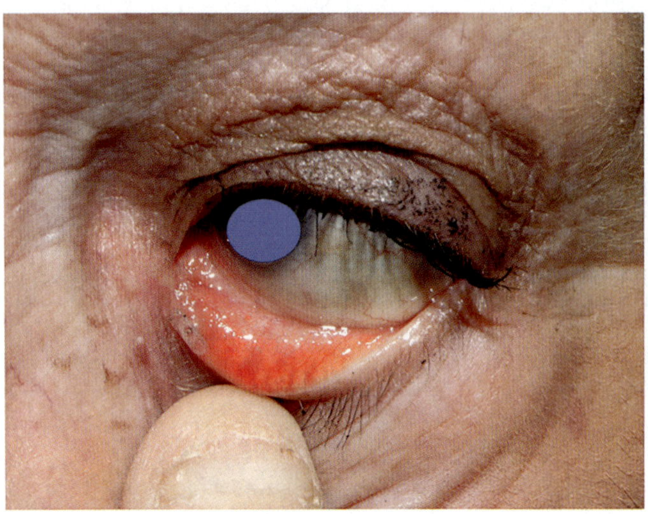

Fig. 13 Monocanalicular stent. Postoperative result 3 months after reconstruction of an inferior canalicular laceration. Note the plate end of the stent inside the punctum.

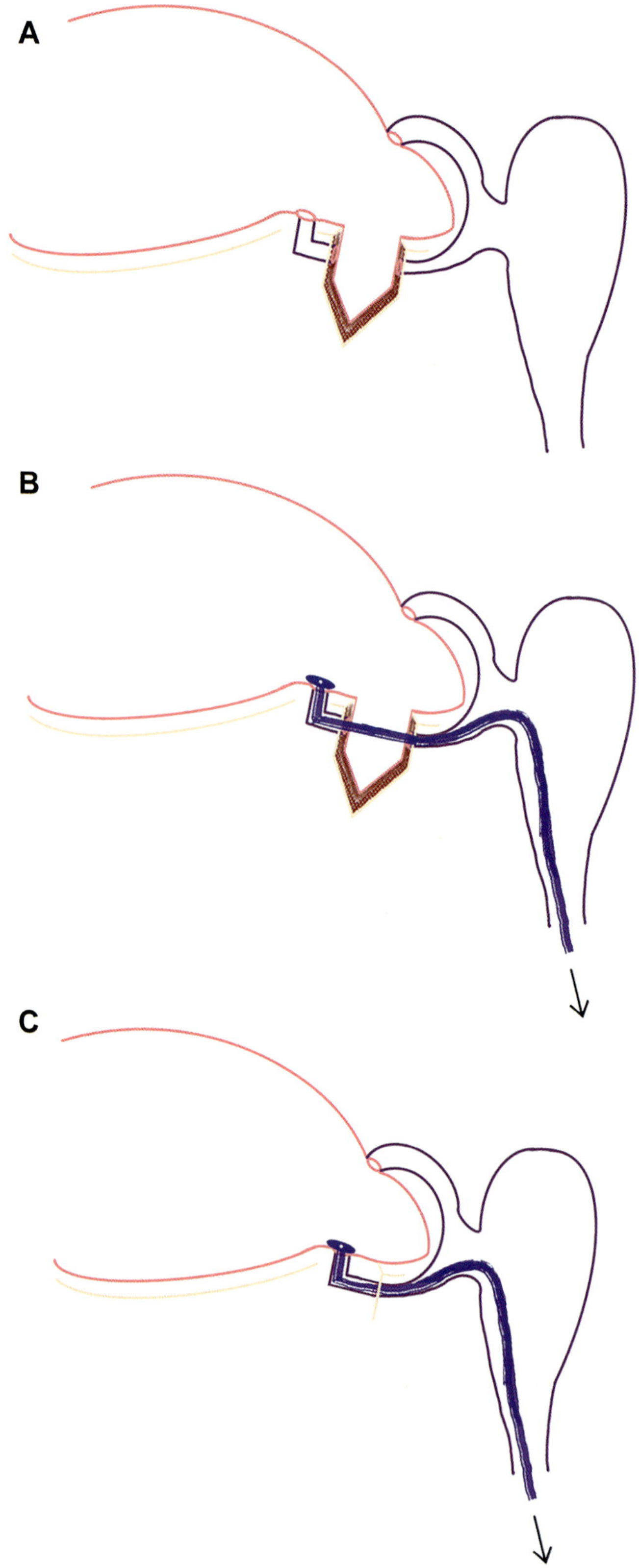

Fig. 14 Schematic representation of monocanalicular stent placement. (*A*) Laceration through the inferior canaliculus. (*B*) Placement of a monocanalicular stent. The proximal plate end sits securely inside the punctum, while the distal end is advanced through the lacrimal sac and nasolacrimal duct and is then retrieved from the nose. (*C*) Pulling on the distal end of the stent pulls the eyelid back into its anatomic position.

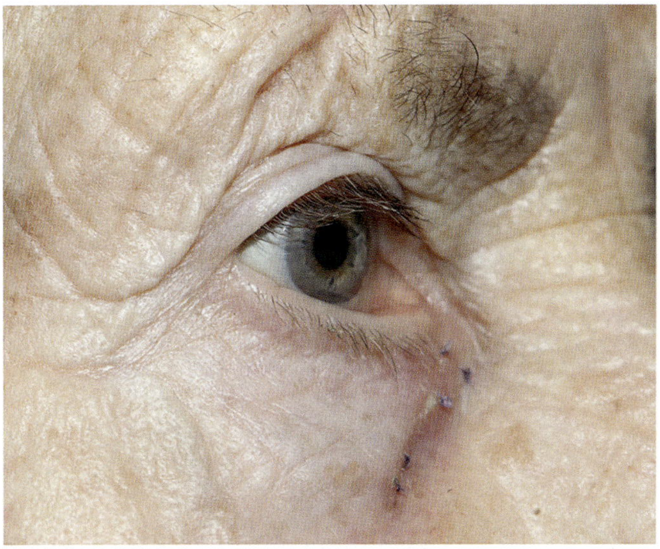

Fig. 15 Medial ectropion. Result 2 weeks after unsuccessful reconstruction of eyelid laceration, including the inferior canaliculus and medial canthal tendon. Note the medial ectropion.

damage to duct and/or nasal mucosa. However, as the proximal end is fixed inside the punctum with the plug, it has the advantage that pulling on the stent now neatly approximates the proximal and distal ends of the cut canaliculus *and* medial canthal ligament (Fig. 14). Not only does this aid in the repair of the canaliculus, but it also pulls the eyelid back into its original anatomic position, which may prevent postoperative structural abnormalities, such as medial ectropion (Fig. 15). The advantage of a monocanalicular stent without a probe is that it does not have to be retrieved from the nose and can therefore be used under local anesthesia. Whichever stent is used, it is generally left in situ for approximately 2 to 3 months, unless ocular irritation or other complaints occur.

- Wound closure: After placement of a stent, 2 Vicryl 6-0 sutures are placed alongside the cut canaliculus. The canthal ligament can be reattached with Vicryl 5-0. The skin is closed with either nonabsorbable sutures, such as Prolene 6-0, or fast-absorbing sutures, such as Vicryl Rapide 6-0.

Traumatic injury to the nasolacrimal duct

Another frequent cause of epiphora after periocular trauma is obstruction of the nasolacrimal duct by fracture of the surrounding bones, such as may occur in naso-orbital-ethmoidal (NOE) fractures. Besides epiphora, obstruction of the nasolacrimal duct may lead to dacryocystitis. The obstruction in these cases may be treated by external or endonasal dacryocystorhinostomy at a later stage. Other signs of NOE fracture include epistaxis and cerebrospinal fluid leakage. As mentioned, the medial canthal ligament is attached to the bones that are involved in NOE fractures. Therefore, a displaced NOE fracture may also cause lateral displacement of the medial canthal tendon, a characteristic feature that is often overlooked at the initial assessment (Fig. 16). Reconstruction of the fragments and/or the medial canthal tendon at primary trauma repair (preferably) may prevent this cosmetic problem.

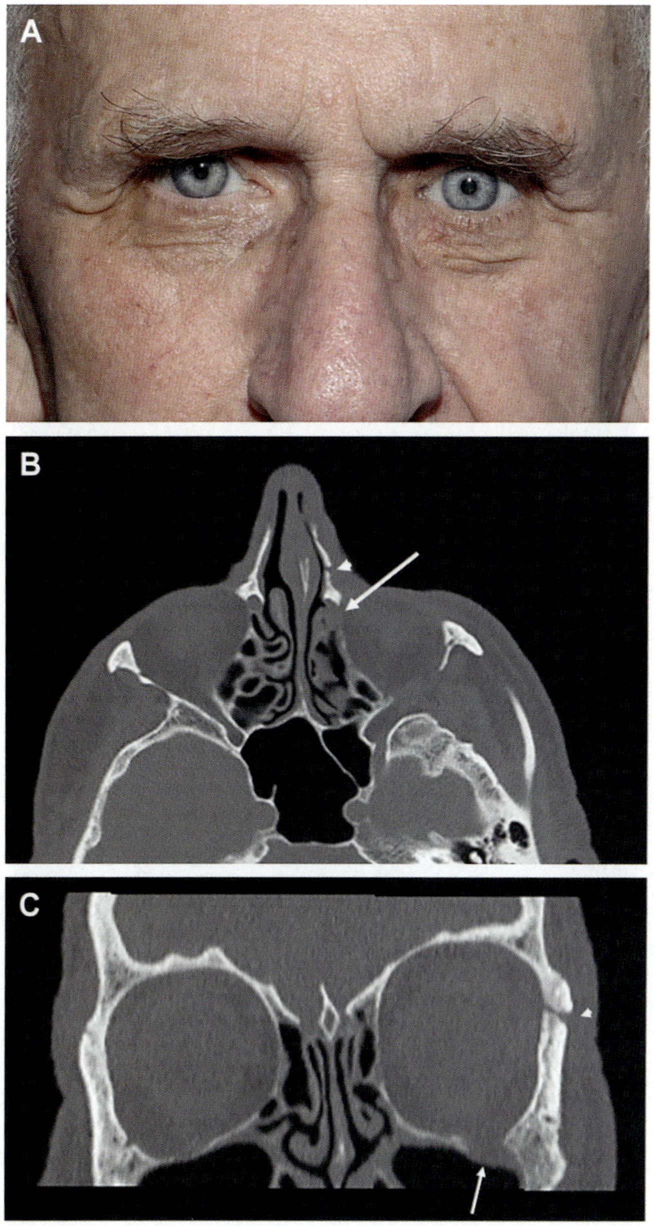

Fig. 16 Nasolacrimal duct obstruction in orbital fractures. (*A*) This patient was referred for epiphora and chronic discharge on the left side only. Patient history reported a head injury with blunt trauma to the left orbit approximately a year earlier, but no orbital imaging was performed at the emergency department of the referring hospital. Note that the left globe is displaced inferiorly, suggesting fracture of the orbital floor. Also note that the medial canthal angle is rounded and displaced laterally, which suggests NOE fracture. (*B*) Axial sections of CT imaging show a fracture of the medial orbital wall at the level of the nasolacrimal duct (*arrow*) and a fracture at the nasomaxillary suture (*arrowhead*). (*C*) Coronal sections of CT imaging show fractures of the orbital floor (*arrow*) and lateral wall (*arrowhead*). ([*B, C*] *Courtesy of* M. Gardeniers, MD, Rotterdam, The Netherlands.)

Acknowledgments

The authors wish to thank Dion Paridaens, Willem van den Bosch, Tjeerd de Faber, and Mayke Gardeniers for their contributions in the figures.

Disclosure

The authors have nothing to disclose.

References

1. Hayreh SS, Kolder HE, Weingeist TA. Central retinal artery occlusion and retinal tolerance time. Ophthalmology 1980;87(1):75–8.
2. Chiang E, Bee C, Harris GJ, et al. Does delayed repair of eyelid lacerations compromise outcome? Am J Emerg Med 2017;35(11):1766–7.
3. Van den Bosch WA. Praktische ooglidchirurgie. Utrecht: Wetenschappelijke Uitgeverij Bunge; 1997.
4. Verhoekx JS, Soebhag RK, Weijtens O, et al. A single- versus double-layered closure technique for full-thickness lower eyelid defects: a comparative study. Acta Ophthalmol 2016;94(3):257–60.
5. Smit TJ, Mourits MP. Monocanalicular lesions: to reconstruct or not. Ophthalmology 1999;106(7):1310–2.

Suggested readings

Kuhn F, Pieramici DJ. Ocular trauma: principles and practice. New York: Thieme; 2002.

Van den Bosch WA, Paridaens D. Available at: www.eyelid-surgery.nl. Accessed October 24, 2020.

Ongoing Debate in Clinical Decision Making in Orbital Fractures

Indications, Timing, and Biomaterials

Leander Dubois, DDS, MD, DMD, PhD [a,*], Jasjit Dillon, MD, DMD, PhD [b], Jesper Jansen, MD, DMD, PhD [a], Alfred G. Becking, DDS, MD, DMD, PhD, FEBOMS [a]

KEYWORDS

• Orbit • Orbital fractures • Indications • Timing • Soft tissues response • Reconstructive surgery • Biomaterials

KEY POINTS

- Trapdoor fracture in children, globe dislocation or trapdoor fracture with a nonresolving oculocardiac reflex, bradycardia, heart block, nausea, vomiting, or syncope are indications for immediate surgery.
- Early enophthalmos, hypoglobus, and severe limitation of eye motility (<15°) are indications for early intervention.
- If there is no enophthalmos present, and the motility of the eye significantly improves within 10 to 14 days, surgery may be not indicated, and clinical findings overrule the computed tomography scan results in all occasions.
- If reconstruction is required, titanium is the current gold standard, because it has many advantages compared with autologous grafts and other alloplastic implants.

Introduction

The orbit is a complex area, because important and delicate anatomic structures are packed together into a small space.[1,2] With its midfacial position and its thin bony walls, the orbit is susceptible to fractures. The trauma mechanism consists of buckling forces applied to the orbital rim and/or the retropulsion of orbital content[3]

Solitary orbital fractures are commonly caused by repulsion, leading to increased intraorbital pressure that is transmitted to all the orbital walls.[3] The lateral wall and orbital roof are relatively strong and can sustain forces more easily, but the orbital floor and medial wall are relatively fragile. This dissipation of force through the 2 thin walls protects the globe, acting as a crumple zone, whereas the stronger roof protects the intracranial structures. In most cases, the increased periorbital pressure results in blowout fracture, where the comminuted orbital wall(s) will be dislocated to the adjacent sinuses (Fig. 1). Occasionally, especially in pediatric patients, the trapdoor phenomenon is seen, wherein the periorbital contents are trapped as soon as the pressure wave decreases and the fracture snaps back into the original position. The viscosity of the bone of children contributes to this phenomenon (Fig. 2). With loss of bony support, the orbital volume may increase, which can potentially result in the protrusion of the orbital contents into adjacent sinuses, with subsequent posterior displacement of the globe (enophthalmos) (arrow in Fig. 1). If most of the impact occurs as a buckling force to the orbital rim, the anterior part of the orbit may be fractured also.[3] The loss of anterior support to the globe may result in vertical displacement of the globe, as well (hypoglobus) (Fig. 3).

Apart from damage to the orbital walls, soft tissues will be disrupted also. If adipose and muscle tissues herniate into the fracture, the suspension system and periorbit will be affected to some extent. Initially, the actual damage may be difficult to assess because of emphysema, swelling, contusion of muscles, and the presence of hematoma (Fig. 4).

For the orbital walls, the goal of reconstruction is to reposition the globe into its original position by placing an orbital implant to recontour the traumatized orbit and restore the pretraumatized anatomy as accurately as possible (Fig. 5). This is mandatory for preventing volume increase of the orbit with clinical sequelae such as enophthalmos and hypoglobus and for adequate support in order to regain proper ocular function and prevent diplopia. On the soft tissue level, the incarcerated tissues also need to be released to restore orbital function. The regenerative capacities of the soft tissues (fat, muscles, septae, nerves) and the amount of damage caused by the surgery itself are highly unpredictable. This unpredictability possibly accounts for persisting debates on the various aspects of orbital fracture management. In the current literature, there is no uniformly accepted guideline for the treatment of orbital fractures.[4]

The shape of the bony orbit and the intricate architecture of the soft tissue pose surgical challenges.[1,5] Orbital reconstruction is performed in a confined space with limited overview in

[a] Orbital Research Group (ACOR), Department of Oral and Maxillofacial Surgery, University Medical Center Amsterdam, University of Amsterdam, Academic Center of Dentistry Amsterdam, Meibergdreef 9, 1105 AZ, Amsterdam, The Netherlands

[b] Department of Oral and Maxillofacial Surgery, University of Washington Seattle, Harborview Medical Center, 1959 NE Pacific Street, Box 357134, Seattle, WA USA

* Corresponding author.

E-mail address: l.dubois@amsterdamumc.nl

Atlas Oral Maxillofacial Surg Clin N Am 29 (2021) 29–39

https://doi.org/10.1016/j.cxom.2020.10.004

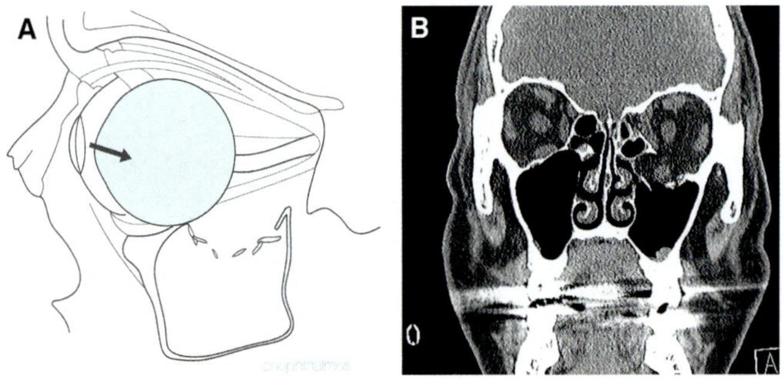

Fig. 1 Blow-out fracture. (*Courtesy of* Leander Dubois, MD, DMD, PhD.)

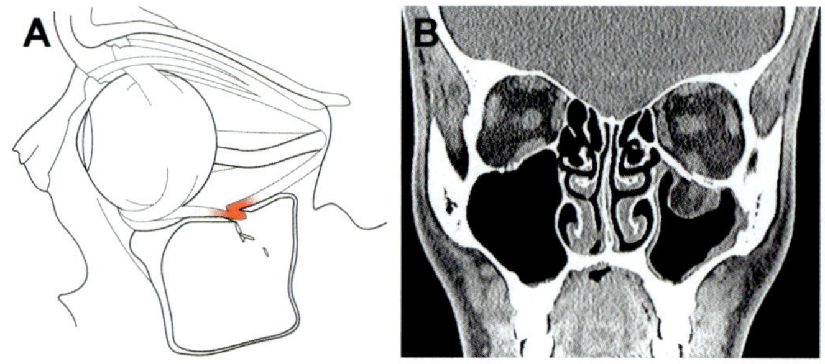

Fig. 2 Trapdoor fracture. *(Courtesy of* Leander Dubois, MD, DMD, PhD.)

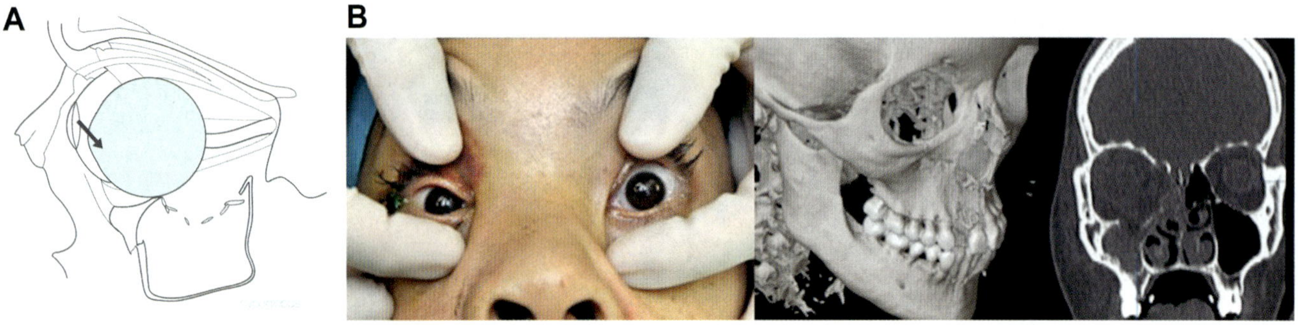

Fig. 3 Loss of vertical support causing a hypoglobus. *(Courtesy of* Leander Dubois, MD, DMD, PhD.)

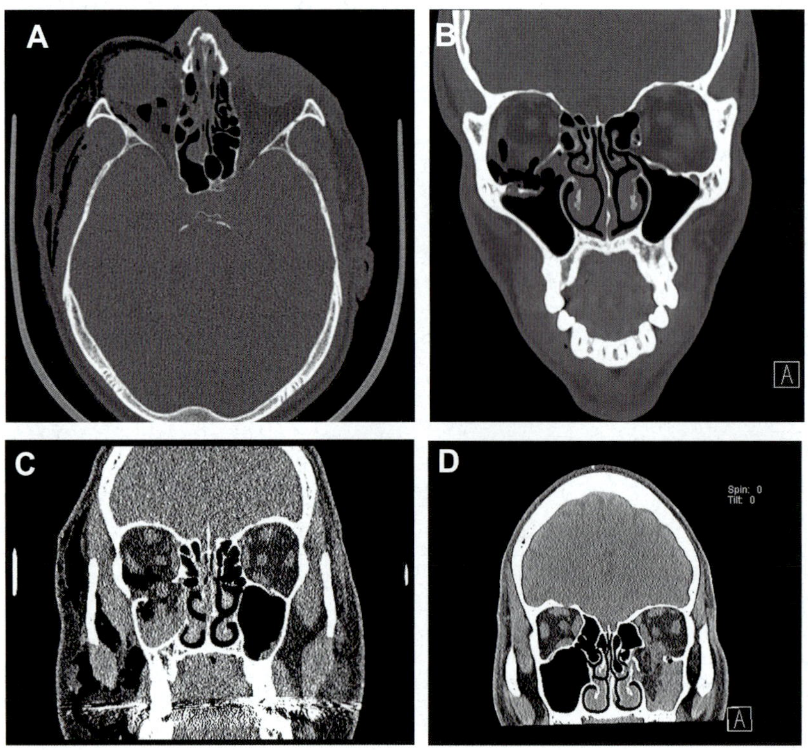

Fig. 4 CT images of (*A*) swelling, (*B*) emphysema, (*C*) swelling of muscles, (*D*) intramuscular hematoma. *(Courtesy of* Leander Dubois, MD, DMD, PhD.)

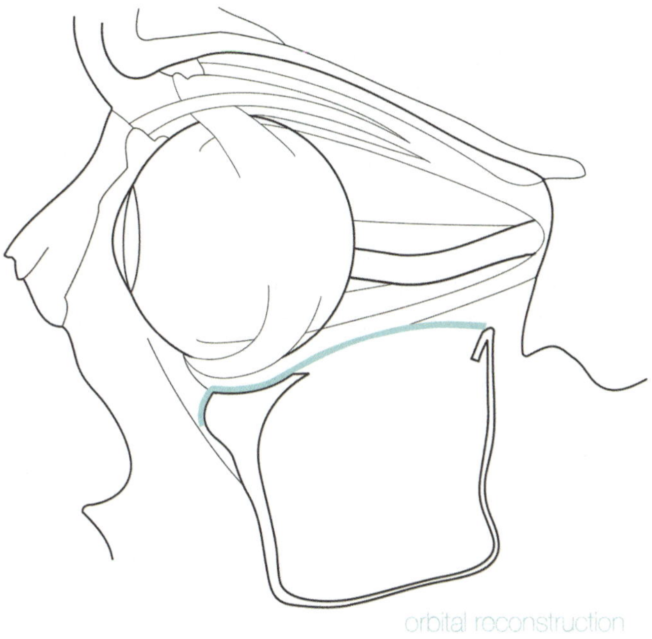

Fig. 5 Reconstruction of the orbital contours. *(Courtesy of* Leander Dubois, MD, DMD, PhD.)

close proximity to vital and delicate structures. Iatrogenic damage and surgical complications are not uncommon.[4,6] The key to successful treatment of orbital wall fractures may be found by carefully selecting the appropriate indications.[4,6,7]

Even if anatomic reconstruction has been achieved, functional rehabilitation does not always follow automatically, as both traumatic and surgical damage to soft tissue contents may induce scarring, entrapment, and fat atrophy. Therefore, persistent diplopia and enophthalmos are believed to be common complications after orbital fracture repair.

Controversies in orbital reconstruction

In orbital fracture management, the most controversial dilemmas are indication, optimal timing, and biomaterials. A scientifically substantiated answer to key questions in orbital reconstruction is therefore desired:

- What type of fracture needs to be reconstructed?
- What is the best timing for orbital reconstruction?
- Which materials are most suitable for the different types of orbital fracture?

What type of fracture needs to be reconstructed?

Several publications have shown that most surgeons base their decision regarding orbital fracture repair on clinical findings, and such data are increasingly obtained from computed tomography (CT) scans.[4,8,9] From a clinical perspective, the presentation of patients with orbital fractures is variable (Fig. 6). The most relevant clinical (nonradiological) symptoms that influence decision making are motility restrictions/diplopia, enophthalmos, and hypoglobus.[4,8,9]

Enophthalmos

Evident enophthalmos and hypoglobus are clear indications for surgery. Hypoglobus is caused by the loss of anterior support and is encountered in less than 5% of the patients with orbital fractures.[10] Enophthalmos is most commonly caused by either an increase in bony orbital volume or a secondary decrease in soft tissue volume caused by fat atrophy or, rarely, a shrinking globe. Enophthalmos is only present in less than 18% of trauma patients with orbital fractures.[10,11] Spontaneous disappearance of enophthalmos can be seen in 50% of the patients with orbital fractures.[11] This results from pseudo-enophthalmos, a phenomenon caused by swelling of the surrounding tissues, resembling an enophthalmos (Fig. 7). Nevertheless, enophthalmos, which does require treatment, is frequently not present immediately after trauma but will occur over time (Fig. 8). A CT scan is the gold standard in imaging for the severity assessment of orbital wall fractures.[12,13] Several studies have suggested that defects of at least 2 cm^2 can cause clinically significant enophthalmos.[12–15] According to Christensen and colleagues[8], who performed among 442 American oral and maxillofacial surgeons, the defect size had the greatest influence on the surgeon's decision to operate, despite absence of enophthalmos. The same trend has been shown by several systematic reviews: clinicians base their

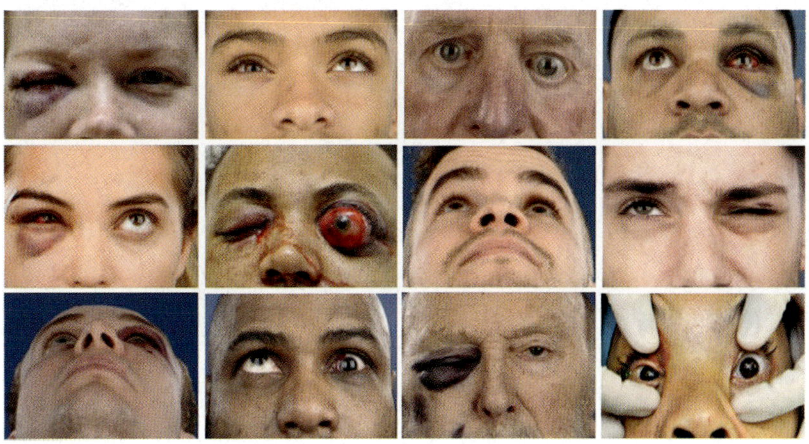

Fig. 6 Clinical presentation of patients with orbital fractures. *(Courtesy of* Leander Dubois, MD, DMD, PhD.)

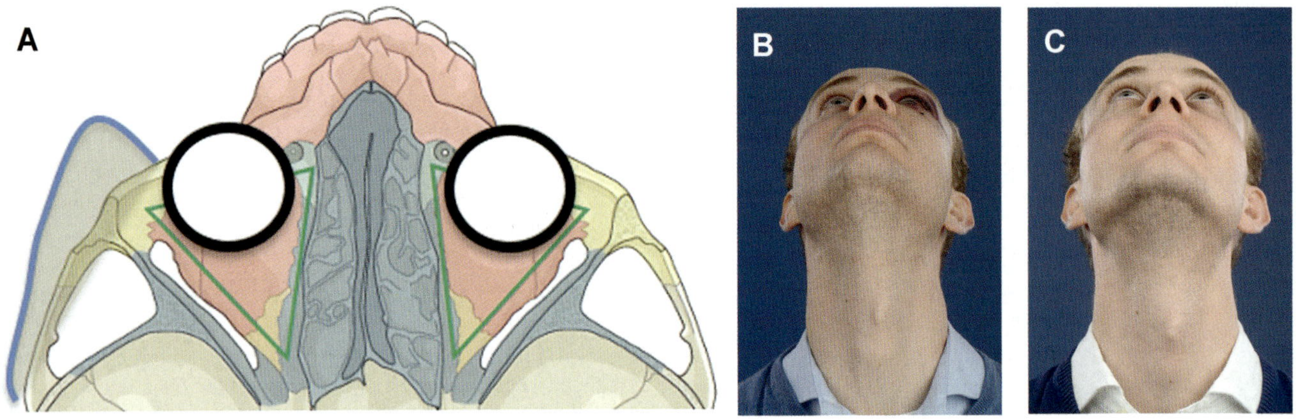

Fig. 7 Pseudo-enophthalmos caused by swelling of the surrounding tissues (*A*). 5 days after trauma (*B*). Months after trauma (*C*).

decision for surgery in almost half of the cases on CT findings.[4,8–10,14] Specifically, a fracture greater than 50% of the surface area was the primary indication for orbital reconstruction in 19% to 30% of the cases.[4,10,14] Although, other radiological observations such as herniated volume, orbital volume ratio, and location of the fracture and inferomedial strut are probably better predictors of enophthalmos (Fig. 9).[16–19]

Accurate quantification of size, location, and complexity of orbital defects is important in the diagnostic process. Nevertheless, accurate measurement or prediction of the defect size remains extremely difficult even on CT,[15,19,20] and the average rate of overestimation is 76%.[20] This overestimation may lead to overtreatment, because a defect size of 1.3 cm^2 is interpreted as greater than 2 cm^2 (Fig. 10A). Interestingly, 30% of the patients with a defect greater than 2 cm^2 have no signs of diplopia, motility disturbance, or enophthalmos.[10] Jansen and colleagues[6] showed that this principle is more evident in single-wall defects. In multiple-wall fractures, the third dimension is increasing the defect size by 27%[20] (Fig. 10B). There seems to be a strong tendency to treat expected problems instead of those that are present. The predictability of the measurements on CT scans is highly questionable in combination with the uncertainty of occurrence of enophthalmos. In terms of indications for reconstruction, defect size should be used cautiously (Figs. 11).

Diplopia and motility disturbances

As previously stated, radiological observations such as defect size and evidence of muscle entrapment are frequently used by most surgeons as strong indications for early intervention.[8,9] Clinical observations such as true muscle entrapment with a positive forced duction test are mainly seen in children (Fig. 12) (76% <15 years) but are relatively rare in adults (Fig. 13).[21] A more common clinical symptom is motility restriction and diplopia caused by a blowout fracture (Fig. 14). The survey of Christensen and colleagues[8] and Aldekhayal and colleagues[9] showed that approximately 4 of 5 surgeons have strong to very strong indications for surgical intervention if diplopia persisted for more than 15 days.

As shown in Box 1, there is a great variability in the extent and causes of diplopia and motility restrictions. This will be further discussed in Yvette Braaksma-Besselink and Hinke Marijke Jellema's article,"Orthoptic Evaluation and Treatment in Orbital Fractures," in this issue. One of the difficulties in clinical decision making is that ocular motility disturbances are commonly caused by muscle edema, hemorrhage, and motor nerve palsy, conditions that cannot be treated surgically, and they are rarely caused by entrapment of the extraocular muscles. In time, most of these deficits may resolve spontaneously. Edema resolves within several days to weeks (Fig. 15), but hemorrhage and motor nerve palsy can even take up to 12 months to recover (Fig. 16). The true dilemma in clinical decision making occurs when the enophthalmos is

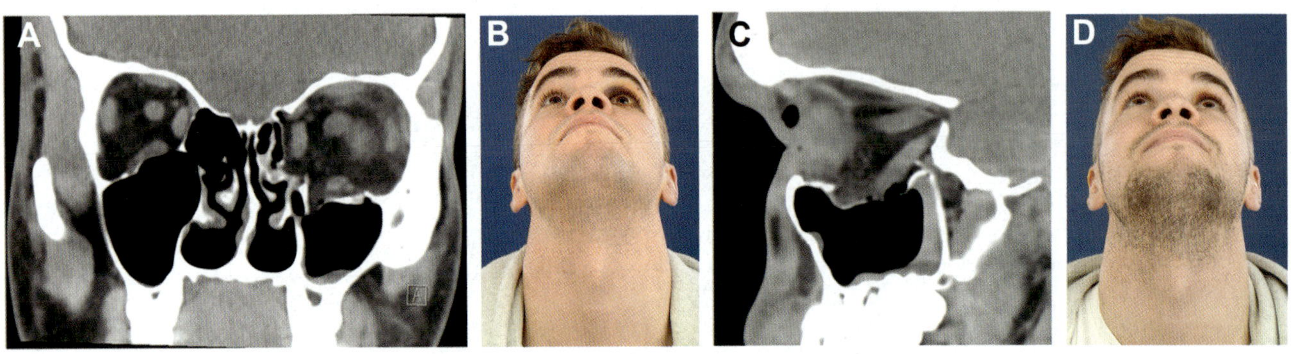

Fig. 8 Clinical presentation of enophthalmos over time. (*A, B*) 6 days after trauma. (*C, D*) 2 weeks later. *(B–D) (Courtesy of* Leander Dubois, MD, DMD, PhD.)

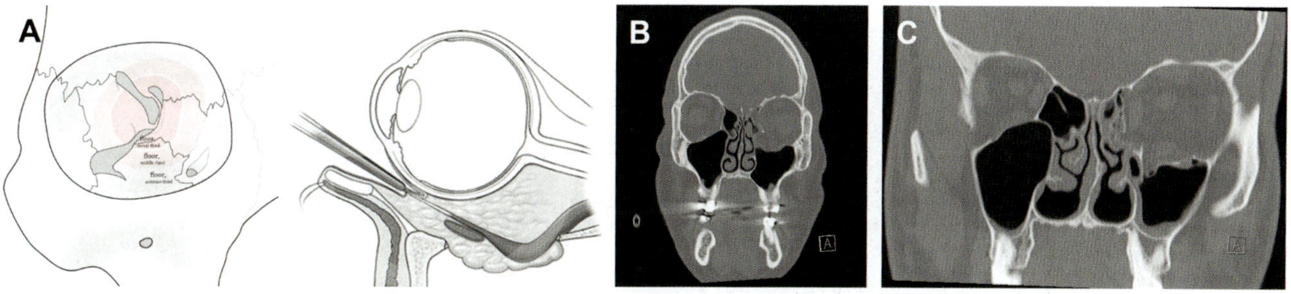

Fig. 9 (*A*) Location of the fracture (anterior fractures), (*B*) significant herniated volume, (*C*) loss of the inferomedial strut in 2 wall fractures. *(Courtesy of* Leander Dubois, MD, DMD, PhD.)

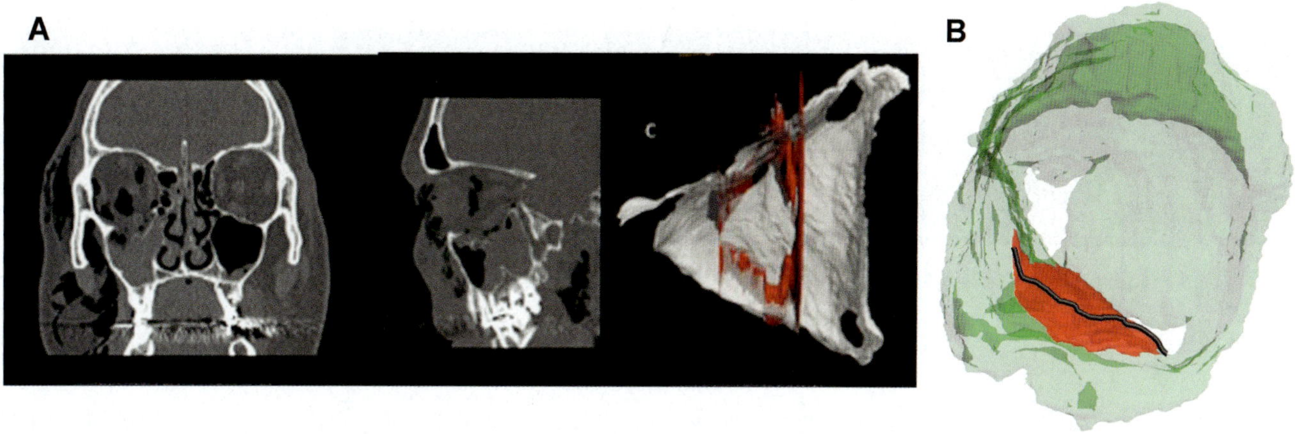

Fig. 10 Illustration of discrepancies between two- and three-dimensional measurements derived from the coronal view, which affects the defect size estimation. *(Courtesy of* Leander Dubois, MD, DMD, PhD.)

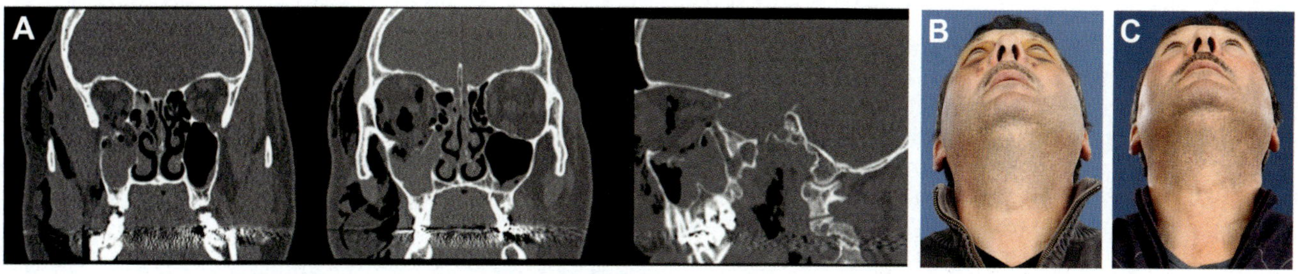

Fig. 11 Clinical example of large defect without enophthalmos (*A*). CT-scan (*B*). 6 days after trauma, (*C*). 1 year after trauma. *(Courtesy of* Leander Dubois, MD, DMD, PhD.)

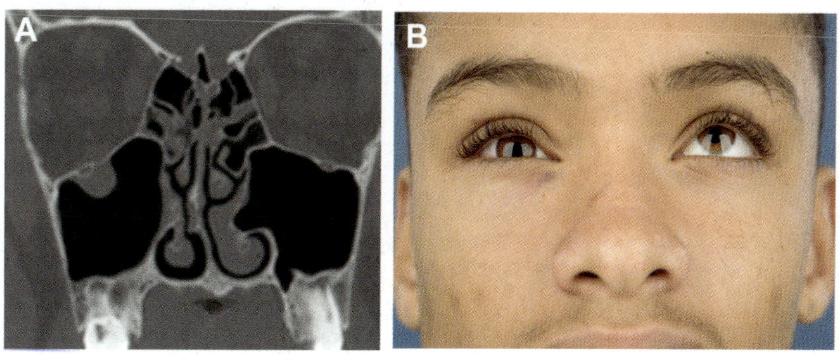

Fig. 12 Clinical example of trapdoor fracture in pediatric patient. *(Courtesy of* Leander Dubois, MD, DMD, PhD.)

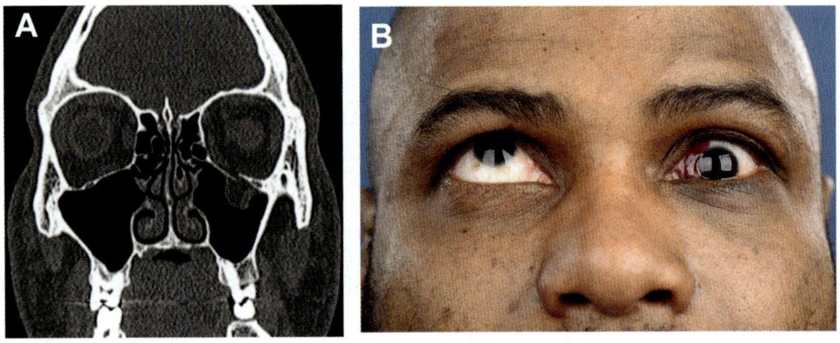

Fig. 13 Clinical example of trapdoor fracture in adult. *(Courtesy of* Leander Dubois, MD, DMD, PhD.)

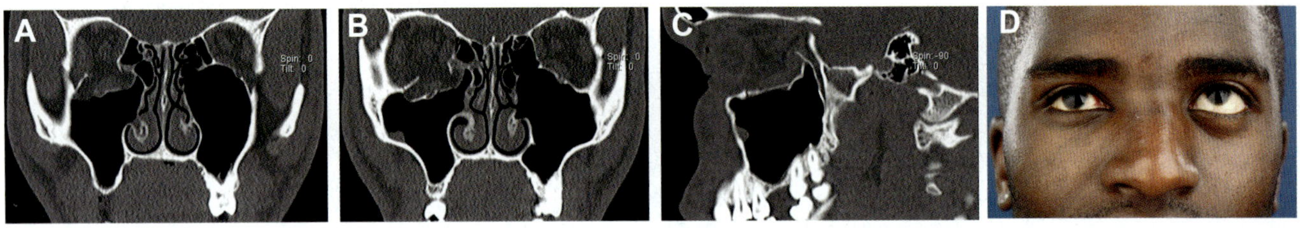

Fig. 14 Absolute motility restriction due to blow-out fracture in adult. *(Courtesy of* Leander Dubois, MD, DMD, PhD.)

minimal or absent and motility has improved, but diplopia persists.

In most studies, diplopia and motility restrictions are subjective observations occurring shortly after trauma and which are not objective or accurate standardized consecutive measurements performed by an orthoptist.[22,23]Other groups stress the importance of quantitative evaluation of ocular motility[6,24,25] and the use of a Hess screen test, interpretation of ductions, and the field assessment of binocular single vision (BSV) can be extremely helpful. Using these measurements, improvement of ocular motility and diplopia can be objectively assessed over weeks or even months after trauma.[25,26] Alhamdani and colleagues[24] and Jansen and colleagues[7] have shown that in minor diplopia (BSV <80), orbital reconstruction can worsen the clinical outcome, and even with moderate diplopia (BSV 60–80), surgery appears to have limited effect on the amount of diplopia. Nevertheless, in severe diplopia (BSV <60), orbital reconstruction has a significant effect on the outcome.

These findings stress the importance of standard orthoptic evaluations during follow-up, especially if diplopia is the only clinical symptom.

What is the best timing for orbital reconstruction?

In many fields of trauma surgery, an increasing body of evidence is emphasizing the importance of optimal timing of surgery.[7] The timing of orbital reconstruction is a determining factor with respect to the potential occurrence of postoperative orbital complications.

In orbital trauma surgery, a general distinction can be made among immediate (within hours), early (<2 weeks), and late surgical interventions (>2 weeks).

There is consensus on the indications for immediate repair, which include vision-threatening symptoms such as retrobulbar hematoma, significant globe displacement (Fig. 17) and (pediatric) trapdoor fractures with muscle entrapment (Fig. 18A) with risk of ischemia and fibrosis, and oculo-cardiac reflex. Without immediate intervention in these cases, permanent damage to the orbital soft tissue and functional impairment are likely to occur. However, except for the trapdoor phenomenon in children, these indications are extremely rare.

Delayed reconstruction (>2 weeks) has some theoretic disadvantages. As a result of the trauma mechanism, there is

Box 1. List of causes of diplopia

- Emphysema
- Muscle edema
- Hemorrhage
- Hematoma formation in the extra-ocular muscles
- Motor nerve palsy (cranial nerves III, IV, and VI, and their respective neuromuscular junctions and target muscles)
- Entrapment of the inferior ocular muscles[a]
- Entrapment of surrounding soft tissues[a]
- Disruption of the orbital septae
- Lack of support of the orbital contents[a]
- Fibrosis of the orbital contents (ligaments and septae)
- Fibrosis of the extra-ocular muscles
- Related to neurotrauma/intracranial

[a] Could be treated surgically.

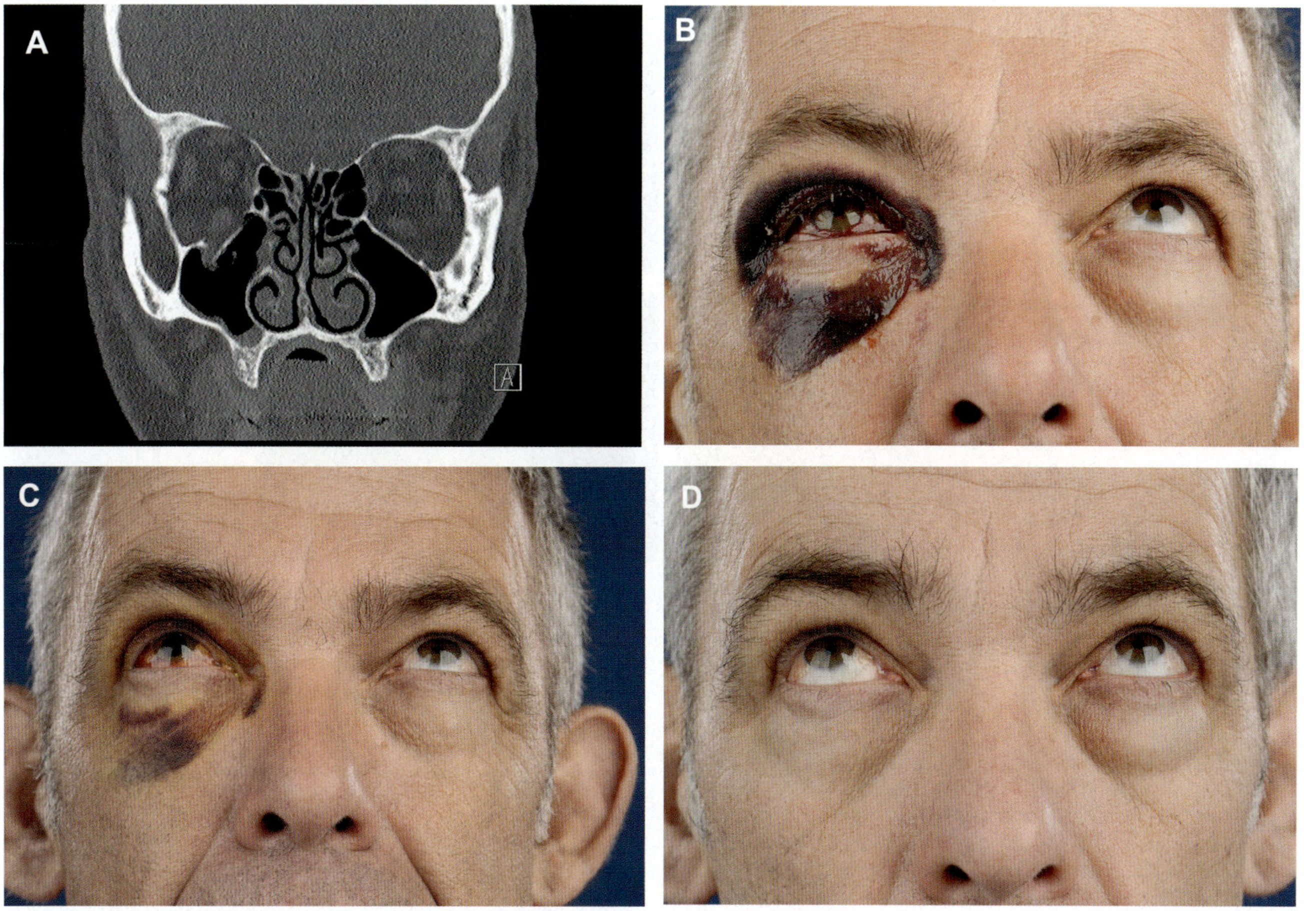

Fig. 15 Clinical example of improvement of motility restrictions caused by swelling (*A*). CT-scan (*B*). 3 days after trauma, (*C*). 2,5 week after trauma (*D*). 1 year after trauma. (*Courtesy of* Leander Dubois, MD, DMD, PhD.)

some initial contusion, hematoma formation, and disruption of the intraorbital tissues. As delayed reconstruction can be considered a second trauma to contents of the orbit, some authors believe that early correction may prevent fibrosis.[27–30]

However, which fractures require early intervention? Diplopia and motility disturbances tend to resolve over time, and enophthalmos mainly occurs in due time. Hence, it is prudent to conclude that small asymptomatic fractures do not need surgery, whereas larger fractures with early enophthalmos require early orbital reconstruction. Most authors agree that a trapdoor fracture without muscle entrapment (Fig. 18B) but with significant motility restrictions requires early surgery.[7] What is the effect on the clinical outcome if surgery in large blowout fractures with proper ocular function

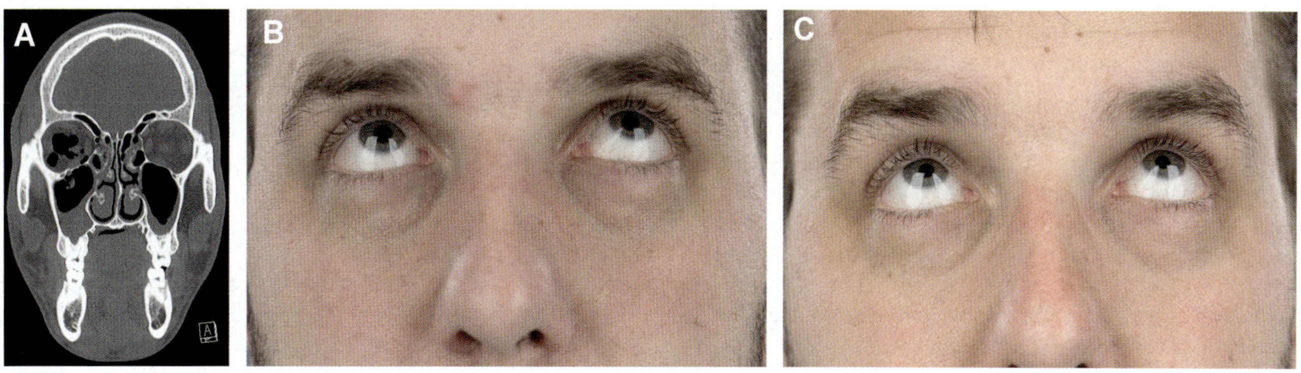

Fig. 16 Clinical example of improvement of motility restrictions caused by neurologic damage (n. VI paresis) (*A*). minor dislocated fracture (*B*) 3 months after trauma (*C*). 12 months after trauma. (*Courtesy of* Leander Dubois, MD, DMD, PhD.)

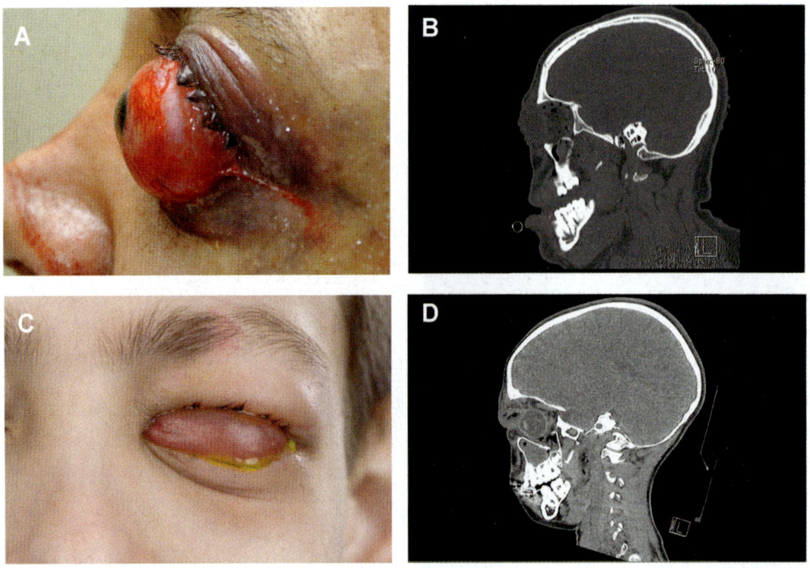

Fig. 17 Globe dislocation. (*A*, *B*) Extreme proptosis. (*C*, *D*) Dislocated globe into adjacent maxillary sinus. (*Courtesy of* Leander Dubois, MD, DMD, PhD.)

that develop enophthalmos over time is postponed? Is it possible to predict the cause of early post-traumatic diplopia (fracture-related, edema, hematoma formation, scarring, motor nerve palsies), and when and how does surgery affect the postoperative clinical outcome? The answers to these questions will help in determining the type of orbital fractures suitable for delayed surgery. If the delay itself of an orbital reconstruction does not affect the clinical outcome, it is surely safer to wait and observe if enophthalmos will occur and if diplopia will resolve, rather than risk complications because of surgery. The size of the fracture does not necessarily correlate to late enophthalmos, and severe diplopia could still resolve without intervention.[6,30,31] A systematic review revealed that even if an early surgical approach was chosen, enophthalmos still persists in 30% of the cases.[31] As a consequence of this, overtreatment of patients with early surgery may be the case, and spontaneous recovery might have occurred over time. Several systematic reviews showed that the literature is not conclusive on whether early surgery is better than delayed surgery for orbital wall fractures. Some authors reported good outcomes after late orbital reconstructions.[32] Hence, the focus of the debate on optimal timing has shifted from the indications for early intervention toward the question of which patients are eligible for delayed repair or may be better treated with nonsurgical treatment. The proposed treatment schedule, which is based on the literature, is presented in Table 1.

Which materials are most suitable for the different types of orbital fracture?

Various implant materials are used to reconstruct an orbital wall fracture. The goal of orbital reconstruction is to restore the pretraumatized orbital anatomy and function primarily for the correction of enophthalmos, hypoglobus, and diplopia. Implant materials must have certain material characteristics to achieve this. The ideal material should have good stability and fixation, should have an ideal architecture or have

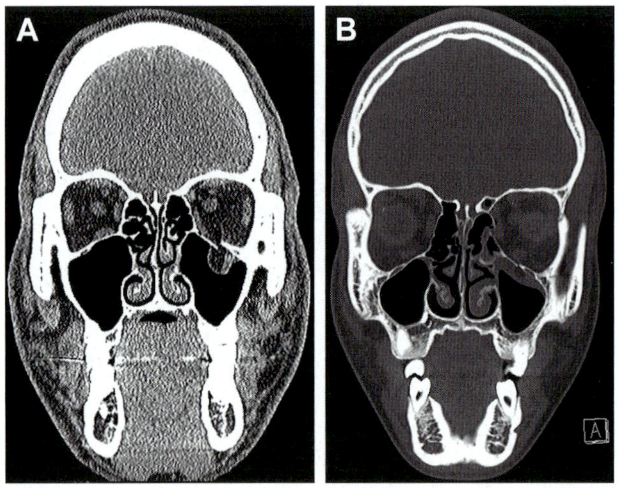

Fig. 18 Trapdoor with (*A*) and without (*B*) muscle entrapment (CT). (*Courtesy of* Leander Dubois, MD, DMD, PhD.)

contouring abilities to restore volume and shape, is biocompatible, is able to facilitate fluid drainage, has no donor site morbidity, is radiopaque, and is readily available at acceptable costs.[33] However, there is no perfect material available. Autologous bone grafts have long been considered the gold standard based on their biocompatibility; however, the use of autologous bone grafts has disadvantages, with donor site morbidity, difficulty of shaping the graft, and unpredictable resorption rates being the major ones. Resorbable materials have been suggested as alternatives because of their more predictable resorption rates, lack of donor site morbidity, and high levels of customizability and control (thermoplastics), but several studies showed lack of rigidity and stability over time, particularly in larger fractures.[33–35] Titanium implants have become widely used and accepted as favorable material because of their high compliance to most of the previously

Table 1 Indications for reconstruction

	Immediate	Early	Delayed
Timeframe	Within 24 h	1–14 d	<14 d
Indications	Diplopia with CT evidence of an entrapped muscle or periorbital tissue associated with a nonresolving oculocardiac reflex: bradycardia, heart block, nausea, vomiting, or syncope White-eyed blow-out fracture. Young patients (<18 y), history of periocular trauma, little ecchymosis or oedema (white eye), marked extraocular motility vertical restriction, and CT examination revealing an orbital floor fracture with entrapped muscle or perimuscular soft tissue Significant globe displacement with vision-threatening emergency	Early enophthalmos/hypoglobus causing facial asymmetry Symptomatic diplopia with positive forced ductions, evidence of an entrapped muscle or perimuscular soft tissue on CT examination	Symptomatic diplopia without proven entrapment on CT examination, negative forced ductions, and insignificant clinical improvement over time Late-onset enophthalmos/hypoglobus

demands mentioned. Titanium implants are available as titanium meshes for intraoperative bending as well as preformed 3-dimensional plates, and lately, they can be customized to patient specifications (Fig. 19). To date, most research are focused on the clinical outcome of allogenic and (non-)resorbable alloplastic materials. Table 2 presents the main groups of biomaterials used for implants as well as their main advantages and disadvantages.

Summary

There is consensus that a trapdoor fracture in a pediatric patient, a severely dislocated globe and a trapdoor fracture with a nonresolving oculocardiac reflex, bradycardia, heart block, nausea, vomiting, or syncope are strong indications for immediate surgery. Most authors agree that early reconstruction is required when there is entrapment of the orbital contents with an absolute motility restriction (adult) or early significant enophthalmos or hypoglobus (>2 mm), but others recommend expectative policy for other uncertain indications. Hence, if the motility of the eye significantly improves within 10 to 14 days, surgery may be not indicated. Favorable results of using a nonsurgical approach have been published over the years.[6,24,31,36] Clinical findings should overrule CT results. The soft tissues are the unpredictable factor in fracture management. An anatomic orbit does not automatically become a perfectly functioning orbit. Surgery will not necessarily heal the already inflicted damage to the soft tissues. If surgery is required, then preoperative planning, navigation, and intraoperative imaging may be help in improving the anatomic bony outcome. Treat what harms, not what is expected to occur. The clinical outcome of each patient whose treatment is guided by a protocol provides accurate feedback for reconstructive decisions ("Evidence-Based Decision Making in Orbital Fractures: Implementation of a Clinical Protocol" by Peter J. J. Gooris, Jesper Jansen, J. E. Bergsma, Leander Dubois).

Disclosure

The authors have nothing to disclose.

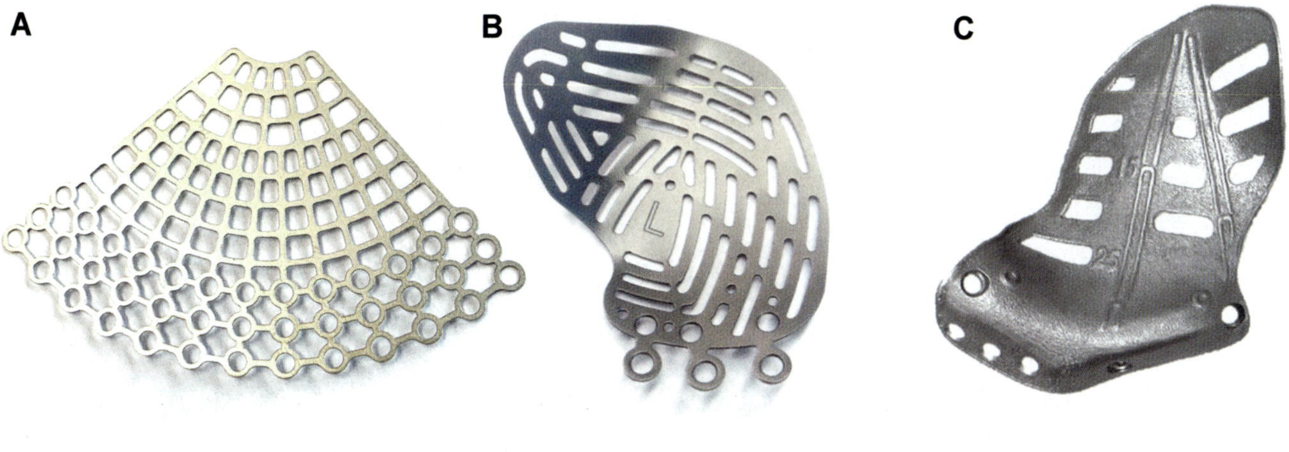

Fig. 19 Shape factor of the orbital implant a. free-handed bending, b. preformed, c patient specific implant. *(Courtesy of* Leander Dubois, MD, DMD, PhD.)

Table 2 Advantages and disadvantages of commonly used biomaterials

	Stability	Contouring	Biological Behavior	Drainage	Donor-Site Morbidity	Radiopacity	Availability	Cost-Effectiveness
Titanium meshes (flat)	Stability +++ Fixation ++	++ Contouring - Possible sharp edges	++ Allows tissue ingrowth - Poor dissection of periorbita in secondary reconstruction	+ Permeable	+	+	+	+
Bone graft	Stability ++ Fixation +	+ Variability in thickness/ smooth surface adequate in 3-wall fractures - Remodelling/difficult to shape	+++ Maximal biocompatibility/ periorbita readily dissects off bone in secondary reconstruction	-	- Donor site needed: Harvest time/pain/ scarring/ complications	+	+/−	+/−
Porous polyethylene sheets	Stability +/− Lack of rigidity when thin fixation +/−	+ Eased by artificial sterile skull/smooth edges	++ Allows tissue ingrowth	-	+	- Not visible on postoperative imagery	+	+
Composite of porous polyethylene and titanium mesh	Stability ++ Fixation ++	+ Eased by artificial sterile skull adequate in 3-wall fractures	++ Allows tissue ingrowth	-	+	+	+	+/−
Resorbable materials	Stability +/− Stable over time? Fixation +/−	+ Smooth surface and edges/ handling (thermoplastics) - Nonthermoplastics - Degradation of material with risk of contour loss	+/− Sterile infection/ inflammatory response	- In case nonperforated: less drainage than uncovered titanium mesh	+	- Not visible on postoperative imagery	+	+
Preformed orbital implant	Stability +++ Fixation ++	++ + Minimal contouring Necessary/smooth surface	++ Allows tissue ingrowth	+ Permeable	+	+	+	+/−

References

1. Cornelius CP, Mayer P, Ehrenfeld M,, et al. The orbits-anatomical features in view of innovative surgical methods. Facial Plast Surg 2014;30:487–508.
2. Koornneef L, Los JA. A new anatomical approach to the human orbit. Mod Probl Ophthalmol 1975;14:49–56.
3. Schaller A, Huempfner-Hierl H, Hemprich A, et al. Biomechanical mechanisms of orbital wall fractures – a transient finite element analysis. J Craniomaxillofac Surg 2013;41:710–7.
4. Dubois L, Steenen SA, Gooris PJJ, et al. Controversies in orbital reconstruction - I. Defect-driven orbital reconstruction: a systematic review. Int J Oral Maxillofac Surg 2015a;44:308–15.
5. Gooris PJJ, Muller BS, Dubois L, et al. Finding the ledge: sagittal analysis of bony landmarks of the orbit. J Oral Maxillofac Surg 2017;75:2613–27.
6. Jansen J, Dubois L, TJJ Maal, et al. A nonsurgical approach with repeated orthoptic evaluation is justified for most blow-out fractures. J Craniomaxillofac Surg 2020;48(6):560–8. Mar 30:S1010-5182(20)30077-9.
7. Dubois L, Steenen SA, Gooris PJJ, et al. Controversies in orbital reconstruction - II. Timing of post-traumatic orbital reconstruction: a systematic review. Int J Oral Maxillofac Surg 2015;44:433–40.
8. Christensen BJ, Zaid W. Inaugural survey on practice patterns of orbital floor fractures for American oral and maxillofacial surgeons. J Oral Maxillofac Surg 2016;74:105–22.
9. Aldekhayel S, Aljaaly H, Fouda-Neel O, et al. Evolving trends in the management of orbital floor fractures. J Craniofac Surg 2014;25: 258–61.
10. Gunarajah DR, Samman N. Biomaterials for repair of orbital floor blowout fractures: a systematic review. J Oral Maxillofac Surg 2013;71:550–70.
11. Tang DT, Lalonde JF, Lalonde DH. Delayed immediate surgery for orbital floor fractures: less can be more. Can J Plast Surg 2011;19:125–8.
12. Manson PN, Grivas A, Rosenbaum A, et al. Studies on enophthalmos: II. The measurement of orbital injuries and their treatment by quantitative computed tomography. Plast Reconstr Surg 1986;77:203.
13. Raskin EM, Millman AL, Lubkin V, et al. Prediction of late enophthalmos by volumetric analysis of orbital fractures. Ophthal Plast Reconstr Surg 1998;14:19.
14. Burnstine MA. Clinical recommendations for repair of isolated orbital floor fractures: an evidence-based analysis. Ophthalmology 2002;109:1207–10.
15. Ploder O, Klug C, Backfrieder W, et al. 2D- and 3D-based measurements of orbital floor fractures from CT scans. J Craniomaxillofac Surg 2002;30:153–9.
16. Choi SH, Kang DH. Prediction of late enophthalmos using preoperative orbital volume and fracture area measurements in blowout fracture. J Craniofac Surg 2017;28:1717–20.
17. Schönegg D, Wagner M, Schumann P, et al. Correlation between increased orbital volume and enophthalmos and diplopia in patients with fractures of the orbital floor or the medial orbital wall. J Craniomaxillofac Surg 2018;46:1544–9.
18. Ahmad Nasir S, Ramli R, Abd Jabar N. Predictors of enophthalmos among adult patients with pure orbital blowout fractures. PLoS One 2018;13:e0204946.
19. Goggin J, Jupiter DC, Czerwinski M. Simple computed tomography-based calculations of orbital floor fracture defect size are not sufficiently accurate for clinical use. J Oral Maxillofac Surg 2015; 73:112.
20. Dubois L, Jansen J, Schreurs R, et al. How reliable is the visual appraisal of a surgeon for diagnosing orbital fractures? J Craniomaxillofac Surg 2016;44:1015–24.
21. Alinasab B, Ryott M, Stjarne P. Still no reliable consensus in management of blow-out fracture. Injury 2014;45:197–202.
22. Tahiri Y, Lee J, Tahiri M, et al. Preoperative diplopia: the most important prognostic factor for diplopia after surgical repair of pure orbital blowout fracture. J Craniofac Surg 2010;21: 1038–41.
23. Su Y, Shen Q, Lin M, et al. Predictive factors for residual diplopia after surgical repair in pediatric patients with orbital blowout fracture. J Craniomaxillofac Surg 2016;44:1463–8.
24. Alhamdani F, Durham J, Greenwood M, et al. Diplopia and ocular motility in orbital blow-out fractures: 10-year retrospective study. J Craniomaxillofac Surg 2015;43:1010–6.
25. Bianchi F, De Haller R, Steffen H, et al. Does vertical incomitance predict the diplopia outcome in orbital fracture patients? A prospective study of 188 patients. J Craniomaxillofac Surg 2019;47: 305–10.
26. Hwang K, Huan F, Hwang PJ. Diplopia and enophthalmos in blowout fractures. J Craniofac Surg 2012;23:1077–82.
27. Safi AF, Richter MT, Rothamel D, et al. Influence of the volume of soft tissue herniation on clinical symptoms of patients with orbital floor fractures. J Craniomaxillofac Surg 2016;44:1929–34.
28. Zimmerer RM, Ellis E, Aniceto GS, et al. A prospective multicenter study to compare the precision of posttraumatic internal orbital reconstruction with standard preformed and individualized orbital implants. J Craniomaxillofac Surg 2016; 44:1485–97.
29. Hawes MJ, Dortzbach RK. Surgery on orbital floor fractures. Influence of time of repair and fracture size. Ophthalmology 1983;90: 1066–70.
30. Kunz C, Sigron GR, Jaquiéry C. Functional outcome after nonsurgical management of orbital fractures - the bias of decision-making according to size of defect: critical review of 48 patients. Br J Oral Maxillofac Surg 2013;51:486–92.
31. Beigi B, Khandwala M, Gupta D. Management of pure orbital floor fractures: a proposed protocol to prevent unnecessary or early surgery. Orbit 2014;33:336–42.
32. Scawn RL, Lim LH, Whipple KM, et al. Outcomes of orbital blow-out fracture repair performed beyond 6 weeks after injury. Ophthal Plast Reconstr Surg 2016;32:296–301.
33. Dubois L, Steenen SA, Gooris PJJ, et al. Controversies in orbital reconstruction - III. Biomaterials for orbital reconstruction: a review with clinical recommendations. Int J Oral Maxillofac Surg 2016;45:41–50.
34. Cordewener FW, Bos RR, Rozema FR, et al. Poly(ll-lactide) implants for repair of human orbital floor defects: clinical and magnetic resonance imaging evaluation of long-term results. J Oral Maxillofac Surg 1996;54:9–14.
35. Van Leeuwen A, Ong SH, Vissink, et al. Reconstruction of orbital wall defects: recommendations based on a mathematical model. Exp Eye Res 2012;97:10–8.
36. Everhard-Halm YS, Koornneef L, Zonneveld FW. Conservative therapy frequently indicated in blow-out fractures of the orbit. Ned Tijdschr Geneeskd 1991;135:1226–8.

Orthoptic Evaluation and Treatment in Orbital Fractures

Yvette Braaksma-Besselink, CO, MMedSci, Hinke Marijke Jellema, CO, MMedSci, PhD*

KEYWORDS

• Orthoptic evaluation • Binocular single vision • Diplopia • Eye motility • Mechanical strabismus • Prisms

KEY POINTS

- Be aware of a combination of mechanical, neurogenic, and sensory causes of diplopia.
- Check for factors influencing the absence of diplopia, such as trauma-related visual problems, abnormal head posture, or preexistent strabismus.
- The severity of the trauma does not always correlate with the impairment of motility or with the degree of diplopia.
- Always prescribe monocular eye movement therapy.
- Treat patients in the first period after trauma with press-on prisms or different types of occlusion, and plan follow-ups as is deemed necessary according to the diagnosis.

Introduction

Orbital fractures are common in facial trauma and are reported in as many as 40% of craniofacial trauma. There is no real consensus with regard to standardized examination or protocolled treatment to determine either the necessity or type of treatment.[1] Surgical indication, meaning possible orbital repair surgery, is predicated on criteria, such as enophthalmos, restriction of extraocular muscles, type and size of the fracture's defect, degree of diplopia, and clinicoradiological findings.[1–3]

Type of diplopia

Disturbances in ocular motility in orbital fractures may have different causes, but, typically, the diplopia is incomitant in pattern. Incomitant strabismus causing the diplopia is complex; the deviation is different in the various gaze positions. This makes the choices in multifaceted treatment complex.[4]

Medial wall and orbital floor fractures are the most common fractures. Medial wall fractures often give rise to horizontal diplopia. Vertical diplopia is reported more frequently and a common symptom in orbital floor fractures (Case 1) (Fig. 1). In a majority of cases, this leads to a limitation of elevation and in a lesser degree to limitation of depression.[5,6]

Mechanisms causing diplopia in orbital fractures

Strabismus resulting in diplopia may occur in 88% of the patients with orbital fractures. The cause of strabismus may be diverse, often involving multiple mechanisms. One of the causes may lie outside of the orbit due to damage to one of the cranial ocular motor nerves or central/peripheral damage due to contrecoup effect of the brain (stem).[7] Acquired neurogenic palsies frequently are seen in head trauma. Because the fourth nerve is one of the longest of cranial nerves, it is the most vulnerable of the 3 cranial nerves involved in eye movements (third, fourth, and sixth).[7]

Another cause of strabismus may be damage to the ocular muscle itself: swelling, hemorrhage, or even incarceration of the muscle, although actual entrapment of the muscle is uncommon and seen only in posterior floor fractures. Strabismus is not necessarily caused by damage to the ocular muscle itself; it may be due partly to the herniation of orbital fat and connective tissue into the surrounding sinus with subsequent traction on the muscle sheaths.

There also might be a combination of paralytic and mechanical damage causing strabismus[8] as well as a sensory cause, meaning that a change in visual acuity disrupts binocular functioning[9] or even decompensation of preexisting strabismus. Be aware of a combination of mechanical, neurogenic, and sensory causes of diplopia.

Role of orthoptic examination

To assess which of the mentioned mechanisms, discussed previously, is causing diplopia, it is essential to incorporate an orthoptic examination in the initial referral patterns.[4] Unfortunately, only a few articles regarding orbital fractures include a quantitative (orthoptic) evaluation of ocular motility.[4,5,10,11] Not all patients present themselves with typical patterns of diplopia[12] and there is no significant relation between the severity of injury and eventual ocular motility outcome (Case 1).[5,6] Diplopia not always is the first concern of patients, initially noticed, or observed at all.[13] Preexisting strabismus and suppression can be reasons for atypical presentation (Case

Funding: None.

Department of Ophthalmology, Amsterdam University Medical Centers, University of Amsterdam, Meibergdreef 9, Amsterdam 1105 AZ, the Netherlands

* Corresponding author.

E-mail address: h.m.jellema@amsterdamumc.nl

Atlas Oral Maxillofacial Surg Clin N Am 29 (2021) 41-50

https://doi.org/10.1016/j.cxom.2020.10.002

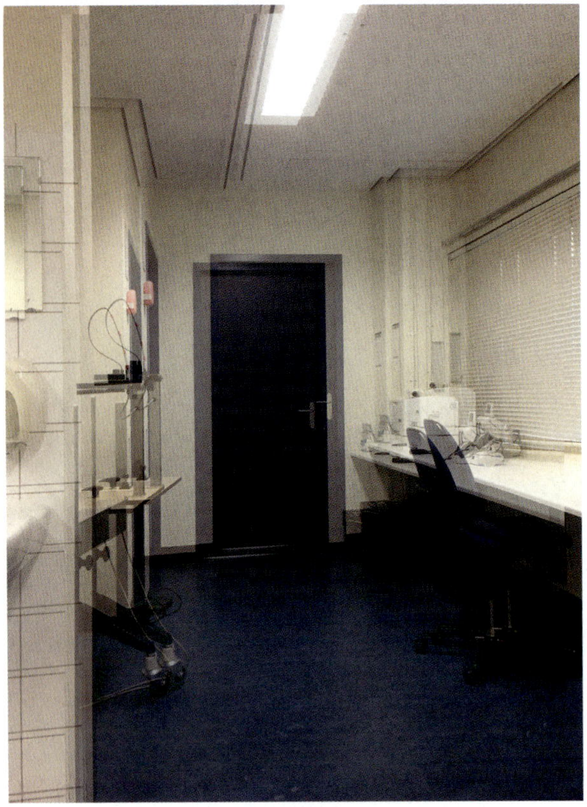

Fig. 1 Vertical diplopia.

2). Suppression is an alteration in visual perception that prevents one of the images to be consciously seen. This results in the absence of diplopia in the presence of strabismus. Other reasons of absence of diplopia are visual field defects, macular problems, vision loss, and neglect. The severity of the trauma does not always correlate with the impairment of motility or with the degree of diplopia.

Timing and frequency of orthoptic examination

There is overall agreement on the necessity of sequential measurements over the first 4 months to 6 months in the presence of acquired orthoptic abnormalities.[13] In cases of a neurogenic cause, spontaneous improvement may occur over a time period of 6 months to 9 months. Strabismus secondary to ophthalmologic abnormalities might resolve as vision increases; decompensated strabismus also might resolve spontaneously. Residual diplopia in conservatively treated patients is reported globally, with a significant range, from 15% to 82%.[1]

Independent of the type of injury, the strabismus is likely to change in the first weeks to months as edema resolves[13] (Case 3); 7 days to 10 days after trauma, examination is performed more easily because the initial edema often is resolved partially or mostly. Through orthoptic examination, it can be determined if and to what degree diplopia is improved spontaneously and orbital reconstruction may be prevented.[6] One study of Gosse and colleagues[6] found no correlation between the type of incomitance and the likelihood of spontaneous recovery; thus, care must be taken in formulating a prognosis in the early stages after trauma.

Strabismus also may occur secondary to orbital reconstruction; an orthoptic examination is advised prior to orbital surgery in cases of suspicion of orthoptic abnormalities to document possible change.[14] In cases of iatrogenic causes of diplopia after orbital reconstruction, orthoptic evaluation is strongly suggested.[14] The motility post–orbital surgery can change over a period of time up to 9 months,[6] so continued follow-up is recommended.

Orthoptic follow-up may lead to different conclusions than primary orbital surgical outcome or may even lead to decisions of further surgery, such as strabismus surgery.

Additionally, it is important to state that after a proper diagnosis, only those with complaints have to be followed-up on.[1]

Orthoptic assessment is important and may play a crucial role in decision making. Each patient must be evaluated individually, however, and the leading practitioner must decide the necessity of orthoptic evaluation based on presentation, severity of trauma, and complaints during the treatment process to avoid excessive examination.

Children

In cases of an orbital trauma under the age of 8 years, there is a substantial risk for amblyopia. Especially in long-standing strabismus, suppression can arise, which eliminates diplopia but may lead to amblyopia (impaired/delayed visual development, which is permanent if not treated on time). If an orthoptic examination in adults is elective and based on the judgment of the leading physician, an orthoptic examination in a child with orbital fracture(s) is mandatory, at least at some point during the treatment period.

Choice of orthoptic examination

Taking history, general impression, and ophthalmologic examination

Patients with orbital trauma often present with periorbital ecchymosis, periocular edema, hemorrhage, enophthalmos, and/or proptosis. When assessing a patient with orbital trauma and possible ocular injury, it is important to determine which ocular structure(s) may be involved. It is imperative to determine whether the injury involves only the orbit or whether the injury may involve the bulb, optic nerve, retina, or other ophthalmic structures. Ocular injury may be indicated by a patient report of monocular diplopia; thus, it is important to distinguish this from binocular diplopia (Box 1). When double vision persists on closing 1 eye, there also is at least monocular diplopia requiring further ophthalmologic examination.

Ocular injury, orbital and retrobulbar hemorrhage, optic nerve damage, retinal injuries, and penetrating eye trauma all constitute ophthalmic emergencies that may threaten vision and require an immediate consult with an ophthalmologist.[15] Previous studies have found rates of ocular injury in the context of orbital fractures in the range of 26% to 40%. Ocular trauma is further discussed in detail in Gijsbert J. Hötte and Ronald O.B. de Keizer, article "Ocular injury and emergencies around the globe," in this issue.

Box 1. Overview of the major causes of monocular and binocular diplopia

Monocular Diplopia	Binocular Diplopia

• Structural abnormalities cornea
• Structural abnormalities lens
• Structural abnormalities retina
• Refractive error
	• Disrupted fusion
	  ○ Head trauma
	  ○ Visual acuity changes
	• Strabismus
	  ○ Preexisting/ decompensation
	  ○ Acquired
	  ○ Incomitant eye movements
	    ■ Mechanical
	    ■ Neurogenic

It is important to be aware of an abnormal head posture (AHP). The advice is to exclude possible preexisting strabismus, which may be the cause of the AHP. An adopted AHP may mask strabismus and may downplay the extent of complaints. A head posture abnormality may be subtle and easily missed. Be aware of factors influencing the absence of diplopia such as trauma related visual problems, AHP, or preexisting strabismus.

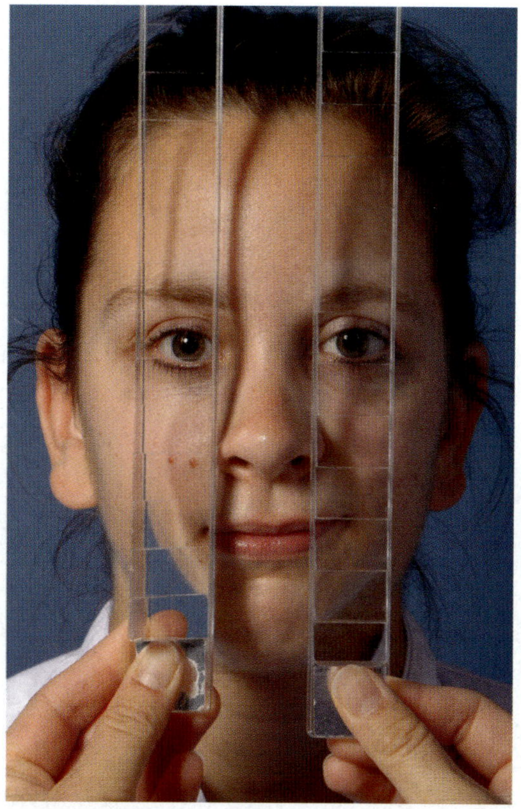

Fig. 2 Horizontal and vertical prisms held in front of the patient's eyes perceiving single vision.

Binocular single vision

Binocular single vision (BSV) is a unique quality, a combination of 2 images of the same size, color, brightness, and focus to be projected on identical places in both retinae. It is preferable to test the quality of BSV in a natural testing environment, on near or distance fixation. In cases of absent diplopia but present strabismus, regular examinations often are used to determine further treatment cannot be interpreted as normally would be cone. It thus is imperative to determine the extent of binocular function in patients.

Superimposition

In patients with diplopia, the first impression of the capacity of BSV is to adjust horizontal and/or vertical prisms held in front of the patient's eyes (Fig. 2) in that specific amount in which the patients achieves a single image. This aspect of BSV is called superimposition. Be aware of any possible disruption of superimposition or fusion, such as macular off detachment[9] or cyclotorsion (tilted image).

Fusion

When superimposition is reached, fusion measurement gives the investigator information about the quality of BSV. Increasing amounts of prisms (see Fig. 2) are held in front of a patient's eye. The patient's binocular system corrects double vision until a threshold is reached in which the maximum amount of fusion is determined and the patient perceives a double image. The total amount of prisms is called the fusion range. With knowledge about the horizontal and vertical fusional amplitude (range), (Fresnel) prisms can be prescribed to create single vision and to minimize the use of the total fusion ability and thus minimize complaints. A good capacity of fusion is a positive prognostic factor in patients prior to strabismus surgery.

Field of binocular single vision

With the field of BSV, the presence or absence of diplopia in all directions of gaze is quantified. For quantifying the field of BSV, different devices are available. In literature, the Goldmann perimeter routinely is used (Fig. 3). This device does not reflect, however, a patient's general viewing condition, because fusion is limited. Measuring the field of BSV (Fig. 4) with the Harmswand or the Maddox screen is performed in more natural viewing conditions.

While measuring the field of BSV, either the patient is asked to follow a light in different directions until double vision is reported or the head is moved while the eyes fixate on a light. Although a field of BSV gives us a way of quantifying double vision, the test outcome may differ significantly from the patient's subjective experience in normal life.

Scoring of the field of BSV can be done with help of the Sullivan core.[16] With this score, the field of BSV is quantified from 0 (no BSV) to 100 (maximum BSV) (Fig. 5). Quantifying the field of BSV is helpful for research purposes but also helps informing the patients about the progress of the disease.

Eye position and motility

The amount of strabismus in primary position and other directions of gaze can be measured with different devices. For the primary position, the prism cover test in near and distance

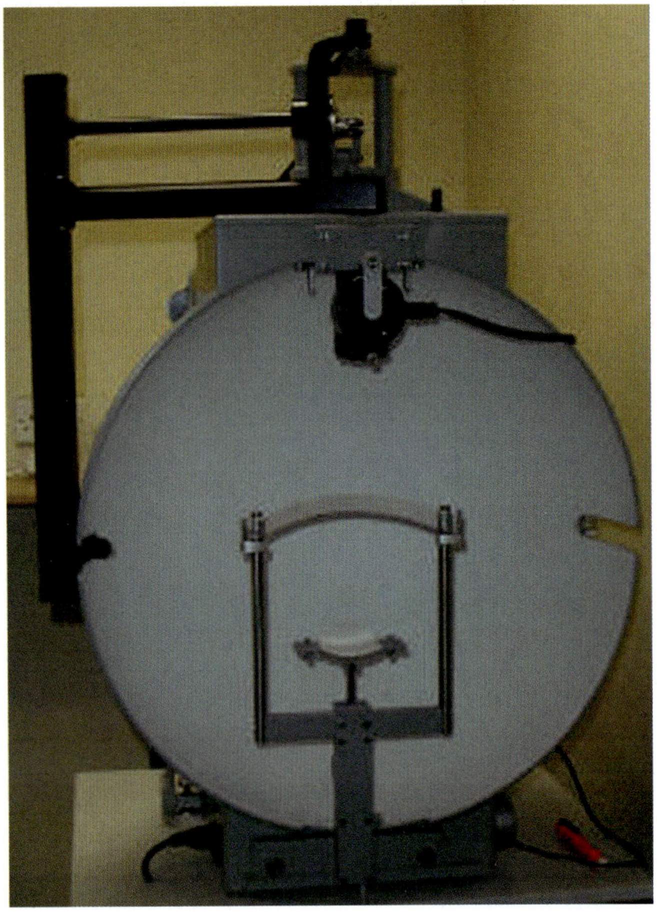

Fig. 3 Goldmann perimeter.

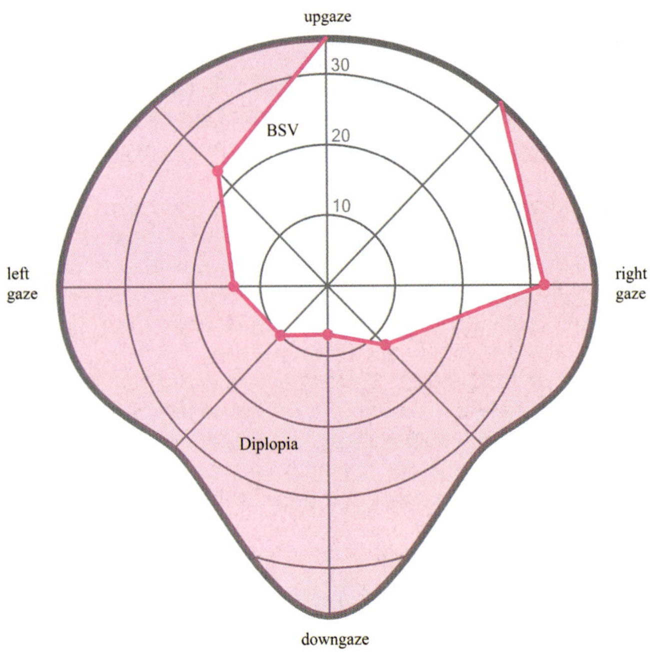

Fig. 4 Example of the field BSV. BSV, binocular single vision.

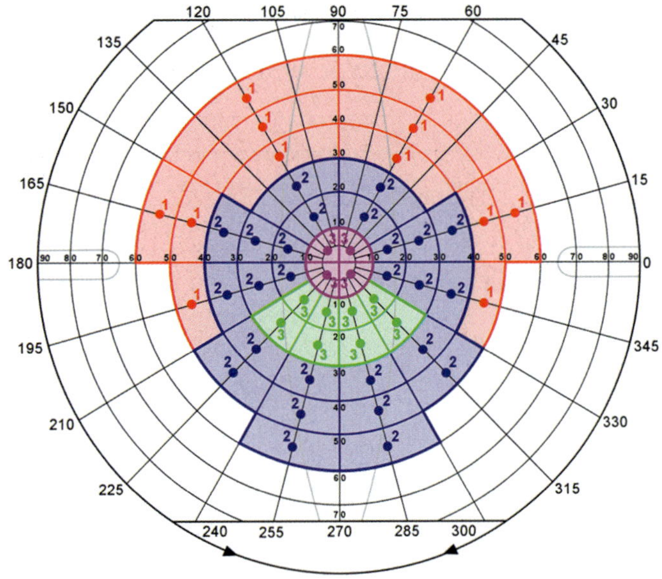

Fig. 5 Field of BSV vision for Goldmann with quantification score of Sullivan.[16]

fixation is used most commonly. A common feature found in patients with traumatic strabismus is the presence of primary and secondary deviation. A secondary deviation means that the amount of strabismus increases when the patient is forced to fixate with an eye that is affected either by mechanical or neurologic restrictions. The eye with the limitation can be identified easily on a motility chart, where the eye movements measured in 9 directions of gaze are visualized. Examples are a Lancaster red-green, a Hess screen, or an Amsterdam motility scheme; the outcome of the diagrams of the aforementioned types of examination, will show a smaller field of measurements for the affected eye (Fig. 6). Alternatively, the cover test in combination with a prism bar can be used in all 9 directions of gaze as well as the Hess-Weis deviometry.[4]

Ductions

Ductions, meaning monocular eye movement, should be evaluated carefully. Quantifying ductions can be performed in different ways. In general, muscle function is graded on a scale from +4 to −4. This quantification, however, is observer dependent and less precise compared with a deviometer like the Goldmann[17] or motility meter (Fig. 7).[10,18]

Ductions generally are measured in 4 positions of gaze: abduction, adduction, elevation, and depression. One article[10] quantified ductions in the field of action of the 6 extraocular muscles, as suggested by Haggerty and colleagues.[19]

Cyclotorsion

A majority of patients with diplopia do not experience torsion (tilted image) or do not describe it as such. This is the reason why it is strongly recommended to measure cyclotorsion in all patients with a history of trauma. Measurement of torsion is helpful in identifying oblique muscle weakness and paretic causes, such as a fourth nerve palsy. An excyclotorsion of greater than or equal to 10° is suspect for a bilateral fourth

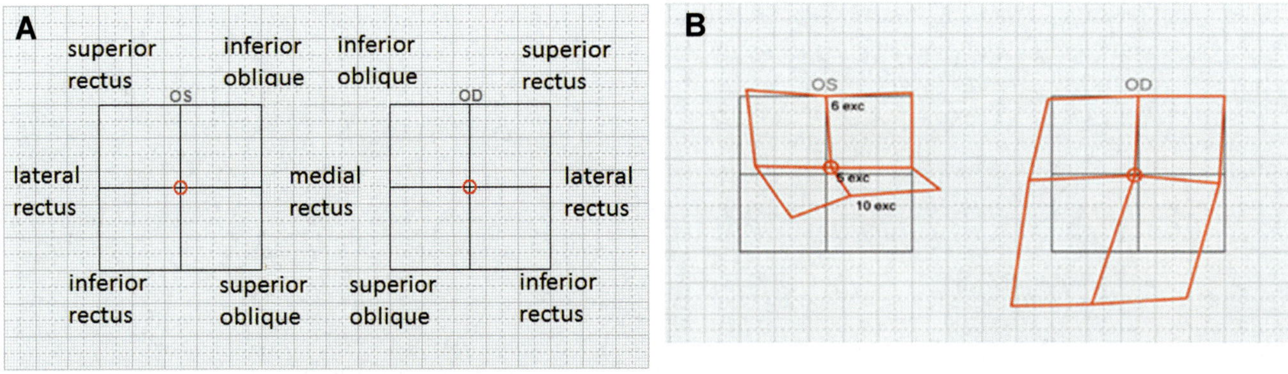

Fig. 6 Amsterdam motility scheme showing the eye movements in nine directions of gaze. (*A*) Muscle actions in each direction. (*B*) Patient example with in red the eye position of the patient. Patient with traumatic fourth nerve palsy left > right and an orbital floor fracture of the left side. exc, excyclodeviation; OD, right eye; OS, left eye.

nerve palsy.[7] Incyclotorsion can be found secondary to orbital injury or repair.[20]

Measurement can be carried out with the Harms tangent screen or Franceschetti cycloforometer of (Fig. 8) in the different directions of gaze. The Maddox double rod test (frame with 2 red glasses) has proved less accurate when measuring more than 10° to 12° out of primary position of gaze.

Orthoptic treatment

In general, all patients are advised to perform monocular eye movement therapy to prevent scarring and maximize ductions. There is no literature, however, which subscribes the efficacy of such treatment.

The primary diplopia after trauma and/or new-onset diplopia after repair of the orbital fracture almost always is incomitant and a challenge for treatment. As in all types of treatment, it is important to quantify the primary complaint of the patient and treat accordingly if possible.

The goal of the nonsurgical treatment is to achieve and maintain BSV in primary position and downgaze (reading position), depending on the complaint/profession of the patient.[13,21] If sufficient BSV is present or the complaints are minor, then conservative treatment is preferred. If not, prisms can be used to regain BSV. Prisms preferably are prescribed as press-on prisms (Fig. 9), because the strabismus may vary over time. If prisms are insufficient, occlusion of 1 eye (Fig. 10) can be advised by means of occlusive foils or an occlusive contact lens.[21] Treat patients in the first period after trauma with press-on prisms or different types of occlusion.

Strabismus surgery

Surgical procedures can be performed only if the measurements are unchanging over time. This can take many months

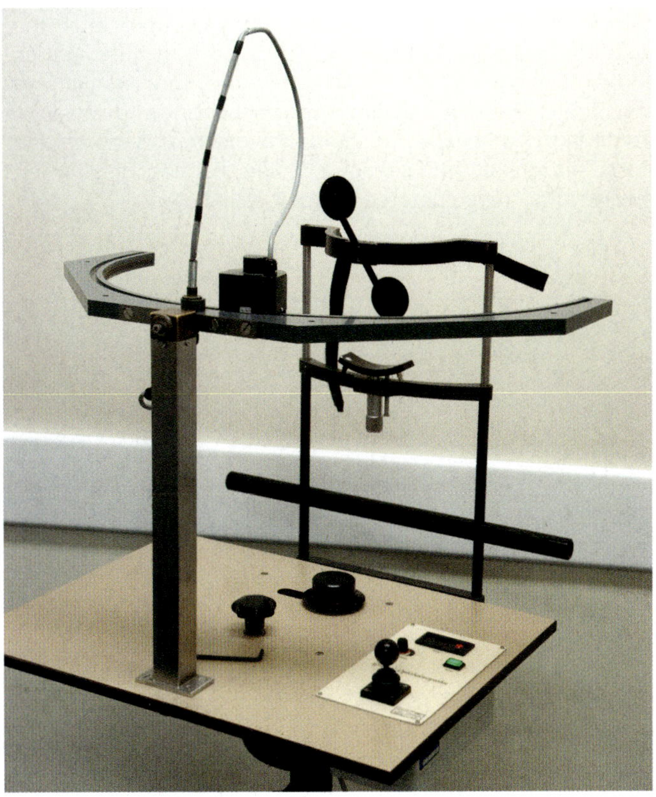

Fig. 7 Motility meter.

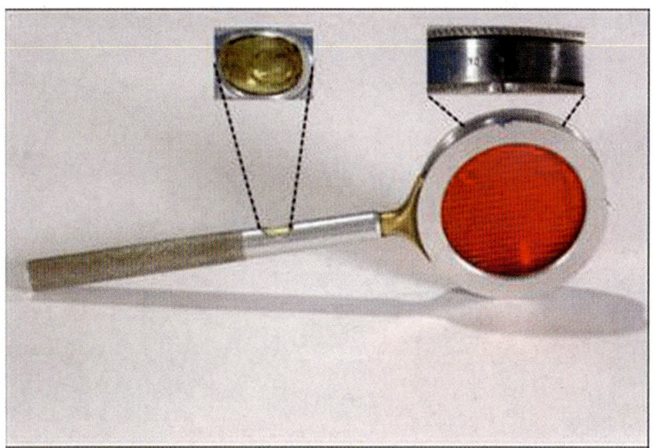

Fig. 8 Cycloforometer of Franceschetti.

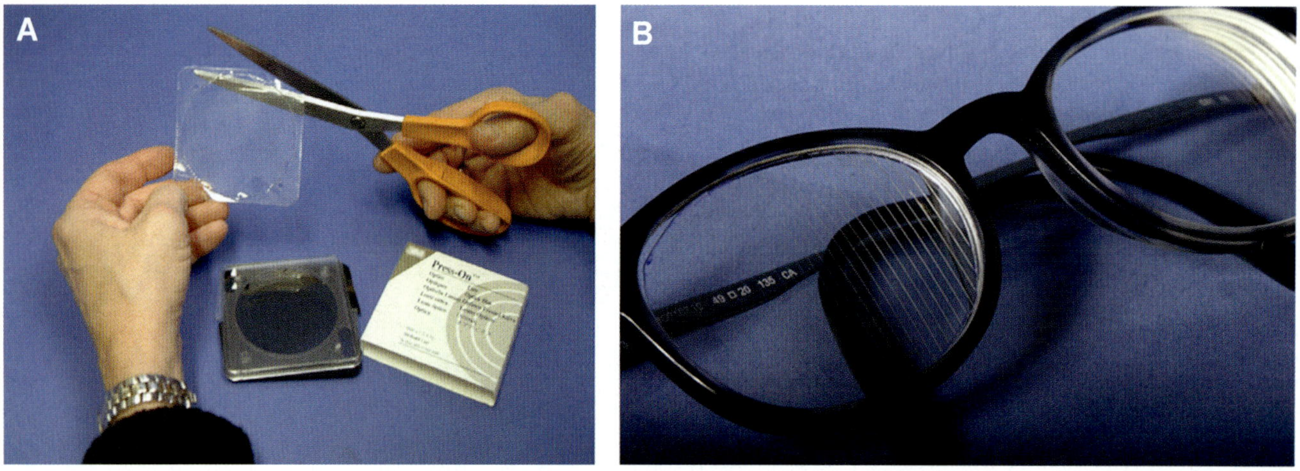

Fig. 9 (*A*) Press-on prisms. (*B*) Adjusted to the right lens.

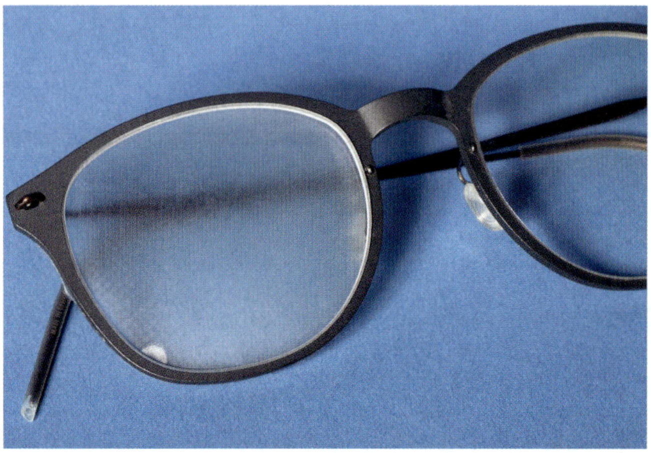

Fig. 10 Occlusion on the right side of the spectacle glass.

following the repair of the orbital fracture if the cause is a mechanical one. In general, the time to stability is even longer in cases of a paralytic strabismus.[21]

The primary goal of surgery is to regain BSV in primary and reading gaze or to expand the field of BSV in another field of gaze (Fig. 11).

In a retrospective case series of blowout fractures of Gosse and colleagues,6 8 of 80 patients (10%) eventually needed strabismus surgery, 5 patients of whom achieved comfortable BSV.

Surgically, the treatment depends on whether there is a paretic or mechanical form of strabismus,[21] but only a few options are possible. Even in cases of strabismus due to orbital surgery, the removal of an orbital implant does not improve the motility.[14] Generally, the only solution is to place a Faden posterior fixation suture in the overacting eye muscle on the noninjured contralateral eye (Fig. 12). This is in the direction of the damaged muscle to achieve more concomitant eye movements. The goal is to limit the overshooting of the healthy muscle in the other eye, which is an overcompensation of the limited movement on the fractured side. Patients may prefer, however, not to be operated on their sound eye.

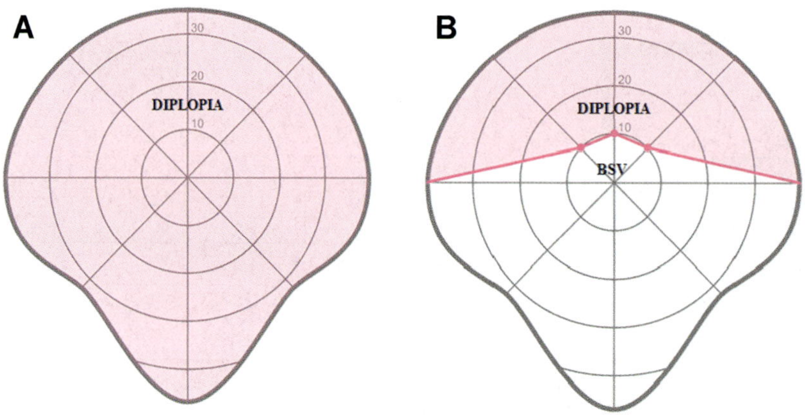

Fig. 11 Field of BSV measured with the Maddox screen. (*A*) Before surgery and (*B*) after surgery. BSV, binocular single vision.

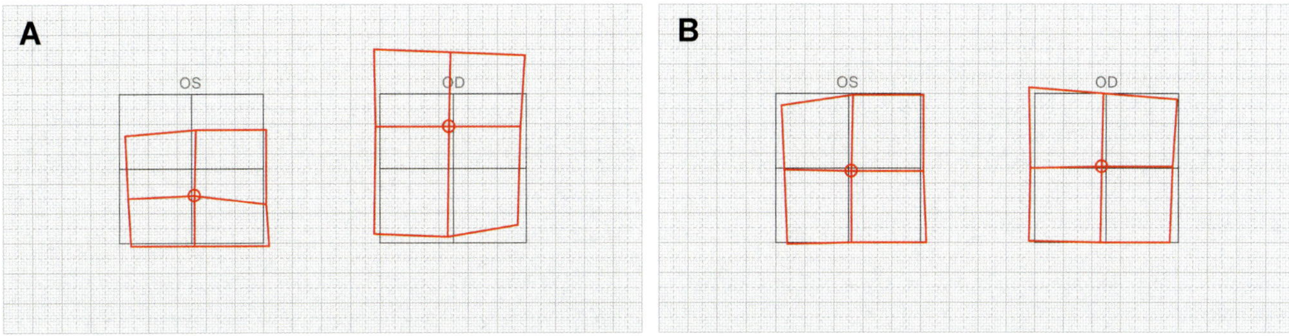

Fig. 12 Eye motility before Faden procedure (*A*) and after procedure (*B*). OD, right eye; OS, left eye.

Pearls and pitfalls

- Check for discrepancies between objective and subjective findings.
- Be aware of other coexisting problems on top of the mechanical causes of the diplopia.
- An orthoptic examination helps in monitoring the recovery process.
- Keep patients comfortable with occlusion and/or prisms until no further change in the orthoptic status are found.
- Diplopia can be treated only by prisms or strabismus surgery.

Conclusion and recommendations

It is agreed that the orbital fracture is a multifactorial problem that requires a multidisciplinary approach. The orthoptic examination is inextricably associated with patients with orbital fractures. It is too simplistic, however, to state that every patient with orbital trauma or an orbital fracture is in (repeated) need of an orthoptic examination. Each case must be individually deliberated to prevent overtreatment.

Cases

Case 1

A 49-year old man with orbital floor fracture due to a soccer accident 2 days ago (Table 1). The CT-scan shows severe herniation of the inferior rectus muscle in the maxillary sinus, including fat (Fig. 13).

Table 1 Details of case 1

	2 Days			10 Days		
Eye position	Straight			Straight		
Ductions		OD	OS		OD	OS
	Elevation	25	29	Elevation	24	29
	Depression	48	61	Depression	60	61
Eye motility	Fig. 14			Fig. 15		
Therapy	Conservative			Conservative		

Abbreviation: OD, right eye; OS, left eye.

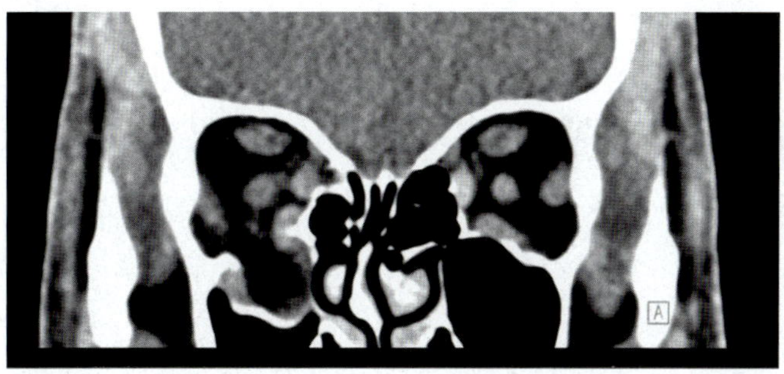

Fig. 13 Orbital floor fracture of the right eye with severe herniation of the inferior rectus in the sinus maxillaris, including fat.

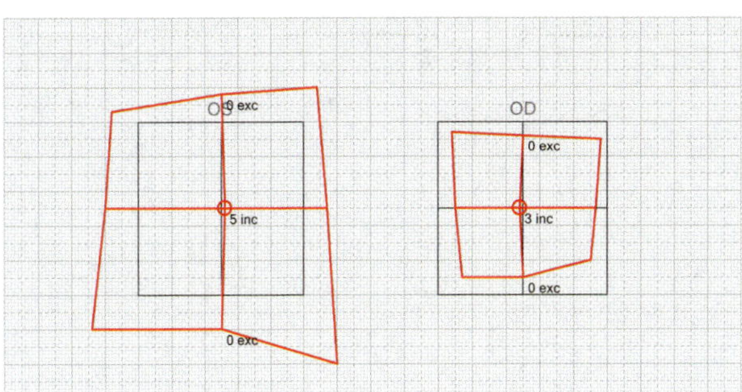

Fig. 14 Eye motility 2 days after trauma (case 1). OD, right eye; OS, left eye.

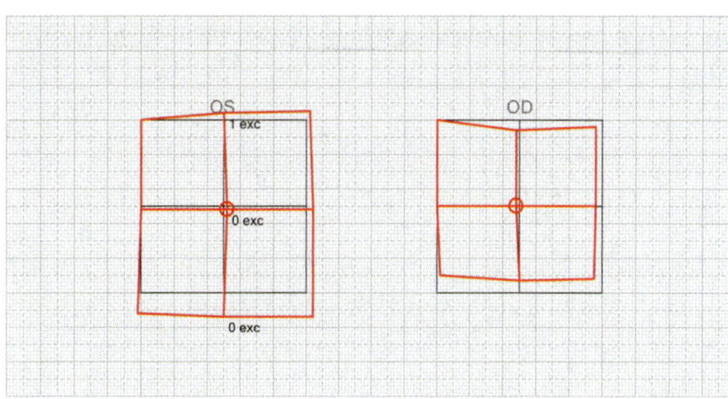

Fig. 15 Eye motility 10 days after trauma (case 1). OD, right eye; OS, left eye.

Case 2

A young man presents to the emergency department after highly energetic trauma. He presents with bilateral epidural hematomas with severe facial trauma. There is an orbital floor fracture on both sides as well as infraorbital extraconal hematomas on both sides. (Fig. 16).

Ophthalmic examination 1 day after trauma:

- No ophthalmologic abnormalities, no signs of optic nerve damage
- Patient reports diplopia only on extreme right and left gaze. He is not hindered by this. He experiences tilted image.
- As a child he was treated for strabismus and amblyopia of the right eye

Eye position: small right exotropia and small right hypotropia (no double vision)

BSV and stereopsis: suppression in primary position.

Binocular eye movements:

- Looking to the right: increase of the right hypotropia, maximal in right upgaze
- Looking up: restriction of elevation

Ductions are shown in Table 2.

Conclusion: manifest and incomitant strabismus due to orbital floor fractures and acquired left fourth nerve palsy. Suppression due to preexistent strabismus.

Therapy: wait and reschedule appointment. Recovery of fourth nerve palsy is less than 6 months.

Table 2 Ductions in case 2

Duction	OD	OS
Abduction	50	44
Adduction	45	45
Elevation	32	54
Depression	54	60

Abbreviation: OD, right eye; OS, left eye.

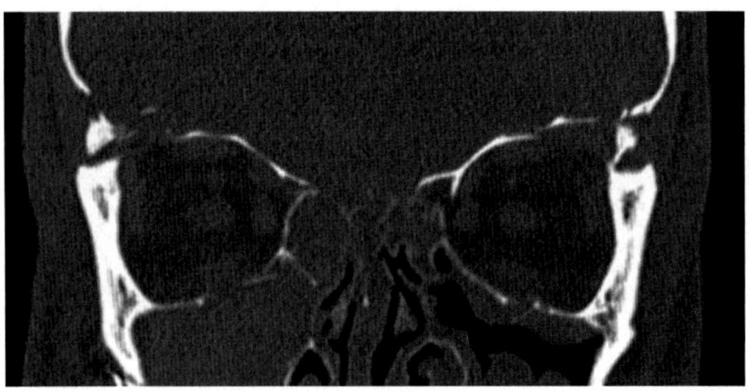

Fig. 16 CT scan of patient showing both orbital floor fractures (case 2).

Case 3

A 55-year-old man with orbital floor fracture of left orbit and herniation of intraorbital fat in sinus maxillaris (Fig. 17, Table 3).

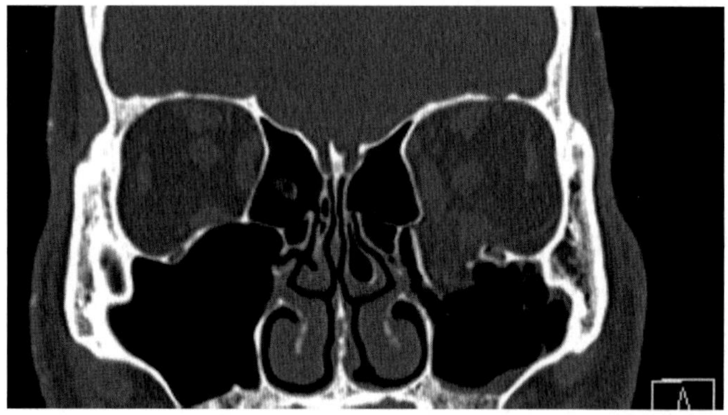

Fig. 17 CT scan showing orbital floor fracture of left orbit (case 3).

Disclosure

The authors have nothing to disclose.

Table 3 Details of case 3

	4 Weeks			8 Weeks			4 Months		
Vision	Right: 1,0 Left: 0,65 due to traumatic uveitis			Right: 1,0 Left: 1,0			Right: 1,0 Left: 1,0		
BSV (Goldmann)	35/100 Fig. 18			66/100 Fig. 19			100/100 Fig. 20		
Eye position Primary position	Small right hyperphoria			No deviation			No deviation		
Eye motility Amsterdam motility scheme	Fig. 21			Fig. 22			Fig. 23		
Duction		OD	OS		OD	OS		OD	OS
	Abduction	46	27	Abduction	46	36	Abduction	46	45
	Adduction	45	38	Adduction	45	41	Adduction	46	45
	Elevation	35	27	Elevation	35	30	Elevation	35	34
	Depression	54	43	Depression	54	43	Depression	54	51
Therapy	Occlusion of left eye Treatment of uveitis			None			Discharge		

Abbreviation: OD, right eye; OS, left eye.

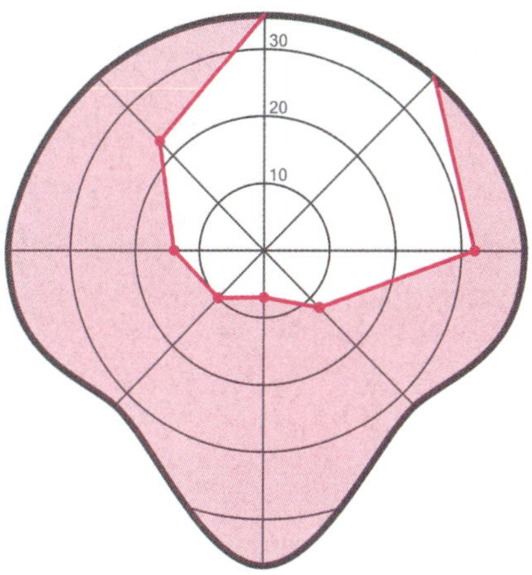

Fig. 18 Field of BSV 4 weeks after trauma (case 3).

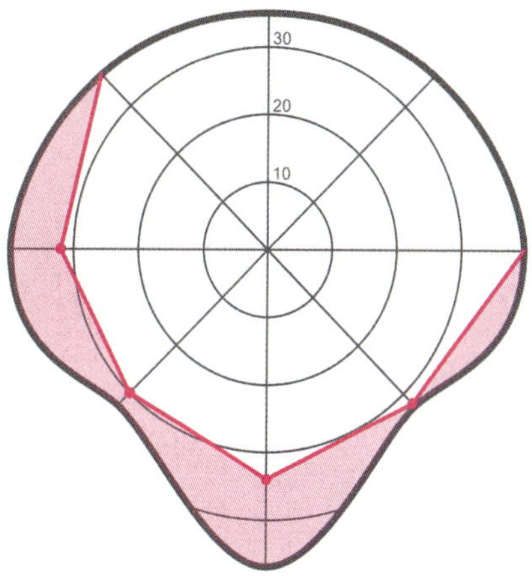

Fig. 19 Field of BSV 8 weeks after trauma (case 3).

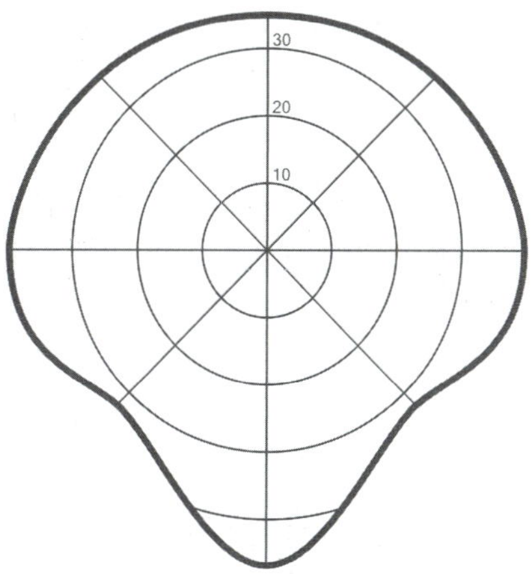

Fig. 20 Field of BSV 4 months after trauma (case 3).

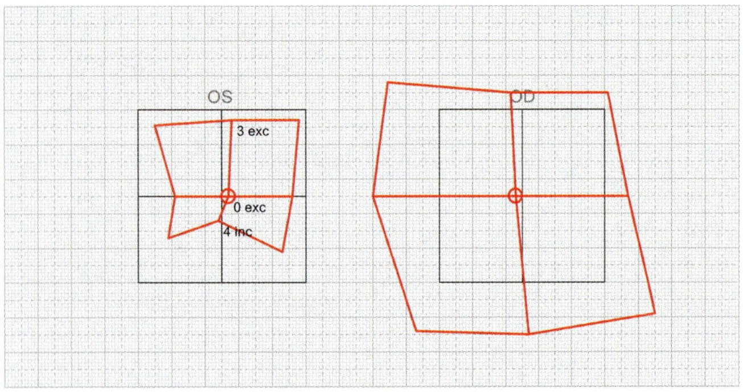

Fig. 21 Eye motility 4 weeks after trauma (case 3). exc, excyclodeviation; OD, right eye; OS, left eye.

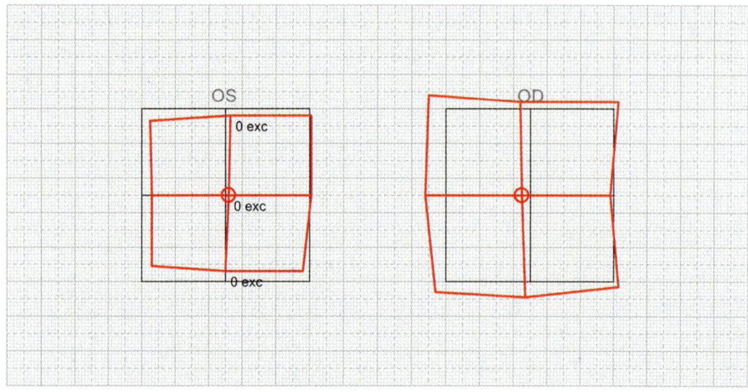

Fig. 22 Eye motility 8 weeks after trauma (case 3). exc, excyclodeviation; OD, right eye; OS, left eye.

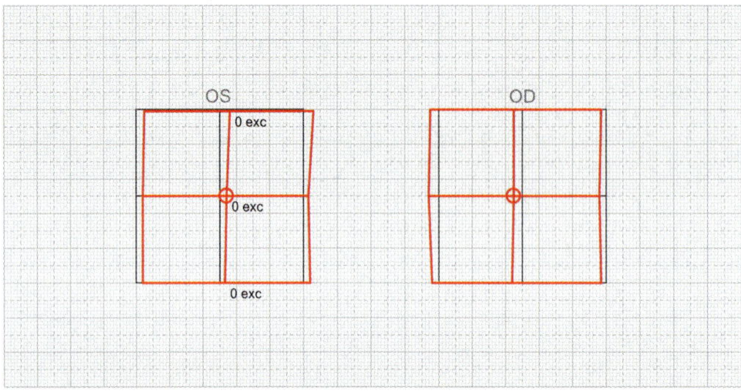

Fig. 23 Eye motility 4 months after trauma (case 3). exc, excyclodeviation; OD, right eye; OS, left eye.

References

1. Steinegger K, De Haller R, Courvoisier D, et al. Orthoptic sequelae following conservative management of pure blowout orbital fractures: anecdotal or clinically relevant? J Craniofac Surg 2015;26(5):433–7.
2. Marano R, Lino PRS, Zanetti F, et al. Is specialized ophthalmologic evaluation necessary afer orbital fractures? A prospective 64-case study. Oral Maxillofac Surg 2019;23:325–9.
3. Dubois L, Jansen J, Schreurs R, et al. How reliable is the visual appraisal of a surgeon for diagnosing orbital fractures? J Craniomaxillofac Surg 2016;44:1015–24.
4. Bianchi F, De Haller R, Steffen H, et al. Does vertical incomitance predict the diplopia outcome in orbital fracture patients? A prospective study of 188 patients. J Craniomaxillofac Surg 2019;47:305–10.
5. Rowe F, Crowley T. Outcome of ocular motility disturbances in orbital injuries. Strabismus 2003;11(3):179–88.
6. Gosse EM, Ferguson AW, Gilmour C, et al. Blow-out fractures: patterns of ocular motility and effect of surigcal repair. Br J Oral Maxillofac Surg 2010;48:40–3.
7. Walonker AF. Diagnostic evaluation of traumatic cranial nerve palsies. Am Orthopt J 2004;54:57–61.
8. Xia Q, Wang Z, Yan J. Surgical management of strabismus in patients with orbital fracture. J Craniofac Surg 2018;29:1865–9.
9. Pritchard C, Ellis GS. Management of central sensory deficits following trauma. Am Orthopt J 2004;54:45–8.
10. Alhamdani F, Durham J, Greenwood M, et al. Diplopia and ocular motility in orbital blow-out fractures: 10-year retrospective study. J Craniomaxillofac Surg 2015;43(7):1010–6.
11. Jansen J, Dubois L, Maal TJJ, et al. A non-surgical approach with repeated orthoptic evaluation is justified for most blow-out fractures. J Craniomaxillofac Surg 2020;48:560–8.
12. Folkestad L, Aberg-Bengtsson L, Granstrom G. Recovery from orbital floor fractures: a prospective study of patients and doctors' experiences. Int J Oral Maxillofac Surg 2006;35:499–505.
13. Arnoldi K, Mattheu J. Diagnosis and nonsurgical management of strabimus secondary to orbital fracture. Am Orthopt J 2004;54: 7–12.
14. Silbert DI, Matta NS, Singman EL. Diplopia secondary to orbital surgery. Am Orthopt J 2012;62:22–8.
15. Ramponi DR, Astorino T, Bessetti-Barrett CR. Orbital floor fractures. Adv Emerg Nurs J 2017;39(4):240–7.
16. Sullivan TJ, Kraft SP, Burack C, et al. A functional scoring method for the field of bincular single vision. Ophthalmology 1992;99:575–81.
17. Gerling J, Lieb B, Kommerell G. Duction ranges in normal probands and patients with Graves' ophthalmopathy, determined using the Goldmann perimeter. Int Ophthalmol 1997;21(4):213–21.
18. Mourits MP, Prummel MF, Wiersinga WM, et al. Measuring eye movements in Graves' ophthalmopathy. Ophthalmology 1994; 101(8):1341–6.
19. Haggerty H, Richardson S, Mitchell KW, et al. A modified method for measuring uniocular fields of fixation: reliability in healthy subjects and in patients with Graves' Orbitopathy. Arch Ophthalmol 2005;123(3):356–62.
20. Roper-Hall G. Diagnosis and management of cetnral motro deficits following trauma. Am Orthopt J 2004;54:49–54.
21. Kerr NC. Management of strabismus following orbital fracture repair. Am Orthopt J 2004;54:24–31.

Primary Orbital Fracture Repair

Simon Holmes, FDS, RCS, FRCS*

KEYWORDS

• Orbital fracture • Orbital reconstruction • Patient-specific implant • Diplopia • Medial wall • Titanium • Mesh • Maxillofacial trauma

KEY POINTS

- Predictable outcomes of complex orbital fracture patterns may be achieved by a structured and evidence-based approach.
- Full anatomic and physiologic assessment of the fracture pattern using computed tomographic data and quantitative orthoptic analysis allows for precise planning of the surgical technique.
- Preseptal transconjunctival access with transcaruncular extension and lateral swinging lid technique allows for ultimate exposure of the fracture complex.
- Incarcerated orbital tissues must be identified and planned for released without surgical duress to the musculature.
- Surgical momentum is progressing toward patient-specific implants for larger and more strategic fracture patterns. Medial and floor reconstruction to the apex can now be achieved.

Introduction

The nature of the problem

Fracture patterns of the anatomic orbit are common in contemporaneous oral and maxillofacial practice and exist in isolation or in concert with adjacent skeletal components. There is variance in complexity according to volume of energy transfer, and clinical heterogeneity in presentation because of soft tissue involvement, some of which may be vision threatening. Predicable outcomes therefore depend on prompt clinical diagnosis augmented by full anatomic description of the fracture configuration in conjunction with formal physiologic assessment. This full clinical data set then will inform prompt surgical management followed by evidence-based indications for surgery, approach, materials and methods used, together with prognostication to manage both surgeon and patient expectation.

Changes within the UK acute trust infrastructure have led to the adoption of major trauma centers, of which the Royal London Hospital was the prototype example, with 30 years of dedicated multidisciplinary trauma experience. This multidisciplinary trauma experience has led to proven increased survival rates in complex high-energy injury mechanisms, and greater survival rates resulting in higher numbers of complex facial injuries coming to surgery. The social demographic of East London, with a substantial history of criminal and even political violence, is well known. The UK Crime statistics indicate 30,000 violent crimes reported per year in East London, representing 19.5% of all crimes *reported*. The map of London in Fig. 1 demonstrates the significantly increased crime levels in the region.

Surgical pathologic condition

Anatomic classification

Classically, orbital fracture patterns were described as either pure or impure. Impure fractures follow failure of the orbital rim, which can either be localized to the inferior orbital rim and associated with the orbital floor or propagate to the orbit from an adjacent facial bone fracture (Table 1).

The distinction of pure and impure of course has surgical significance but seems to be less important in the association with ocular damage, this born out clinically and by finite element analysis, which illustrates that the failure threshold for globe rupture is less than that of bone.

The surgical principle is to convert impure to pure orbital injuries and then treat the floor and medial walls accordingly. The size of the defect and position have both profound influence on surgical complexity and prognostic implications in terms of both aesthetics and function. Most surgeons will agree that fractures toward the posterior floor and upper medial third are more technically challenging and take longer to return to normal function postoperatively. Ahmad proposed a quantitative assessment of orbital fractures by splitting the floor and medial wall into separate thirds, as well as quantifying fracture severity in the rest of the facial skeleton, with recognition of the presence or absence of the posterior medial ledge. Jaquiery classified orbital fractures into 5 types according to surgical complexity, focusing on the size of defect and presence or absence of the posterior bone ledge medial to the infraorbital nerve, which facilitates anatomic dissection, and in addition, seating of the implant (Table 2).

Department of Oral and Maxillofacial Surgery, Royal London Hospital, London, UK

* Corresponding author. Department OMFS, Fourth Floor Dental Institute, Royal London Hospital, Whitechapel, London E1 1BB, UK.

E-mail address: s.holmes@qmul.ac.uk

Atlas Oral Maxillofacial Surg Clin N Am 29 (2021) 51–77

https://doi.org/10.1016/j.cxom.2020.11.004

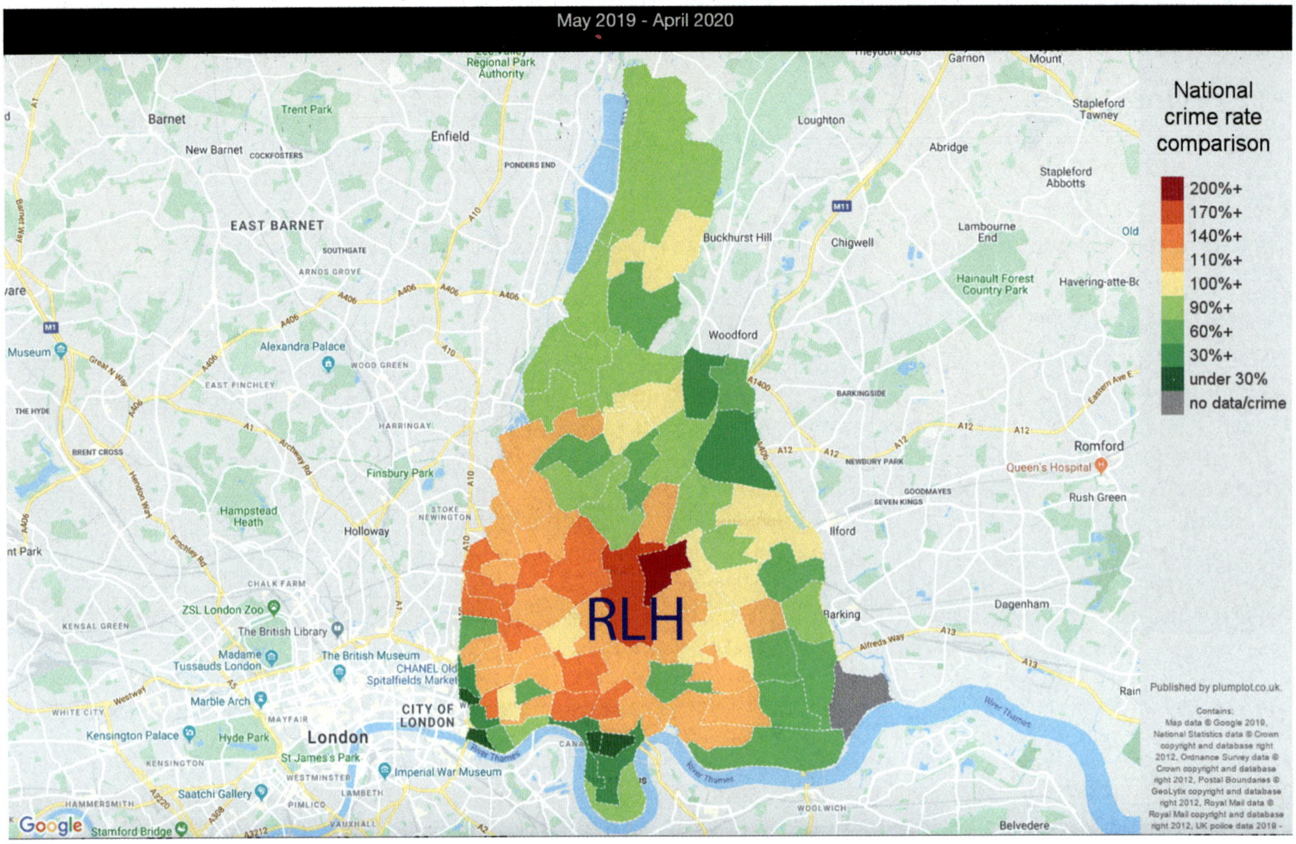

Fig. 1 Map of London demonstrating the significantly increased crime levels in the region. RLH, Royal London Hospital.

Functional classification

Facilitation of binocular single vision requires the integration of a complex neuromuscular system involving 4 cranial nerves and 6 extraocular muscles working in a highly coordinated syncytium. The nuclei of the cranial nerves supplying these muscles are linked by the medial longitudinal fasciculus, which allows coordination with integration of the vestibular nerve. Disruption by intracranial damage can cause internuclear ophthalmoplegia. The muscles themselves are easily damaged or trapped in certain fracture patterns (Table 3).

Fracture progression is influenced by the mechanism and biomechanics of the orbit itself. In paediatric mechanisms, energy transfer commonly produces a linear fracture resulting herniation of the orbital contents with entrapment due to the elastic biomechanical nature of the orbital floor. Linear fracture pattern may occur with comparatively low-energy transfer and produce the so-called white-eye blowout fracture, which could be initially missed in accident and emergency departments. One of the symptoms is persistent postinjury nausea and vomiting, so a computed tomographic (CT) scan of the brain could incidentally expose the orbital fracture. Nevertheless, experience shows that CT scan is not always conclusive, and a trapdoor fracture could be missed easily.

Indications for surgery

The decision to operate follows comprehensive assessment of the fracture pattern in concert with the patient, in which clinical, medical, anatomic, and functional considerations are supported by objective evidence from detailed imaging and formal quantified orthoptic examination. With the exception of a vision-threatening condition that demands immediate surgical treatment, all indications are relative. Ultimately, it is a

Table 1 Classification of orbital floor and wall fractures

Pure	Impure	Roof
Floor	Segmental lower-orbital rim	Isolated
Medial wall	Nasomaxillary	Craniofacial
	Zygomatic	
	Maxillary	
	Nasoethmoid	

Table 2 Jaquiery classification

Stage	Size of Defect (cm^2)	Bone Ledge Medial To Orbital Fissure
I	1–2	Yes
II	>2	Yes
III	>2	No
IV	Entire orbital floor/ medial wall	No
V	Extension to roof	No

Table 3 Neurology of the orbit

Structure	Function	Pathologic Conditions
Oculomotor nerve	Motor to • Medial rectus • Inferior rectus • Superior rectus • Inferior oblique	• Entrapment • Contusion • Snagging • Tearing • Neuromuscular
Trochlear nerve	Motor to superior oblique	• Contusion • Snagging • Tearing • Neuromuscular
Abducent nerve	Motor to lateral rectus	• Contusion • Snagging • Tearing • Neuromuscular
Medial longitudinal fasciculus	Linking all intracranial nuclei	• Head injury • Neurologic pathologic condition

balanced decision between the surgeon and the patient according to individualization of the risk-benefit ratio.

Restoration of anatomy

The aesthetic form of the orbit involves harmony between the soft and hard tissues.

The orbital floor and medial wall have several key strategic landmarks, which maintain globe position. These landmarks have been described by Hammer with reference to the posterior medial bulge (Fig. 2). Note the normal left side in this low orbital axial view (blue arrow) and the fractured right side (right arrow), and the sigmoid nature of the floor in sagittal view (Fig. 3). In this view, the blue zone maintains the vertical height of the globe, and the sigmoid green zone maintains projection.

The concept of orbital volume remains but is, of course, related to the geometry of the bone orbit. It should also be appreciated that the volume comprises all the orbital adnexae, which includes fat and muscle, but in addition, the globe itself.

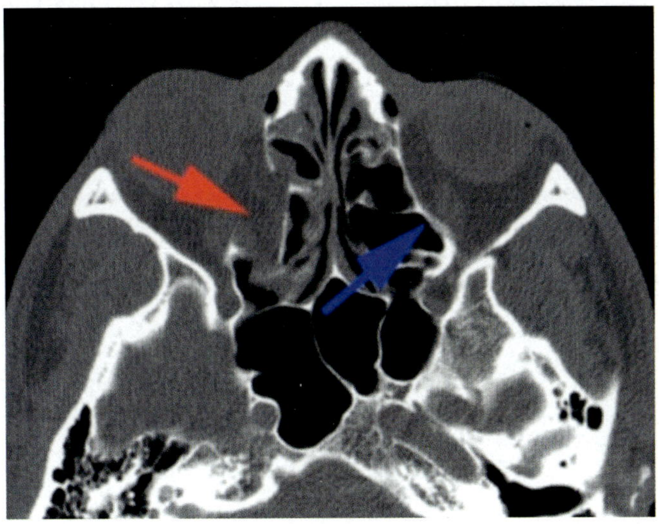

Fig. 2 Axial CT scan at the level of the mid to lower orbit demonstrating Hammer's key area (*blue arrow*). The fracture of the medial orbital wall compromises this (*red arrow*).

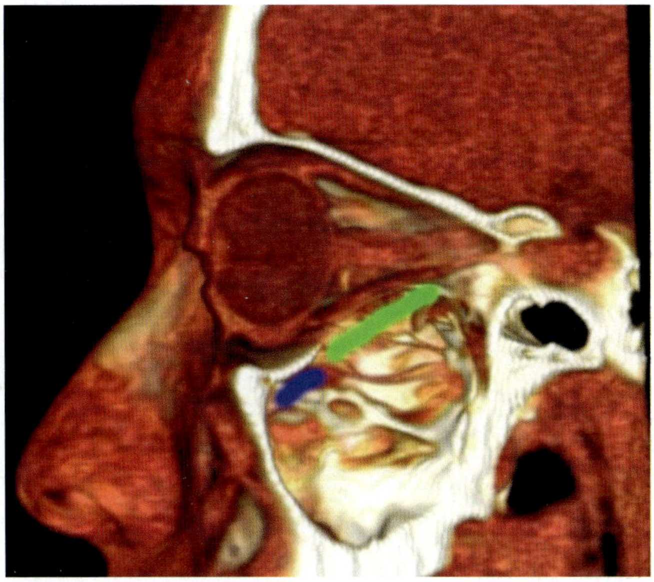

Fig. 3 Sagittal view of an intact orbit. Fractures involving the posterior and middle third of the orbital floor (*green line*) reduce globe projection; fractures of the anterior third (*blue line*) contribute to vertical discrepancy (hypoglobus).

Restoration of function

In order to facilitate free movement of the globe, any trapped tissue within linear fractures, or physical limitation by sharp bone fragments, needs to be removed.

Primary orbital trauma decision making

Decision making for Orbital Reconstruction should follow a logical and stereotypical process which includes appraisal of physical findings, and assessment of hard and soft tissue subunits, with didactic surgical treatment planning (Fig. 4).

Emergency management

The orbit is described as a 4-walled pyramid contained by the orbital septum constrained by the lateral and medial canthal tendons, making the orbital contents vulnerable to compartment syndrome. Although an expanding retrobulbar hematoma is recognized, it must also be appreciated that intraorbital surgical emphysema, cerebrospinal fluid, and displaced bone fragments can be implicated.

Although medical management in the form of acetazolamide, mannitol, and hydrocortisone is described, lateral cantholysis in a timely manner is frequently vision saving.

Fig. 5 demonstrates an axial view of a medial wall fracture (red arrows) and a retrobulbar hematoma (blue arrows).

Physical signs of ocular compartment syndrome

- Ophthalmoplegia
- Tense and proptosed globe
- Loss of red vision
- Loss of visual acuity
- Escalating pain

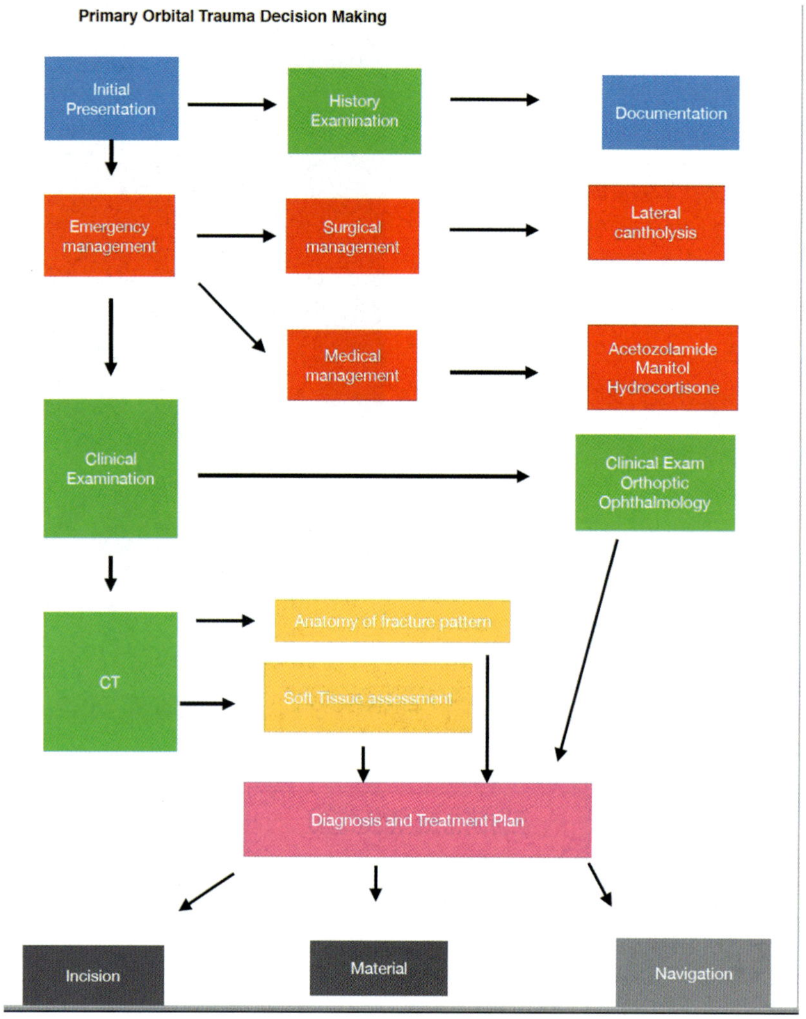

Fig. 4 Pathway and decision making in orbital trauma.

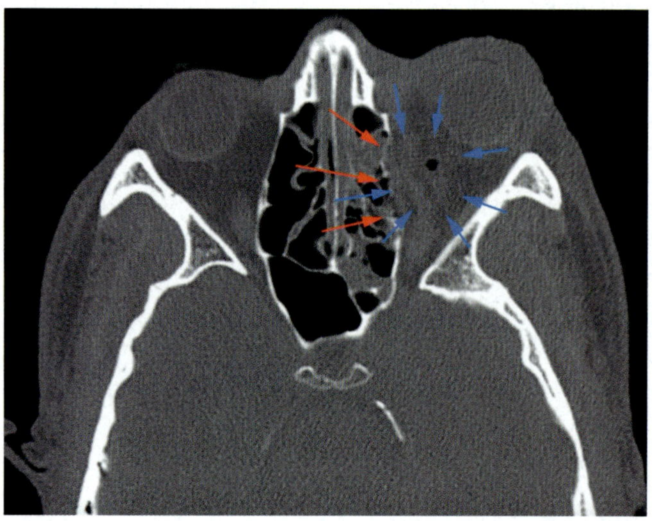

Fig. 5 Axial view of a medial wall fracture (*red arrows*) and a retrobulbar hematoma (*blue arrows*).

The risk of ocular damage in facial injuries has been described many times, and the famous mnemonic device of BAD ACT has been constructed to raise awareness:

B: Blow out
A: Acquity
D: Diplopia
A: Amnesia
CT: Comminuted trauma

These injuries can frequently be difficult to assess because of acute periorbital swelling or may be masked by substance or alcohol abuse and a lowered level of consciousness. High-energy mechanism injured patients with multisystem injuries may mask orbital injuries that are not life threatening (Box 1).

Box 1. Risk factors for ocular involvement

- Significant volume of trauma
- Orbital fracture: increased probability with increasing size
- Multiple fractures: particularly involving orbital cancellous bone
- Impaired consciousness: pain is less of a feature

Diagnosis, quantification, and prognostication of fracture pattern

CT scan analysis is central to diagnosis and planning treatment as well as to prognostication.

The sequential analysis of axial-coronal-sagittal formatted scans with measurement of bone loss and even angulation of fragments can be conducted near the patient with modern PACS systems.

Interpretation will influence the incision with the need for lateral and medial extensions to achieve predictable access, which materials to reconstruct, and risks to anatomic structures.

CT scans can also be interrogated to both diagnose and prognosticate functional deficits because of muscular involvement. The classic description of a trapdoor fracture typically seen in the pediatric or adolescent, otherwise known as the white-eye blowout fracture, is an example.

The CT scans visualized in coronal format demonstrate the region (blue square) of the fracture that is typically close to the infraorbital canal (green arrow) (Fig. 6).

The sagittal view illustrates the small size of the fracture (T), and soft tissue windows may distinguish between muscle and fat prolapse (Fig. 7).

This fracture pattern is not exclusively seen in young patients and is not always confined to the floor. The author has seen this pattern in older patients and affecting the medial wall involving medial rectus and superior oblique.

The scan, soft tissue windows, coronal format demonstrates the fracture (blue arrow) and the superior oblique (red arrows) (Fig. 8).

CT scans may also support orthoptic diagnosis and prognosticate on the possibility of postoperative functional defect. Orthoptic examination is mandatory for all clinical diagnoses of diplopia and will help prognosticate (Table 4).

Diplopia on downgaze is a predictor of the likelihood of postoperative diplopia, although it must be appreciated that the Hess chart only examines to 30° of elevation/depression, so type II and III may be more common than first appreciated.

Radiological predictors of postoperative diplopia included bone spurs in close proximity (blue arrow showing involvement with inferior rectus) (Fig. 9).

Another prognostic indicator is the change in shape of the muscle bellies, seen in coronal section.

This can be seen in both the medial rectus and, in this case, the inferior rectus. Note the ribbon shape of the normal side (blue arrow) compared with the rounder fractured side (red arrow) (Fig. 10).

Choice of material

The function of reconstruction material for primary repair has now become more objective. The choice of material depends on the anatomic and functional deficit (Table 5).

For simple defects, which in essence simply partition the orbit from adjacent anatomy, the polydiaoxanone sulfate (PDS) membrane is a very acceptable choice, easy to use, and well tolerated.

If the fracture size according to local anatomy and relationship to key structures is considered, then treatment planning becomes logical. In the schematic of the right orbit (Fig. 11), floor (light blue defect) and medial wall (blue defect), which do not transgress the white line described by

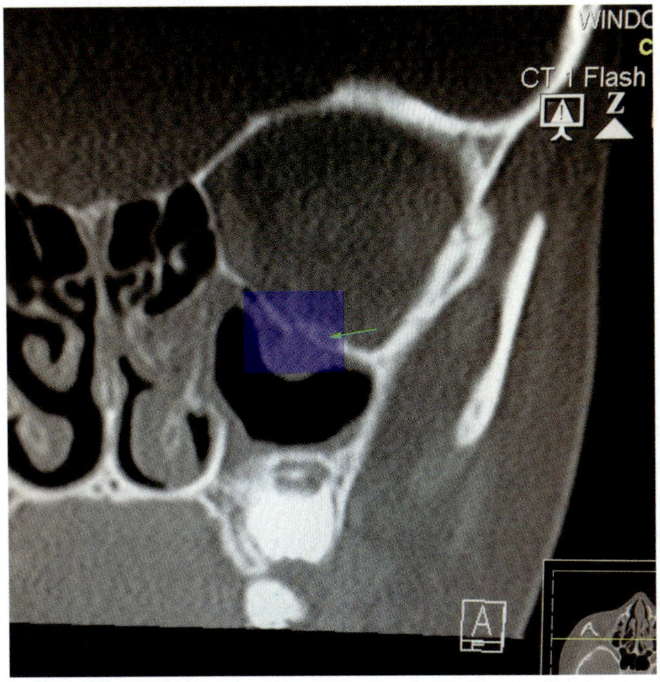

Fig. 6 Coronal CT scan demonstrating region of an orbital floor fracture with herniation of contents (*blue zone*); the infraorbital canal is demonstrated by the green arrow.

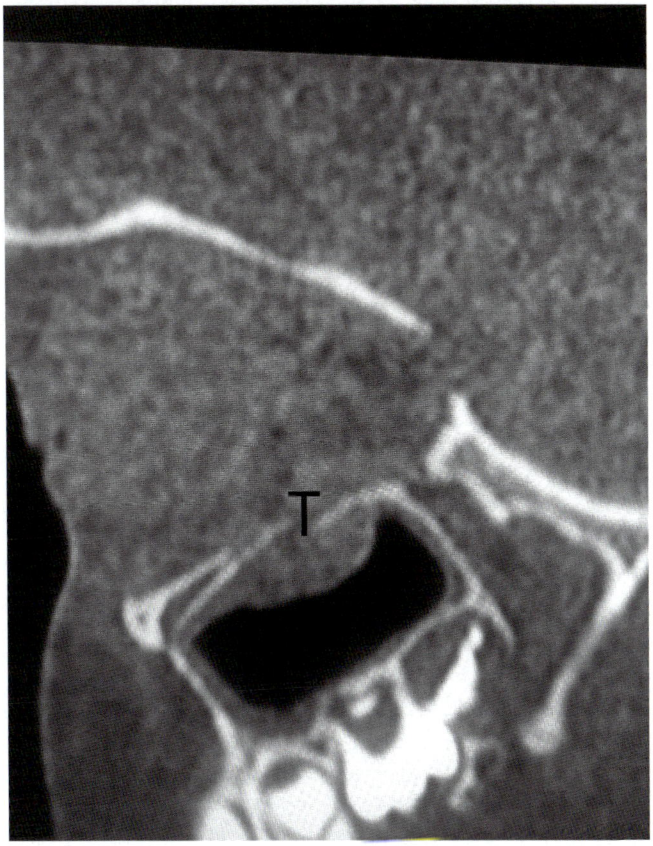

Fig. 7 Sagittal fracture of the orbital floor trapdoor fracture T.

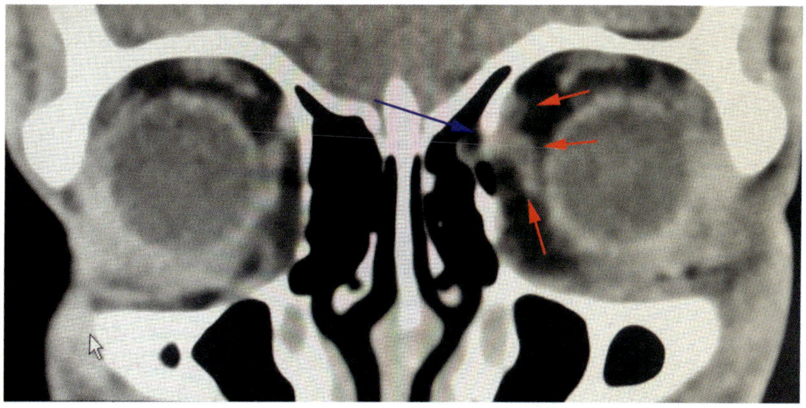

Fig. 8 Coronal CT scan. Soft tissue windows demonstrating a high medial wall fracture (*blue arrow*) with distortion and incarceration of superior oblique (*red arrows*).

Jaquiery, are extremely predictable when reconstructed by preformed plates. The red areas of the apical third have close proximity to the optic nerve, and the high medial wall can be technically challenging to check plate positioning; for that reason, a custom plate with or without support by navigation is required.

The prefabricated plates are deficient laterally (purple zone), and for that reason a second plate (PDS), or alternatively a custom plate, is required.

The anterior ethmoidal and posterior ethmoidal foramina are illustrated but are anatomically inconsistent, and vessels are invariably thrombosed in primary surgery.

The dimensions of a typical prefabricated plate are illustrated in Fig. 12 in millimeters. The plate may be divided according to reconstructive requirements. Moderate defects floor (green), junctional zone (red), and medial wall (yellow) can be reconstructed, but lateral defects (blue) need further support. The footplate needs to remain in only the largest defects and can often be removed, simplifying plate placement.

Timing of surgery

There is anecdotal and published evidence to suggest that pediatric trapdoor defects are best operated on as soon as possible. Although this is the ideal, often presentation is delayed. The author has had good outcomes even in delayed cases. The surgical approach is easiest performed following resolution of chemises and lower-eyelid swelling, which occurs between 4 and 10 days after injury. The timeframe allows for treatment planning on a semielective pathway and also for fabrication of a custom plate if indicated. After 3 to 4 weeks, fibrous adhesions start to be noticeable, and by 6 weeks, the orbit begins to behave as a revision case.

Table 4 Classification of diplopia

Binocular Diplopia	Upgaze	Downgaze	Postoperative
I	Yes	No	Possible, self-limiting
II	No	No	Likely
III	Yes	Yes	Very likely
Complex	Yes	Yes	Extremely likely

Surgical approach

Historical access to the orbit has undergone a significant evolution to achieve adequate surgical access in a cosmetically privileged region. Modern reconstructive principles have driven the development of more cosmetic incisions around the orbit that deliver at least equivalent, but, in fact, better surgical access. The eyelid can be divided anatomically and philosophically into 2 distinct zones:

- Anterior lamella, which consists of skin and orbicularis oculi
- Posterior lamella, which consists of conjunctiva and tarsal plate

Approaches to the orbit can be described in terms of the position of the initial incision; both techniques separate the

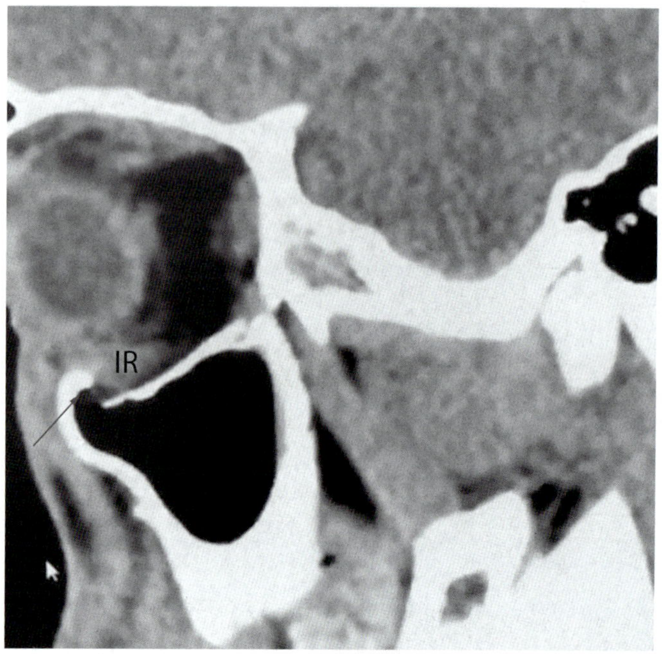

Fig. 9 Sagittal CT scan. Soft tissue windows demonstrating involvement of inferior rectus (IR) with the anterior fracture margin (*arrow*).

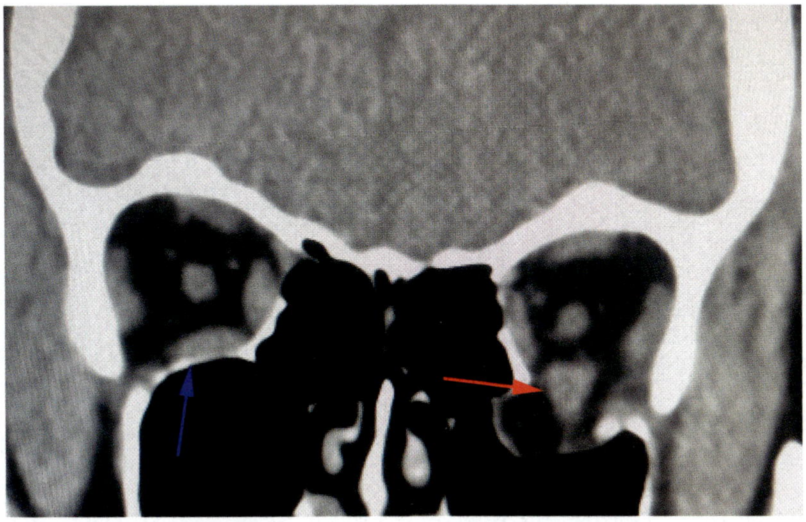

Fig. 10 Coronal CT scan. Soft tissue window demonstrating the normal shape of inferior rectus (*blue arrow*) and the abnormal contour of inferior rectus caused by a floor fracture (*red arrow*).

anterior and posterior lamellae along the plane of the middle lamella, scarring of which is implicated in both the pathologic condition and the secondary correction of ectropion and entropion. Further subclassification of the approaches is indicated in Table 6.

Although it is accepted that good results can be achieved by all the orbital approaches, there is increasing evidence that the posterior lamellar approaches provide for excellent surgical access with superb aesthetic outcomes. In view of the fact that there is no disturbance of the orbicularis oculi muscle, the postoperative bruising and swelling are very much reduced, as is the time to resolution.

Improved lateral exposure with an anterior lamellar approach requires a cutaneous extension that can be very visible postoperatively, and even compromises lymphatic drainage if extensive. In the case of the posterior lamellar approach, the addition of a McCord swinging lid greatly increases the surgical access to the whole orbital floor and lateral wall. Medial exposure through an anterior approach is difficult and may require an additional incision Lynch incision, whereas, in the posterior approach, extension into the transcaruncular zone will achieve a predictable exposure to the whole medial wall.

The surgical exposure resulting from a lateral cantholysis with transcaruncular extension is very satisfactory and highly predictable, allowing access from above the frontozygomatic suture laterally to the skull base medially and well into the posterior third of the orbital floor.

There has been debate about the relative merits of surgical incision of the orbital septum. It must be appreciated that the

Table 5 Justification of choice of orbital reconstruction material

Defect	Defect	Material	Special consideration
Single wall	Trapdoor	Polydiaxanone sulfate	
Single wall, loss contour	Anatomic loss	Preshaped titanium	
Floor, medial wall	Anatomic loss	Preshaped titanium	
Approach, apex	Anatomic loss	Custom-made	Navigation
Approach, skull base	Anatomic loss	Custom-made	Navigation
Large combined defect	Anatomic Loss	2-part custom-made	Navigation

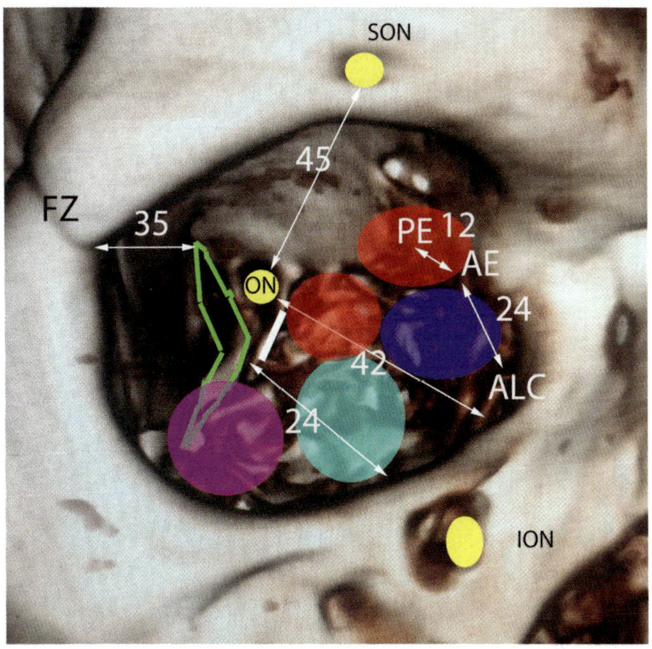

Fig. 11 Three-dimensional image of the right orbit. The anatomic structures with distances are illustrated, and the position of the fracture pattern within the orbit will dictate the strategic choice of material (see text). AE, anterior ethmoidal; ALC, anterior lacrimal crest; FZ frontozygomatic; ION Infraorbital nerve; ON, optic nerve; PE, posterior ethmoidal; SON; superior orbital nerve.

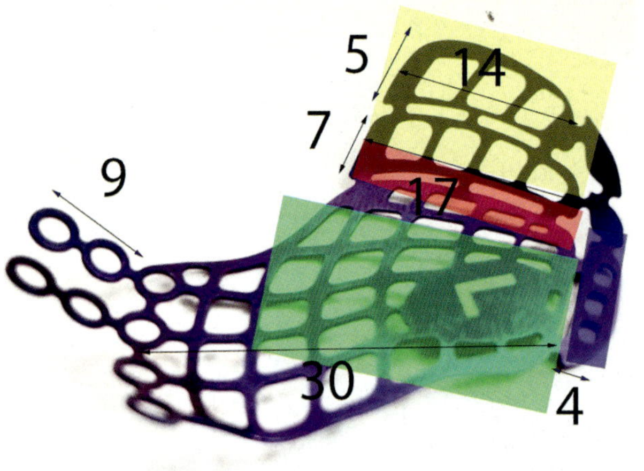

Fig. 12 A typical preformed plate as favored by the author for moderate orbital floor defects with loss of 3D contour. The various regions of the plate are illustrated in color regions, and the dimensions of the components are in millimeters.

Table 6 Classification of orbital approaches	
Approach	Lamellar
Infraorbital	Anterior
Blepharoplasty	Anterior
Lower lid	Anterior
Transconjunctival: retroseptal	Posterior
Transconjunctival: preseptal	Posterior

septum may be violated in more significant orbital trauma, and in those cases, surgical exploration is more challenging, and postoperative results are less predictable. There is increasing understanding in the literature to support this, and the author has practiced the preseptal approach for 15 years with a low-complication and returned-to-theater rate, in a significant quantitative and qualitative trauma practice. It is for this reason that this approach is presented.

The technique

Initial assessment of the approach requires testing the integrity of the medial and lateral canthal tendons (Fig. 13). The shape and integrity of the lateral canthus (blue arrow) are demonstrated here. At this time, the presence or absence of a "crow's foot" can be determined to site the position of the lateral canthal release (red line). Note that the length of the incision is short, and simply enough to access the lateral tarsal plate.

The cantholysis can be planned (blue arrow) (Fig. 13) (red line) and made before the conjunctiva incision, or in a "cut as you go," if during the subsequent dissection further access is required.

A 4/0 suture is placed through the midpoint of the lower eyelid (Fig. 14), and evert the lid over a Desmarres retractor. This view demonstrates the tarsal plate (red arrows) nicely. Note that the tension within the eyelid causes an avascular zone; it is here that the incision is best sited (green arrows). The assistant applies gentle downward traction with both the Desmarres retractor and the suture.

It is extremely important to ensure that there is a low-power setting of the diathermy. The settings required are "10to 10 blend and spray."

The initial incisions are mapped out using a postage-stamp technique (Fig. 15) using the cutting setting. It is important to have the lightest touch on the surgical instrument until just the conjunctiva is incised.

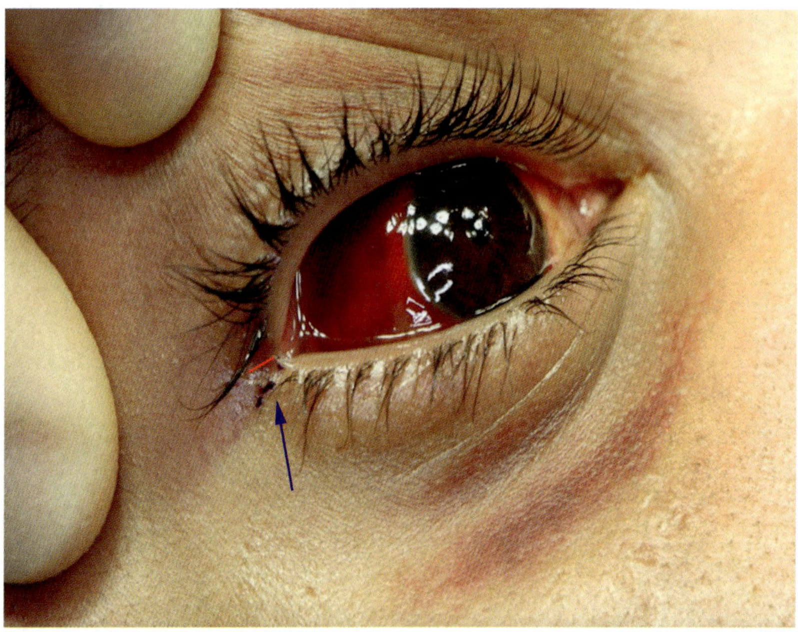

Fig. 13 Preoperative view of patient prepared for a transconjunctival incision with a McCord swinging lid (*red line*), at the lateral canthus (*blue arrow*).

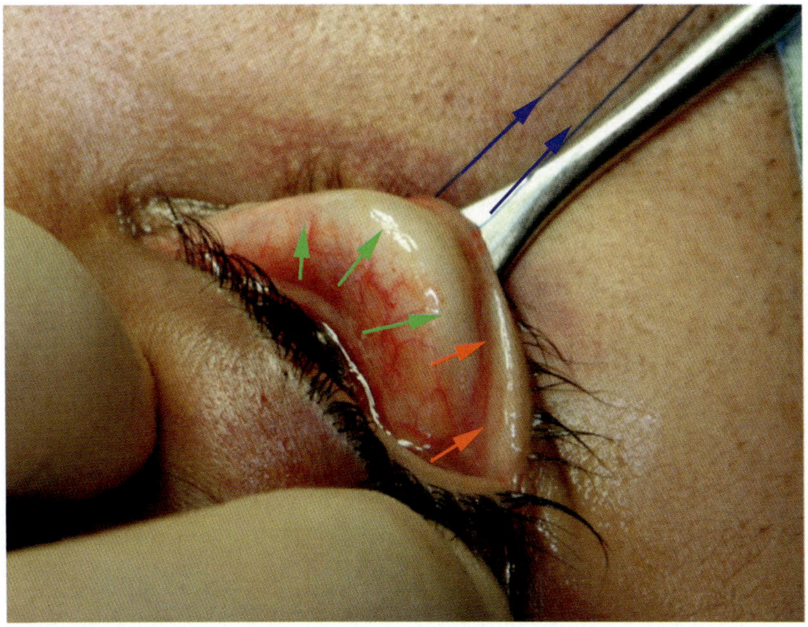

Fig. 14 The conjunctiva is everted over a Desmarres retractor, and the retractor is used to gently retract anteriorly (*blue arrows*). The tarsal plate is indicated by the red arrows. The incision line is sited where the conjunctival arcade blanches (*green arrows*). It is important to leave a cuff of conjunctiva below the tarsal plate.

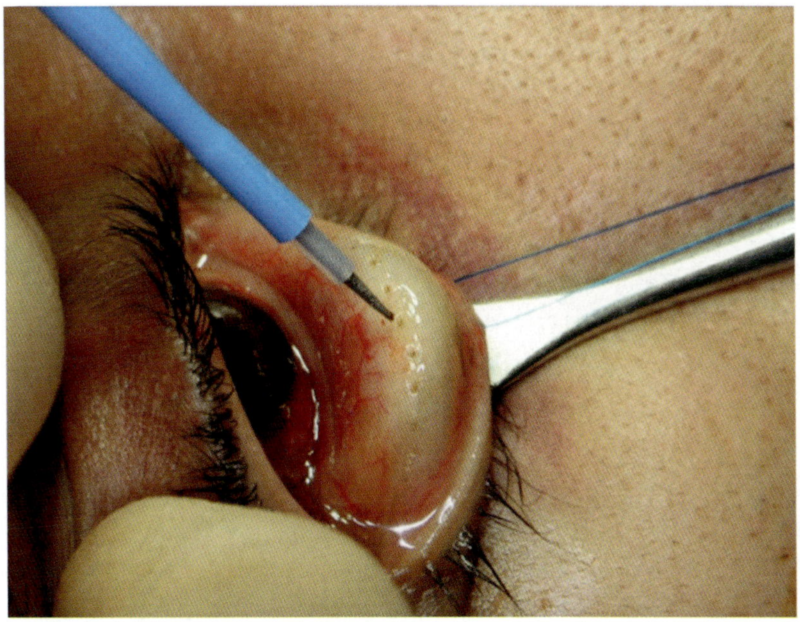

Fig. 15 The conjunctival incision is marked using the cutting setting of the diathermy using a postage-stamp technique. The settings are 10 to 10 blend and spray.

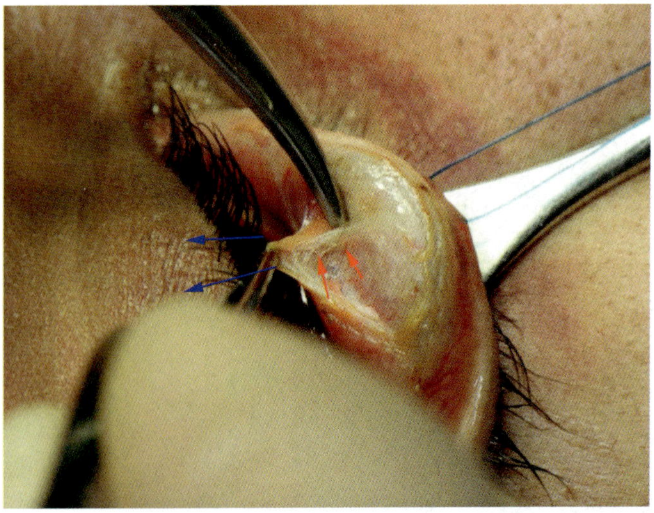

Fig. 16 The surgeon then retracts the free edge of the conjunctiva cranially (*blue arrows*). This demonstrated the middle lamella (*red arrows*). This plane is usually bloodless.

This is then completed by joining each postage stamp, extending to the posterior aspect of the caruncle medially to the lateral canthus posteriorly.

The conjunctiva is then picked up with a small-toothed forceps, and tension is applied cranially (blue arrows) (Fig. 16), leading to exposure of the middle lamella, which can be either incised with the diathermy or sharply cut with scissors.

The free edge of the conjunctiva can then be advanced cranially, and this acts as an eye shield. Note the integrity of the orbital septum (blue arrows) (Fig. 17).

In this case, the skin incision is made with a number 15 scalpel (Fig. 18).

The incision is then clipped with a mosquito forceps for a period of not less than 25 seconds, with the curve extending cranially (Fig. 19).

The lateral tendon is then visualized, and this can be divided along the blue line (Fig. 20). The downward traction (red arrows) allows the tendon to be tight, which greatly facilitates cutting the ligament with a pair of tenotomy scissors.

Downward traction of the lower eyelid is crucial to facilitate separation of the tendon (blue arrows) (Fig. 21).

It is important to ensure that the tendon is freely mobile as demonstrated here (Fig. 22).

A Lacks tongue retractor is then placed on the orbital margin to control the septum. It is crucially important that Lacks retractor remains stable and static. The soft tissues can then be scooped forward using a Mitchell's trimmer to mobilize the orbicularis forward (Fig. 23).

This allows full exposure of the orbital periosteum, which is sharply incised using diathermy (Fig. 24).

The orbit can then be entered laterally, and initial dissection continues along the subperiosteal pocket. The lateral wall is robust, and this is an easily developed plane, "the lateral wall is your friend" (Fig. 25).

Transcaruncular extension

One of the many advantages of the preseptal approach is that the surgical plane can readily be identified medially. The dissection is made easier by the use of multiple traction sutures (blue arrows). The mucosa can be cut with scissors along the green retrocaruncular line (Fig. 26).

Subsequently, the orbital periosteum is incised along the rim and the soft tissue retracted along the green arrows and the medial orbit readily entered (blue arrow) (Fig. 27).

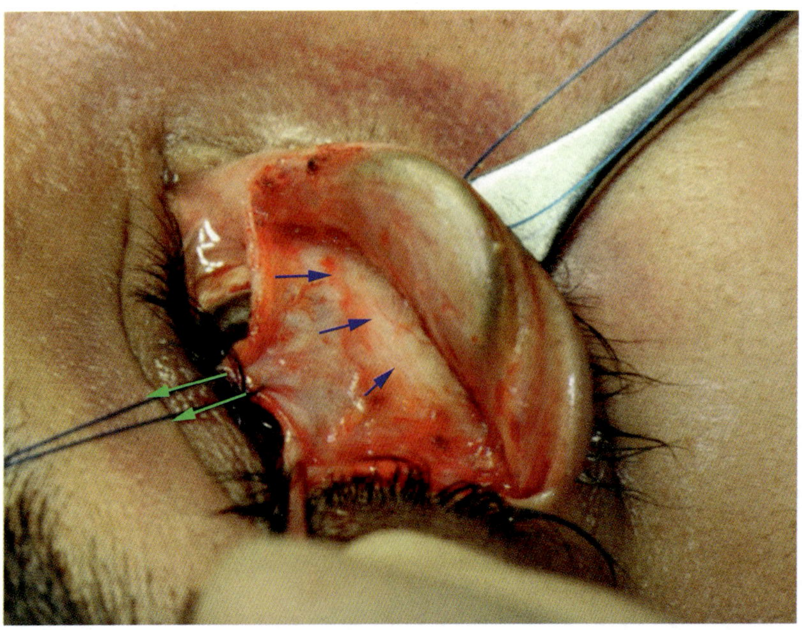

Fig. 17 The free edge of the conjunctiva is then used as a physiologic eye shield by gentle traction (*green arrows*). Note the intact orbital septum, which controls the orbital fat (*blue arrows*).

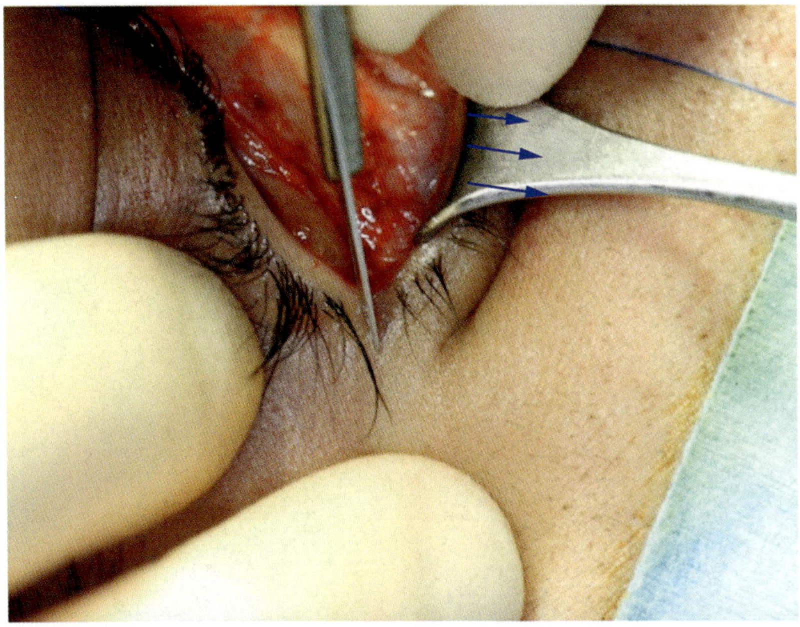

Fig. 18 In this case, the cantholysis is performed following the initial conjunctival incision, in a cut-as-you-go manner. The anterior tension of the eyelid is a key maneuver in facilitating this incision (*arrows*). The cantholysis can be performed before the conjunctival incision. This may be useful in revision cases.

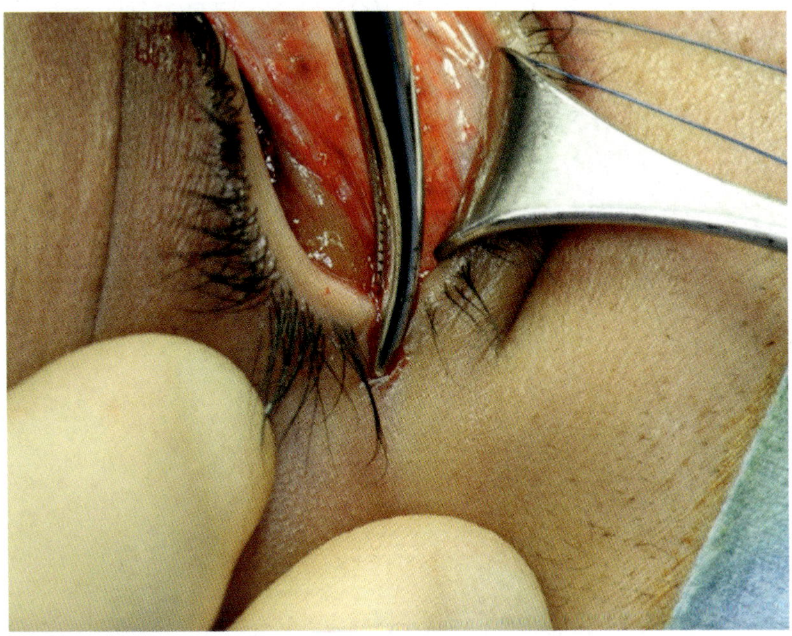

Fig. 19 Following the skin incision, the canthal tendon is clipped with a hemostat for a minimum of 20 seconds.

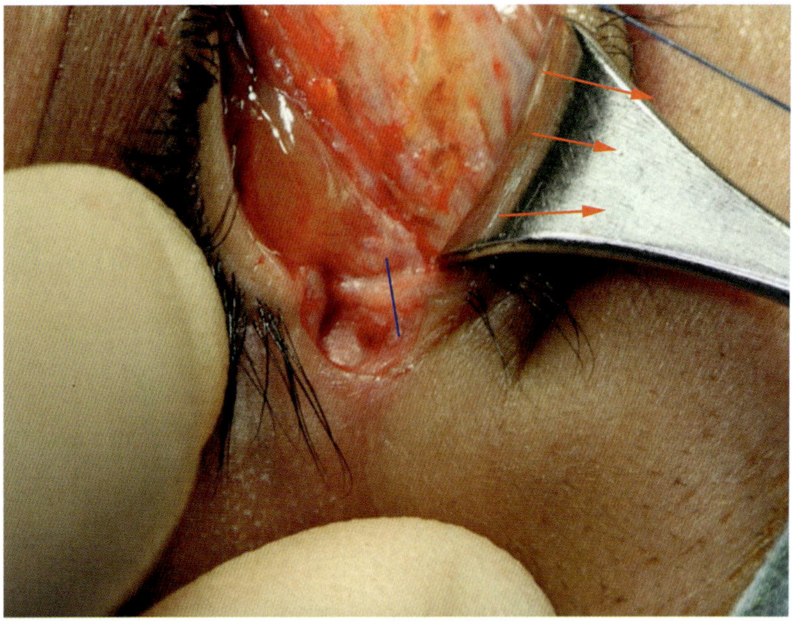

Fig. 20 The canthal tendon is clearly demonstrated and can be cut with a pair of tenotomy scissors along the blue line. The incision is facilitated by the anterior traction (*arrows*).

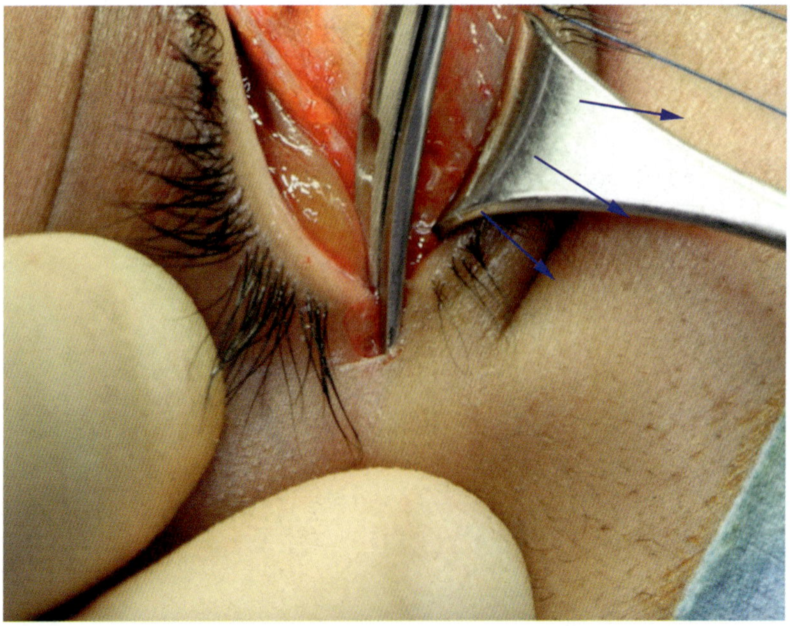

Fig. 21 The curve of the scissors is concave caudally. It is important to maintain traction on the lower eyelid in the direction go the blue arrows.

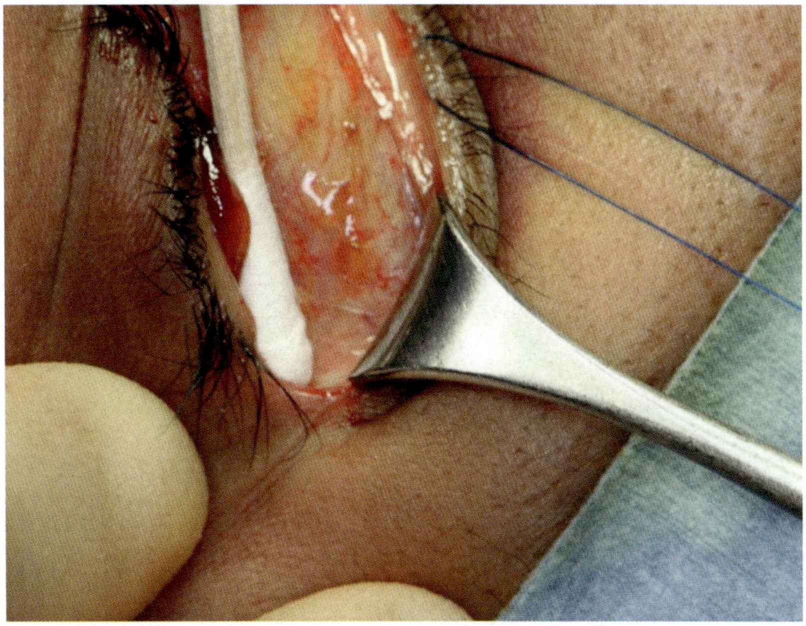

Fig. 22 The freedom of movement of the lateral canthus.

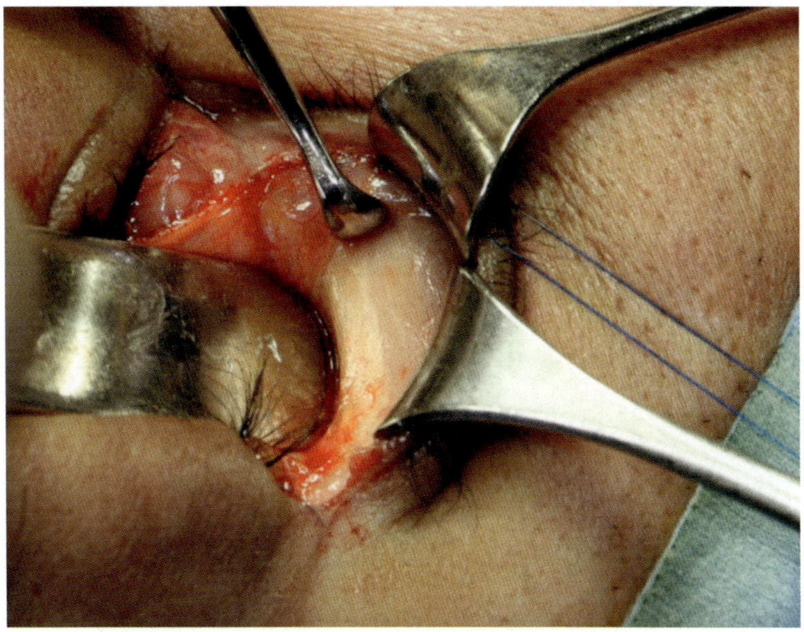

Fig. 23 Orbicularis oculi can now be swept forward off the periosteum. The tissue overlying the orbital rim is tented between the Lacks tongue retractor and the Desmarres.

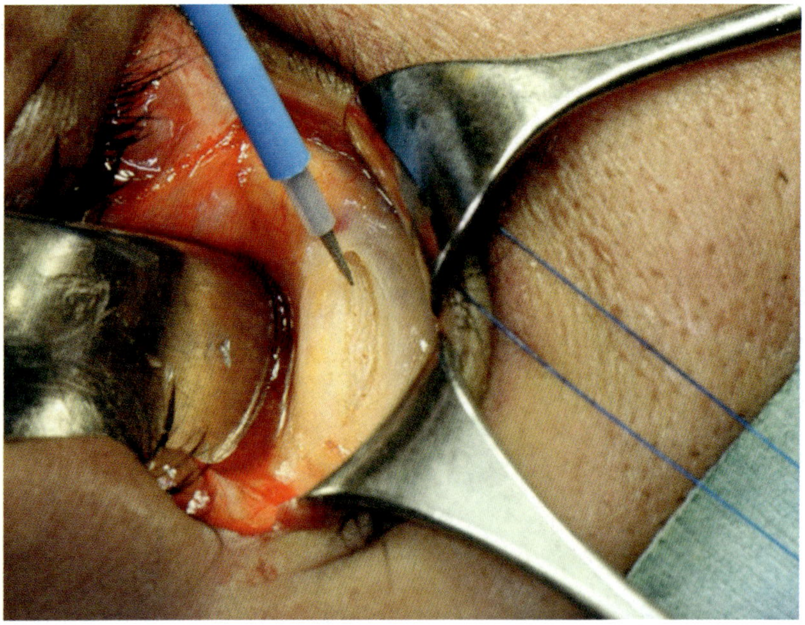

Fig. 24 The infraorbital bone is exposed using a cutting diathermy on coagulation setting.

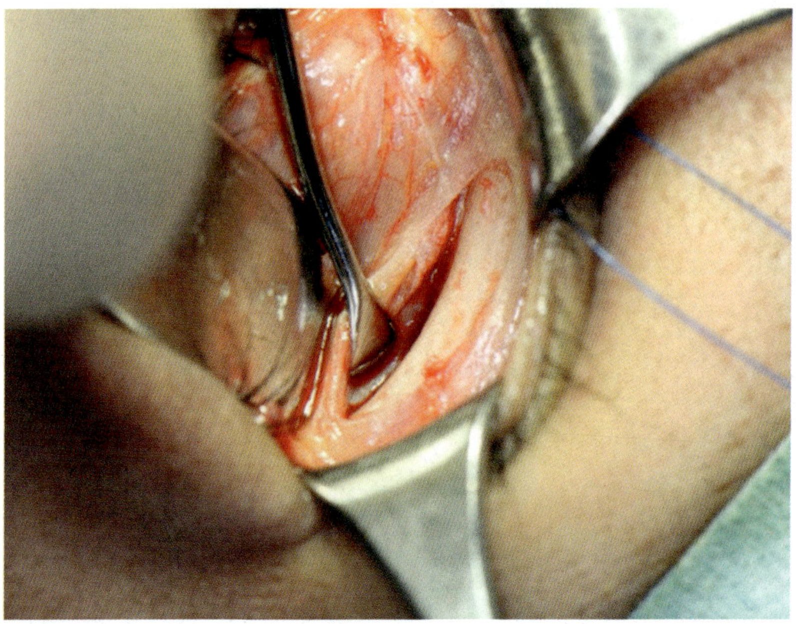

Fig. 25 The approach to the subperiosteal plane is achieved by a lateral vector, "the lateral wall is your friend."

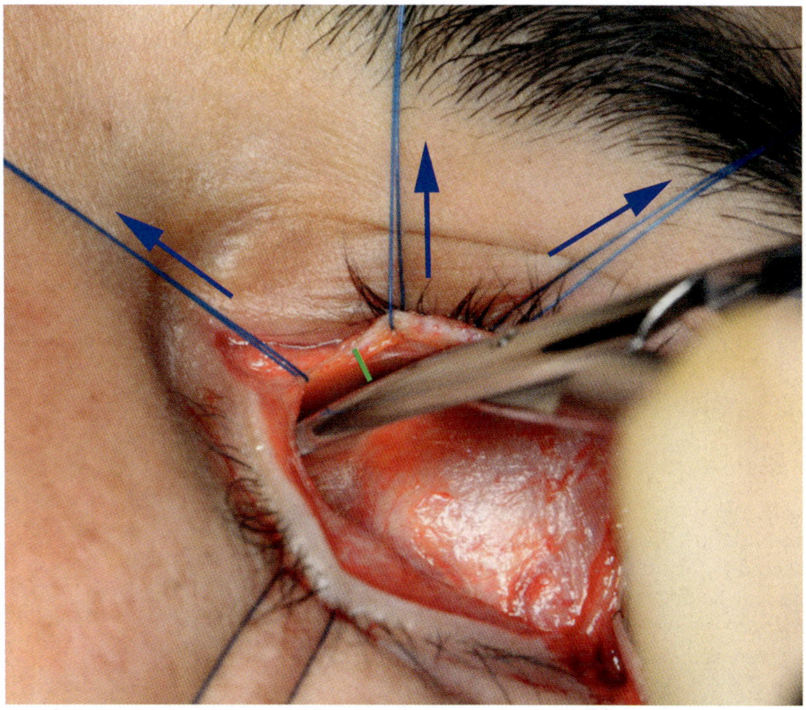

Fig. 26 The preseptal dissection facilitates a straightforward exposure of the medial wall. Note the conjunctival traction sutures(*blue arrows*), which facilitate the approach. The retrocaruncular mucosal incision can be made along the green line.

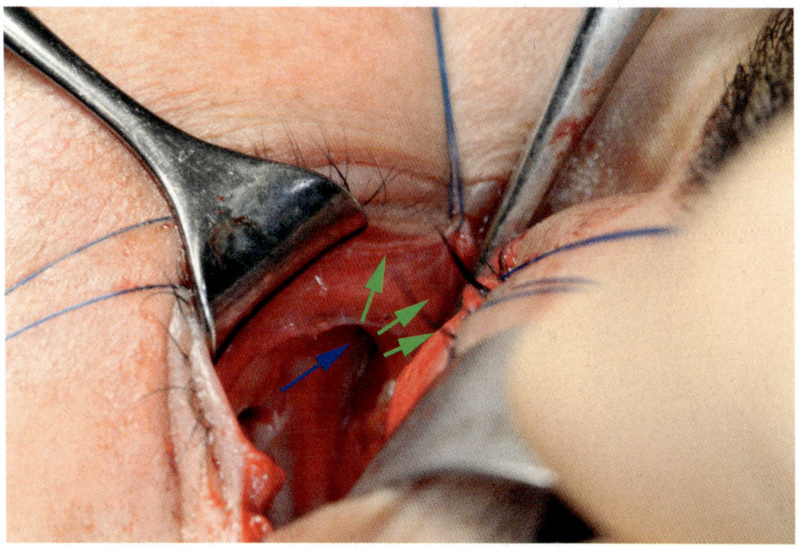

Fig. 27 Following incision to infraorbital periosteum, the plane of the subperiosteal approach to the medial wall is now straightforward (*blue arrow*). A quarter Langenbeck retractor along the free edge (*green arrows*) would greatly facilitate progress.

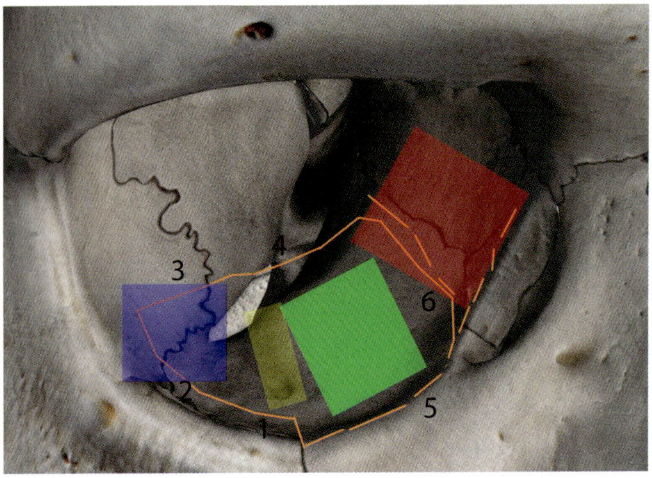

Fig. 28 The "zones of surgical bleeding." The orange line indicates the stepwise progression in a strict numerical order (1-6). Each region must be fully dissected to facilitate onward progress. Laterally (*Blue zone*), the bone may be perforated by a branch of the maxillary artery; the yellow zone may contain branches of the infraorbital vessels, and the green and red zones may contain branches of the antral mucosae. The anterior and posterior ethmoidal vessels represent a theoretic risk.

Dissection

The approach to the orbit follows a stereotypical route (Fig. 28). Following subperiosteal access at the inferior orbital rim (1), the dissection proceeds laterally (2). The sphenozygomatic region allows a firm surface to develop the surgical plane. Following bipolar diathermy in the inferior orbital fissure (4), the posterior orbit is dissected to the palatine bone; this is the ledge that Jaquiery references.

The medial dissection then proceeds (6). The medial tissue can usually be delivered by traction (indicated by the dotted lines).

The clinical view shows the fracture margins (blue arrows) (Fig. 29) and the herniated contents. Should there be a sharp bone edge, then this is best removed with a "Mitchell's trimmer" to enlarge the hole. The contents should be delivered very gently.

The plate can then be gently insinuated between the bone and the soft tissues and fixed with screws.

Control of hemorrhage

Preseptal dissection is crucial to help avoid bleeding in a potentially closed space.

Operative bleeding can be managed according to the operating site (Fig. 28).

1. Lateral bleed (blue zone): This is usually from the zygomaticofacial vessel; the vessel can be diathermied, and the foramen can be packed with bone wax.
2. Inferior orbital vessel tributary (yellow zone): This manifests as a small leak; the bleeding point can readily be identified, and bipolar cautery will normally arrest it.
3. Maxillary floor (green zone): This manifests as a persistent and slow ooze. This is managed by use of a ribbon gauze soaked in 1:1000 adrenaline placed in the bleeding point for 2 minutes. This allows for slowing of the bleeding point for diathermy to be used. Occasionally the maxillary antrum itself will need packing, if necessary with removal of the orbital floor to facilitate access. The packing with a saline soaked swab maintained for 2 minutes is usually all that is required.
4. Medial wall (red zone): This manifests as a persistent ooze that is complicated by reduced surgical vision due to the position. This is managed in a similar way to the maxillary sinus using an 1:1000 adrenaline soaked ribbon gauze. This area must be surgically dry to facilitate further surgery and patient safety.

Case example 1: pure fracture

The axial CT scan demonstrates the fracture (blue arrows) (Fig. 30) and the region of the optic canal (yellow area). Note the extensive surgical emphysema.

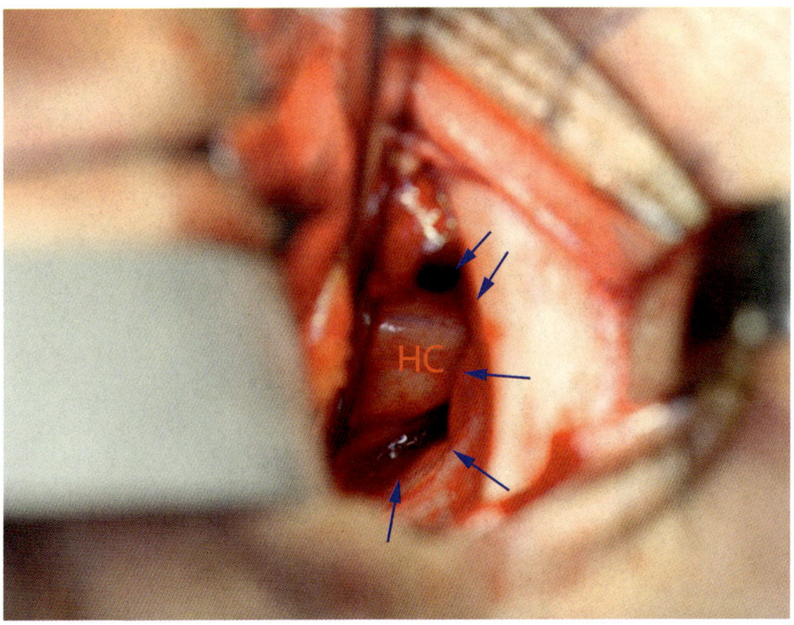

Fig. 29 The margins of the fracture are identified (*arrows*), and the herniated contents (HC) are retrieved.

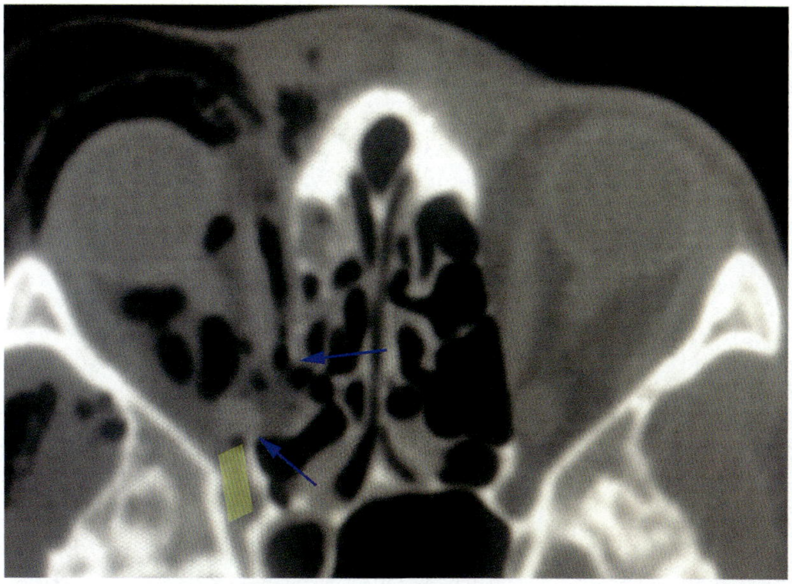

Fig. 30 Axial CT scan demonstrating a fracture in the right posteromedial third of the orbit (*arrows*). Note the extensive surgical emphysema and proximity to the optic nerve (*yellow area*).

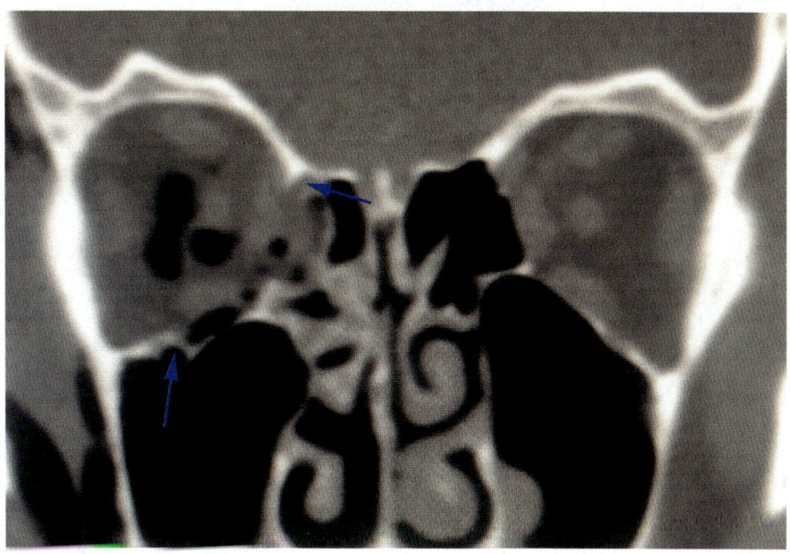

Fig. 31 The coronal CT scan demonstrates the extent of the fracture (*arrows*).

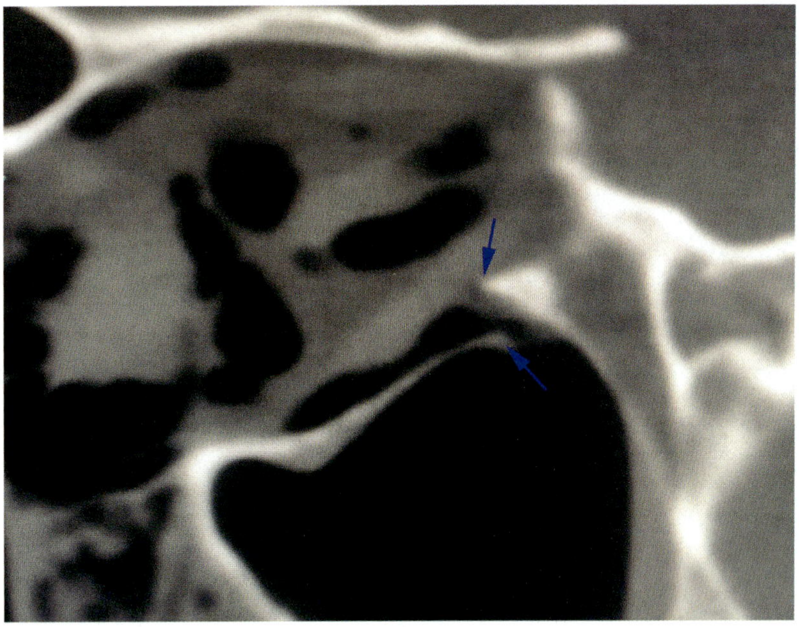

Fig. 32 The sagittal CT view again shows the posterior extent of the fracture (*arrows*).

The coronal view (Fig. 31) and sagittal view (Fig. 32) again demonstrate the defect.

The large defect with proximity to the optic canal and medial extension to the orbital roof could only be managed predictably by a custom-made orbital plate.

The postoperative views indicate a satisfactory position; the margins are indicated by blue arrows (Figs. 33–35).

Case 2: impure orbital fracture

The coronal CT scan demonstrates a fracture extending from the medial wall (blue line) (Fig. 36) through the junctional zone (red line), with the orbital plate cantilevered inferiorly (yellow arrows). The extra bone in the sinus (red arrows) is also noted. The lateral margin of the fracture extends on the body of the zygoma (green line).

The sagittal view shows no credible bone ledge posteriorly, and no anterior orbital margin (blue zone) (Fig. 37).

The 3-dimensional (3D) reconstruction shows the displaced piriform aperture (blue arrows) and the orbital margin (red arrows) (Fig. 38).

The lateral extension precluded a standard plate, and a custom orbital plate was required. At surgery, the precise lateral margin articulation and the landing on the medial wall allowed localization of the orbital margin, and the fragments were fixed to the plate following reconstruction of the piriform aperture.

The postoperative views show accurate placement of the prosthesis (blue arrows) (Fig. 39), with good reconstruction of

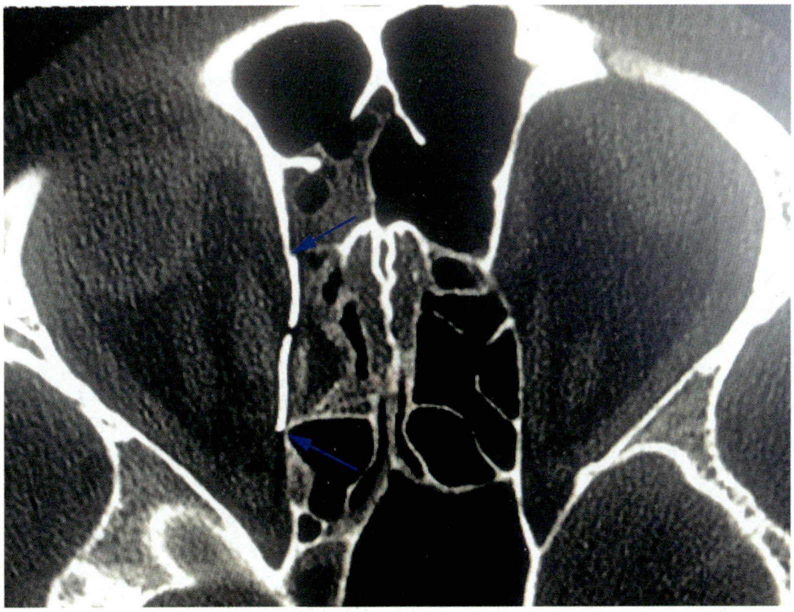

Fig. 33 The axial CT scan shows a good medial wall reconstruction with good fracture margins (*arrows*).

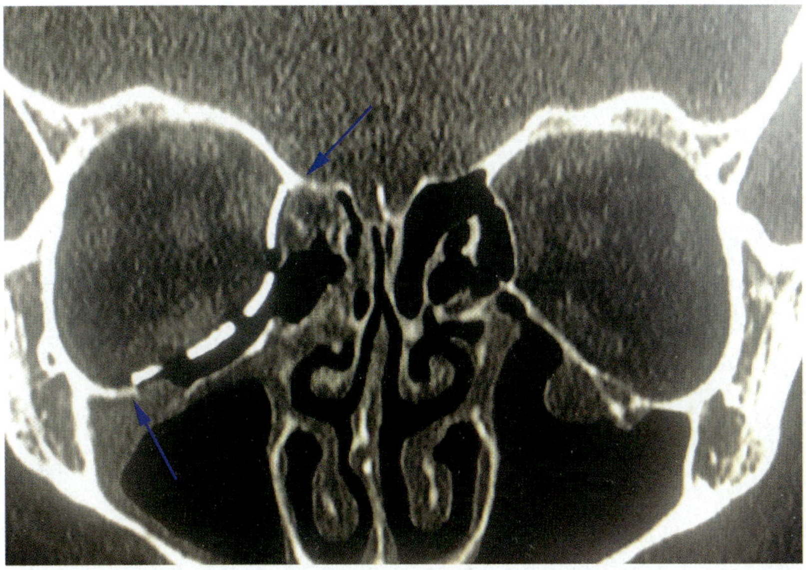

Fig. 34 The coronal CT scan demonstrating accurate reconstruction (*arrows*).

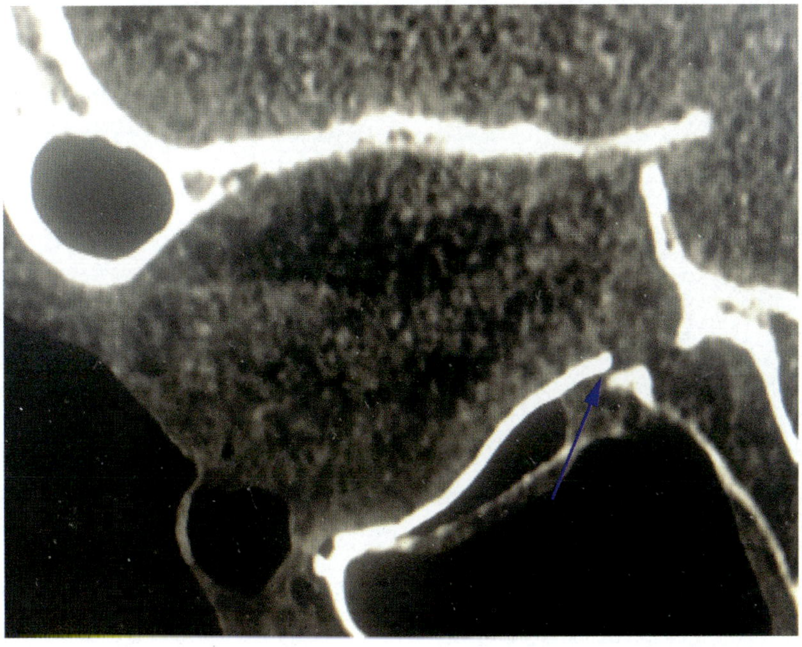

Fig. 35 The sagittal CT scan shows adequate reconstruction of the posterior third (*arrow*) in addition the restoration of the S-shaped contour.

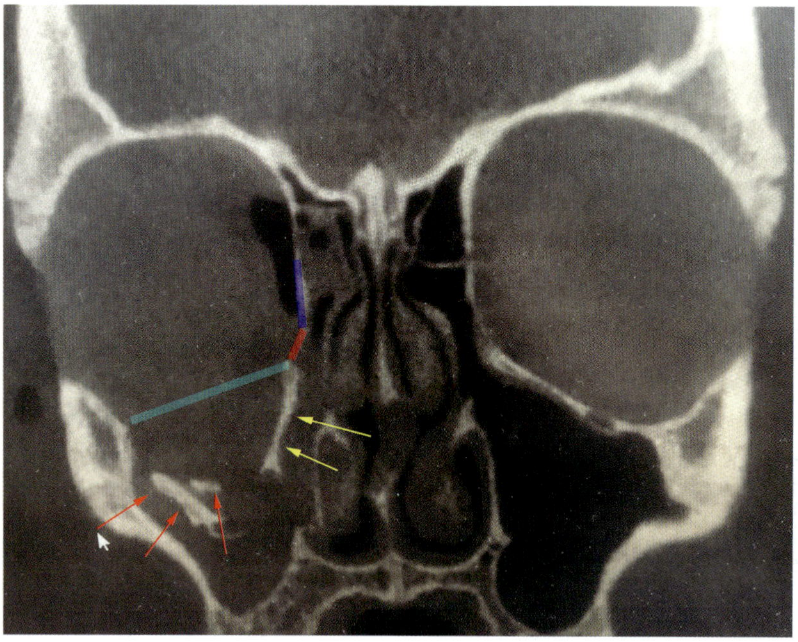

Fig. 36 In this coronal CT scan of an impure blowout fracture, the orbital floor and walls are demonstrated: floor in green, medial wall in blue, and the junctional zone in red. The cantilevered floor is denoted with yellow arrows and the anterior maxillary wall fractures are denoted with red arrows.

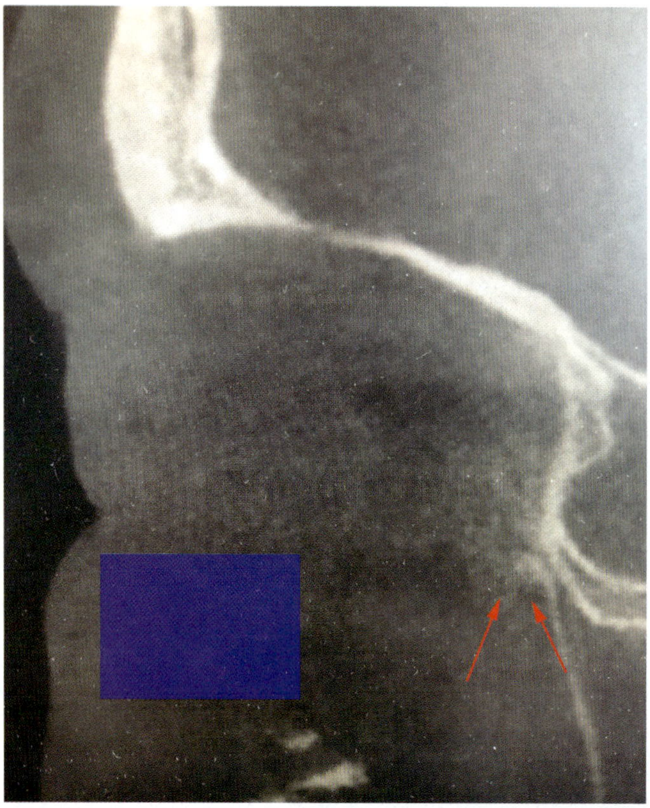

Fig. 37 The sagittal CT scan demonstrates a complete absence of the anterior orbital margin (*blue zone*) but an intact posterior ledge (*arrows*). This ledge is key to the reconstruction.

the intermediate zone (yellow zone) and the lateral extension (red zone and arrows) (Fig. 40).

The sigmoid-shaped blue zone is also reproduced (Fig. 41).

The 3D view in Fig. 42 shows faithful reconstruction of the orbital margin .

Soft tissue closure

Closure of the lateral canthus is normally problem free provided that some simple rules are observed. The lower eyelid is sutured with a 5/0 suture capturing the lateral aspect and is then sutured to the lateral canthus on the medial free edge (blue arrows) (Fig. 43), allowing for approximation of the lid to the globe when tightened.

The gray lines of the eyelids are then approximated using a 6/0 suture, which is tied first. The tension suture is then tied, and any skin incision is closed with the 6/0 suture (Fig. 44).

Fig. 45 provides a postoperative view following lateral canthal repair.

The long suture

Occasionally, particularly in extended dissections, the surgeon may have concerns about postoperative bleeding. There is an option to not tie the suture of the canthus until the following day (Fig. 46).

Postoperative recovery

The patient is nursed head up and given icepacks in the recovery ward to self-apply. The patient is forbidden to blow their nose for 3 weeks.

Eye observations, including

- Pain score
- Visual acuity
- Pupil size and reactivity

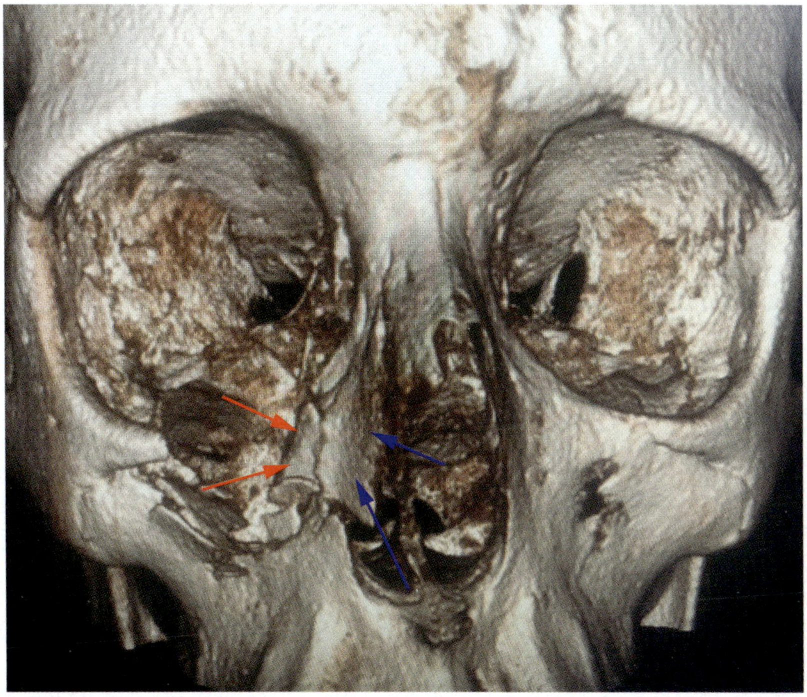

Fig. 38 The nasomaxillary component with the piriform rim (*blue arrows*) and the rim (*red arrows*).

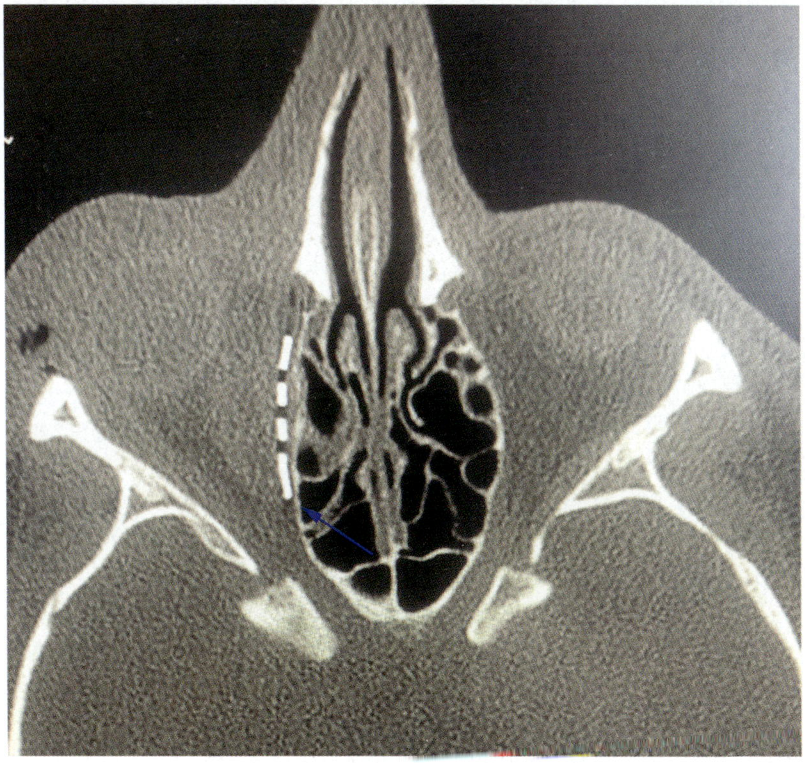

Fig. 39 The axial CT scan shows a strong reconstruction (*arrow*).

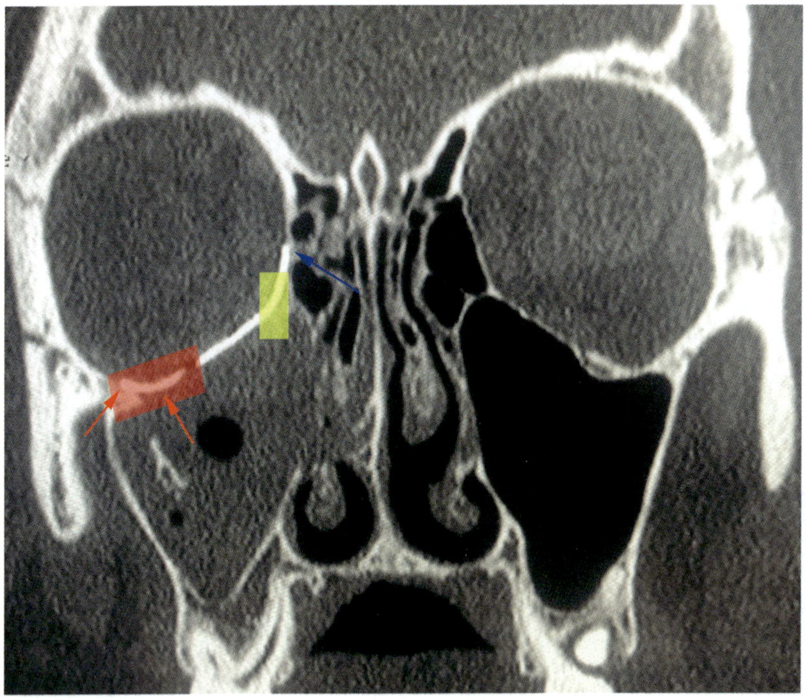

Fig. 40 The postoperative coronal CT scan illustrating key reconstructed zones, for which a custom plate is more predictable. The lateral extent of the fracture (*red zone and arrows*) is often deficient in off-the-shelf plates. The medial articulation is accurate (*blue arrows*), and the curve on the plate around the junctional zone (*yellow zone*) is restored perfectly.

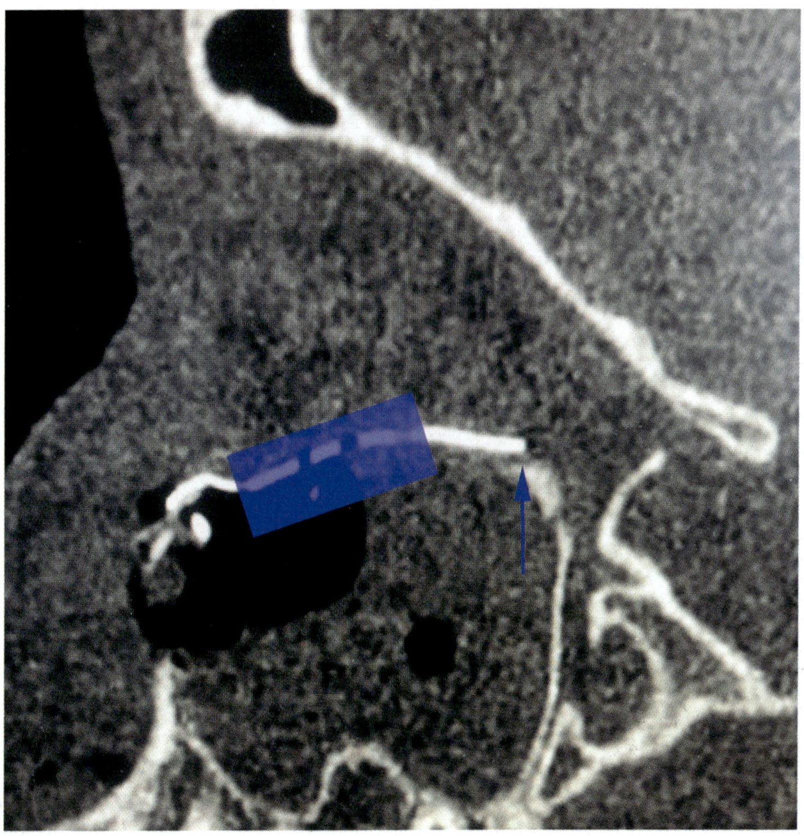

Fig. 41 The sagittal CT scan shows the replication of the S-shaped curvature (*blue zone*) and the posterior margin (*arrow*).

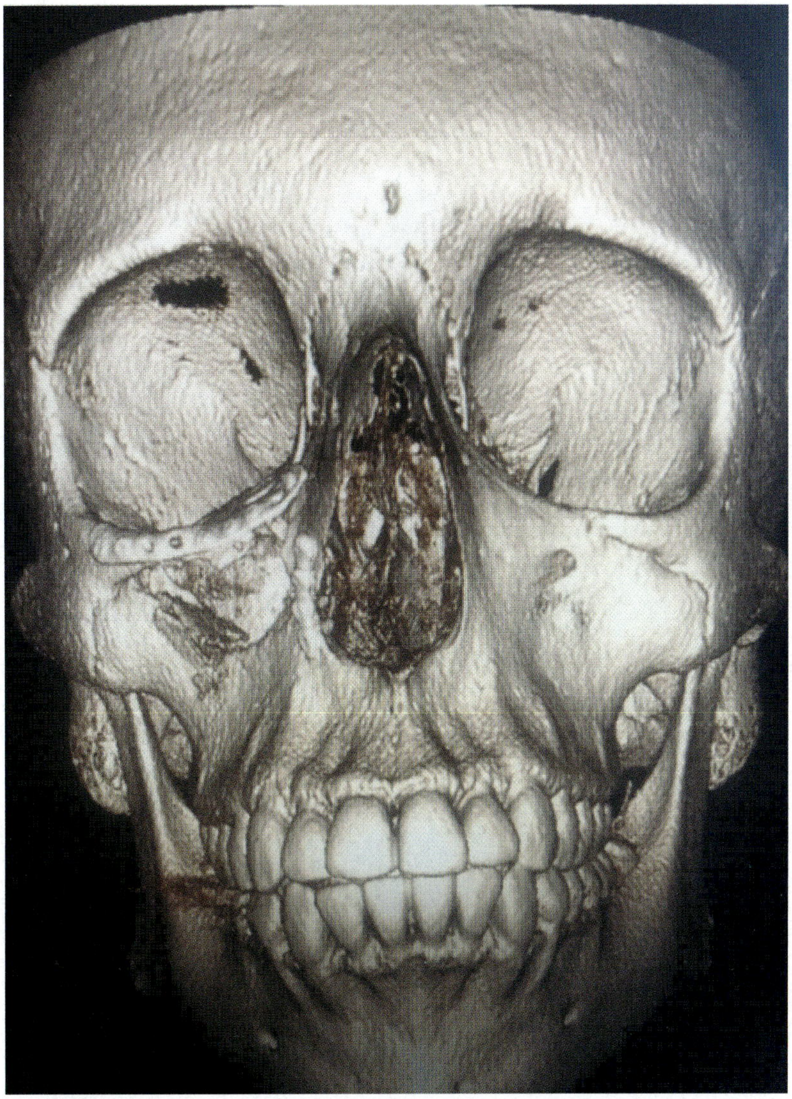

Fig. 42 The 3D reconstruction with accurate piriform aperture and infraorbital reconstruction.

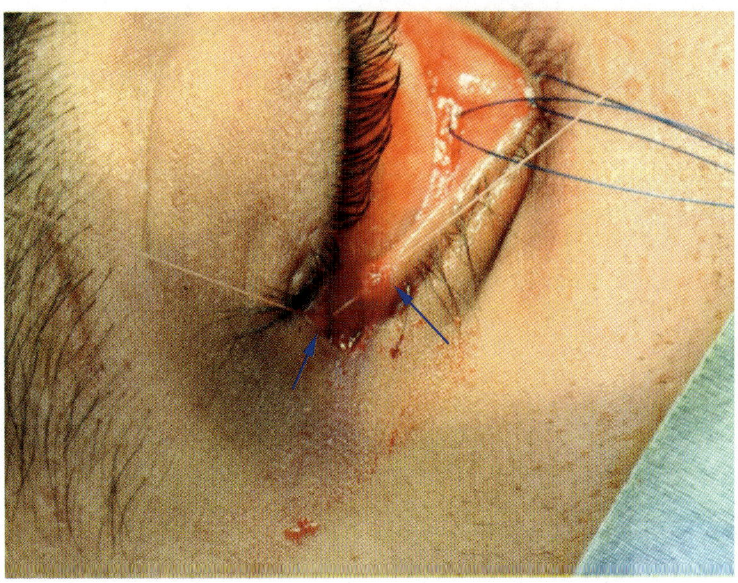

Fig. 43 The canthal tendon should be considered as a tube and a 5/0 Vicryl suture on the outer quadrant of the lid, to the inner quadrant of the lateral canthus (*blue arrows*).

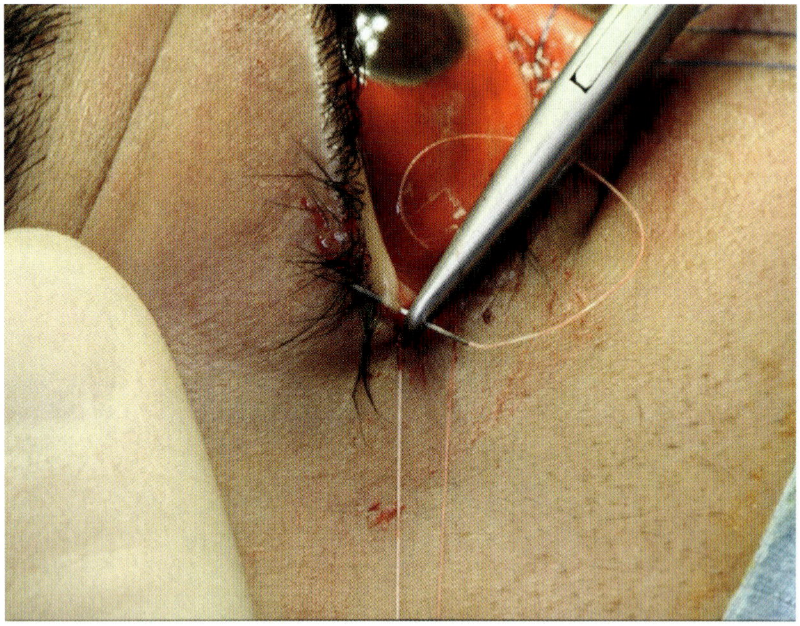

Fig. 44 It is important to approximate the lash line/gray lines well. This is with 6/0 Vicryl.

Are performed every 15 minutes for 2 hours and thereafter every 30 minutes for 2 hours.

Postoperative imaging

Although it is appreciated that there is a movement to reduce the exposure to radiation, when large titanium orbital plates are placed, then postoperative imaging is essential.

The postoperative view of a secondary referral clearly demonstrates poor positioning; the referring surgeon did not take a postoperative view as "the plate seated well"(Fig. 47).

Results

The author's operative clinical practice is presented in Fig. 48 over a 5-year period.

Although orbital access is required for maxillary and cranioorbital surgery, for the purposes of this article, these were excluded. The breakdown into pure and impure fractures is detailed in Fig. 49.

Most impure fractures included zygomatic patterns, nasomaxillary, or those complicated by segmentation of the orbital margin (Fig. 50).

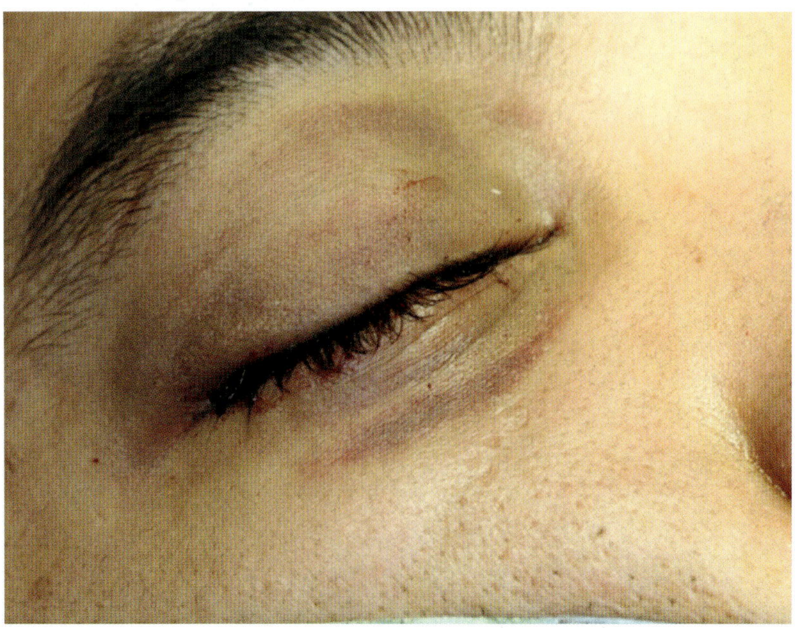

Fig. 45 The finished closure.

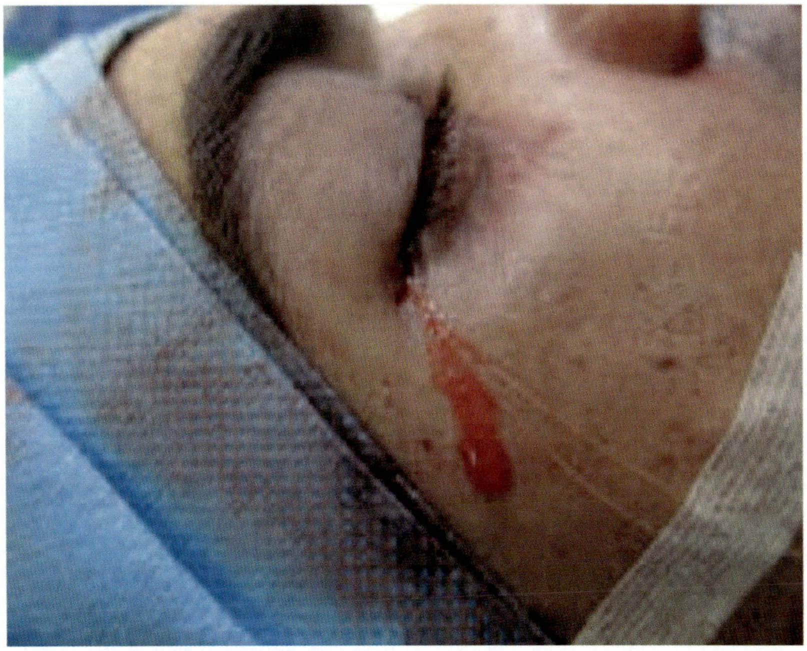

Fig. 46 On occasion in the vulnerable orbit, either technically demanding, difficult to hemostase, or if the patient has a coagulopathy, the suture can be left long and tied on the ward the next day.

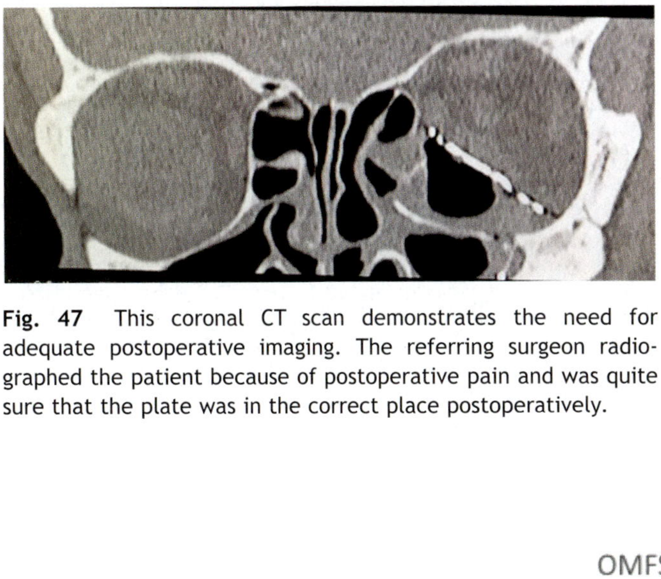

Fig. 47 This coronal CT scan demonstrates the need for adequate postoperative imaging. The referring surgeon radiographed the patient because of postoperative pain and was quite sure that the plate was in the correct place postoperatively.

Outcomes

Using the methodology described in the text in the 5 years, there were a total of 329 pure orbital fractures and 289 impure orbits operated on. Complication rates were low; with no loss of sight, 13 cases returned to theater for plate repositioning, and 3 patients requiring lateral canthal revision.

The author examined a consecutive series of prefabricated plate reconstructions (in preparation) and found that, out of a case series of 79 patients, with 45% involving the medial wall and a mean Jaquiery score of 3.2, with satisfactory plate position in 86%, only 3 cases returned to theater, all of these because the preformed plate was not large enough. No patients required secondary strabismus surgery.

This study has led to the modification of the protocol to lower the threshold for custom plate, leading to greatly increased surgical accuracy approaching 95% in the next 25 cases despite higher Jaquiery scores (in press).

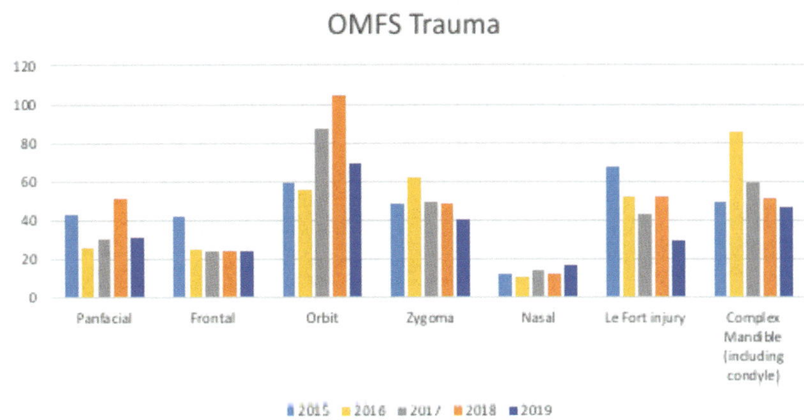

Fig. 48 The author's operative clinical practice is presented here over a 5-year period. OMFS, oral and maxillofacial surgery.

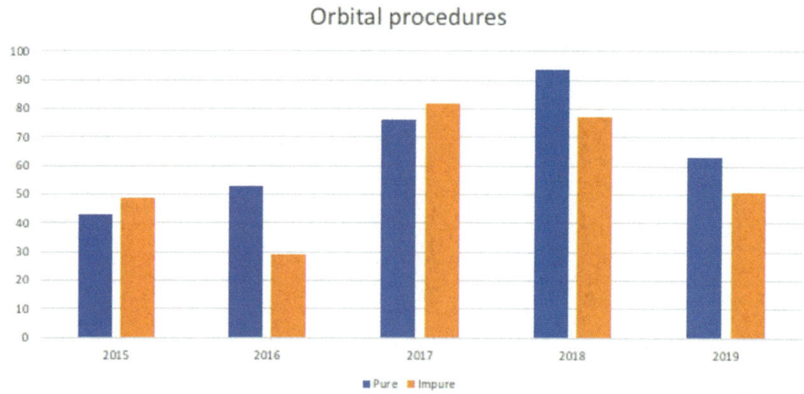

Fig. 49 The numbers of operated pure and impure blowout fractures.

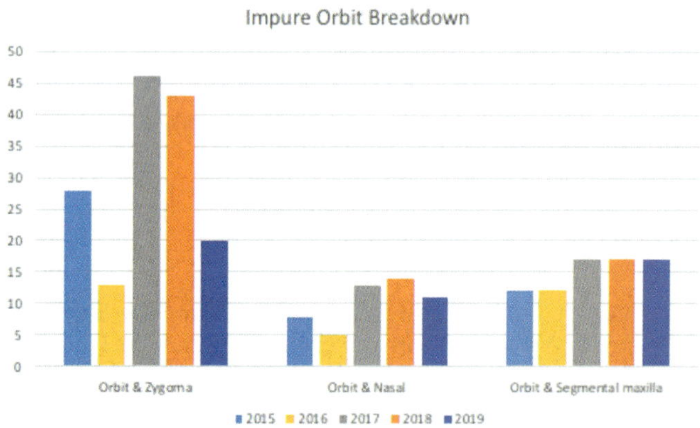

Fig. 50 Classification of impure blowout fractures.

Summary

Orbital surgery can be performed in a predictable manner provided that an ordered diagnostic and surgical protocol can be followed.

A posterior lamellar approach in a preseptal plane with a logical selection of reconstructive material is recommended.

The use of a custom-made prosthesis greatly improves surgical accuracy and facilitates reconstruction in high-medial-wall and apical third fracture patterns without the absolute need for surgical navigation.

Disclosure

The author has nothing to disclose.

Further readings

Ahmad Z, Nouraei R, Holmes S. Towards a classification system for complex craniofacial fractures. Br J Oral Maxillofac Surg 2012;50: 490–4.

Ahmed FKN, Lyne J, Waterhouse N. Buckling and hydraulic mechanisms in orbital blowout fractures: fact or fiction? J Craniofac Surg 2006; 17:438–41.

Al-Sukhun J, Lindqvist C, Kontio R. Modelling of orbital deformation using finite-element analysis. J R Soc Interface 2006;3:255–62.

Boffano P, Kommers SC, Karagozoglu KH, et al. Aetiology of maxillofacial fractures: a review of published studies during the last 30 years. Br J Oral Maxillofac Surg 2014;52:901–6.

Boffano P, Roccia F, Zavattero E, et al. European Maxillofacial Trauma (EURMAT) project: a multicentre and prospective study. J Craniomaxillofac Surg 2015;43:62–70.

Catherine Z, Courvoisier DS, Scolozzi P. Is the pure and impure distinction of orbital fractures clinically relevant with respect to ocular and periocular injuries? A retrospective study of 473 patients. J Craniomaxillofac Surg 2019;47:1935–42.

DavenporT RA, Tai N, West A, et al. A major trauma centre is a specialty hospital not a hospital of specialties. Br J Surg 2010;97: 109–17.

De riu G, Meloni SM, Gobbi R, et al. Subciliary versus swinging eyelid approach to the orbital floor. J Craniomaxillofac Surg 2008;36: 439–42.

Dubois L, Jansen J, Schreurs R, et al. Predictability in orbital reconstruction: a human cadaver study. Part I: endoscopic-assisted orbital reconstruction. J Craniomaxillofac Surg 2015;43:2034–41.

Dubois L, Schreurs R, Jansen J, et al. Predictability in orbital reconstruction: a human cadaver study. Part II: navigation-assisted orbital reconstruction. J Craniomaxillofac Surg 2015;43:2042–9.

Dubois L, Steenen SA, Gooris PJ, et al. Controversies in orbital reconstruction-III. Biomaterials for orbital reconstruction: a review with clinical recommendations. Int J Oral Maxillofac Surg 2016;45:41–50.

Evans BT, Webb AA. Post-traumatic orbital reconstruction: anatomical landmarks and the concept of the deep orbit. Br J Oral Maxillofac Surg 2007;45:183–9.

Gavin clavero MA, Simon sanz MV, TIL AM, et al. Factors influencing postsurgical diplopia in orbital floor fractures and prevalence of other complications in a series of cases. J Oral Maxillofac Surg 2018; 76:1725–33.

Gerber B, Kiwanuka P, Dhariwal D. Orbital fractures in children: a review of outcomes. Br J Oral Maxillofac Surg 2013;51:789–93.

Gooris PJJ, Muller BS, Dubois L, et al. Finding the ledge: sagittal analysis of bony landmarks of the orbit. J Oral Maxillofac Surg 2017; 75:2613–27.

He Y, Zhang Y, An JG. Correlation of types of orbital fracture and occurrence of enophthalmos. J Craniofac Surg 2012;23:1050–3.

Jaquiery C, Aeppli C, Cornelius P, et al. Reconstruction of orbital wall defects: critical review of 72 patients. Int J Oral Maxillofac Surg 2007;36:193–9.

Metzger MC, Schon R, Tetzlaf R, et al. Topographical CT-data analysis of the human orbital floor. Int J Oral Maxillofac Surg 2007;36:45–53.

Mustafa SF, Evans PL, Bocca A, et al. Customized titanium reconstruction of post-traumatic orbital wall defects: a review of 22 cases. Int J Oral Maxillofac Surg 2011;40:1357–62.

Raschke GF, Rieger UM, Bader RD, et al. Transconjunctival versus subciliary approach for orbital fracture repair-an anthropometric evaluation of 221 cases. Clin Oral Investig 2013;17:933–42.

Salentijn EG, Van den bergH B, Forouzanfar T. A ten-year analysis of midfacial fractures. J Craniomaxillofac Surg 2013;41:630–6.

Schaller A, Huempfner-hierl H, Hemprich A, et al. Biomechanical mechanisms of orbital wall fractures - a transient finite element analysis. J Craniomaxillofac Surg 2013;41:710–7.

Scolozzi P, Momjian A, Heuberger J, et al. Accuracy and predictability in use of AO three-dimensionally preformed titanium mesh plates for posttraumatic orbital reconstruction: a pilot study. J Craniofac Surg 2009;20:1108–13.

Young SM, Koh YT, Chan EW, et al. Incidence and risk factors of inferior rectus muscle palsy in pediatric orbital blowout fractures. Craniomaxillofac Trauma Reconstr 2018;11:28–34.

Advanced Diagnostics and Three-dimensional Virtual Surgical Planning in Orbital Reconstruction

Ruud Schreurs, MSc [a,b,c,*], Cornelis Klop, MSc [a,b], Thomas J.J. Maal, MSc, PhD [a,b,c]

KEYWORDS

• Computer-assisted surgery • Orbit • Orbital trauma • Orbital reconstruction • Virtual surgical planning

KEY POINTS

- The first step in advanced diagnostics and virtual surgical planning is the generation of a virtual patient model.
- Information can be added to the virtual patient model through image manipulation for advanced diagnostic purposes.
- The virtual surgical planning is used preoperatively, but can also be used intraoperatively and postoperatively.

Introduction

The principles and limitations of orbital reconstruction have triggered technological developments in the past 2 decades. Because of the complex anatomy of the orbit and limited exposure during surgery, computer-assisted surgery (CAS) is of great added value.[1–5] Several studies have shown that CAS assists the surgeon in achieving a better and more predictable treatment outcome.[1,3,6–8] CAS consists of several preoperative, intraoperative, and postoperative components. Advanced diagnostics and three-dimensional (3D) virtual surgical planning (VSP) ensure a better inspection of the problem and the possible solutions during the preoperative phase.[9,10] This article explains the preprocessing steps required to start VSP, the benefits of advances in diagnostics, and the tools used in VSP.

Imaging and preparation

Several modalities may be encountered in imaging of the orbit and orbital contents: MRI, ultrasonography, and two-dimensional (2D) or 3D radiologic imaging (eg, radiographs or computed tomography [CT]).[11–13] MRI is seldom used as the primary imaging modality after trauma: soft tissue structures can be excellently distinguished, but sensitivity for hard-tissue trauma is low.[11–13] MRI is contraindicated if metallic foreign bodies may be present. Ultrasonography may provide fast evaluation of the globe, but should not be used if a rupture of the globe is suspected because of the pressure exerted on the globe during image acquisition. This pressure may lead to further acute decompensation of the eye and/or intraocular content extravasation.[11–13]

CT is the modality of choice in orbital traumatology.[14–16] CT has higher sensitivity for fracture detection than plain radiography and offers the additional possibility of internal hemorrhage detection. The problem of superimposition on 2D radiographic imaging and missing information of one of the dimensions is overcome by the 3D nature of the data that are produced with CT: the imaging volume is reconstructed and built up in voxels (3D pixels), each with a gray-scale value (Hounsfield unit [HU]) corresponding with the x-ray absorption within the voxel. From the image data, several planes can be reconstructed: a typical multiplanar view is made up by axial, coronal, and sagittal slices. In order to be able to distinguish existing bony ledges of the thin orbital floor and walls in the advanced diagnostics and virtual planning phase, it is recommended to use a maximum slice thickness of 1 to 1.5 mm.[17–19]

An important preparation step in CAS in orbital reconstruction is to create a virtual 3D model of the bony structures and soft tissue of the patient from the basic CT slices. Typically, volume rendering is used to create a fast 3D overview. The original anatomy and fractured orbit can be easily visualized. For planning purposes, a volume render is not sufficient because it cannot be manipulated; a surface model needs to be created for this. Surface rendering is a technique that generates this virtual surface model: voxels belonging to the same anatomical structure can be selected in the image volume (segmentation) and a 3D virtual object is generated based on the selection made. Surface models can be modified and manipulated and are therefore required for VSP. Typical surface models used in the preparation step include at least a surface model of the bony structures (Fig. 1) and the soft tissue exterior.

The generated surface models provide the same fast 3D overview as the volume renders and accurately represent the patient's orbital anatomy and disorder. If required, CT images from different time points or 3D images from different imaging

[a] Department of Oral and Maxillofacial Surgery, Amsterdam University Medical Centres (location AMC), Meibergdreef 9, Amsterdam, AZ 1105, The Netherlands
[b] Academic Center for Dentistry Amsterdam (ACTA), University of Amsterdam, Gustav Mahlerlaan 3004, 1081 LA, Amsterdam, The Netherlands
[c] Department of Oral and Maxillofacial Surgery, Radboud University Medical Centre Nijmegen, Nijmegen, The Netherlands
* Corresponding author.
E-mail address: r.schreurs@amsterdamumc.nl

Atlas Oral Maxillofacial Surg Clin N Am 29 (2021) 79–96

https://doi.org/10.1016/j.cxom.2020.11.003

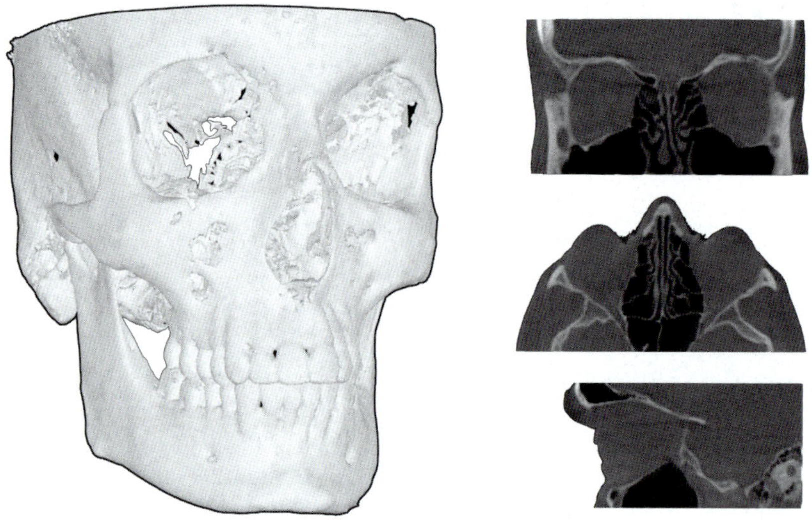

Fig. 1 Multiplanar views of a cone-beam CT scan and the generated hard-tissue surface model. (*Courtesy of* Ruud Schreurs, MSc, Cornelis Klop, MSc, and Thomas J. J. Maal, MSc, PhD.)

modalities (eg, MRI, intraoral scans, cone-beam CT, 3D stereophotogrammetry) can be combined with the CT data using (multimodality) image registration techniques.[20,21] In this way, a CT base image can be augmented with additional 3D data to create a complete and detailed virtual representation of the patient: the virtual patient model (Fig. 2). The integration of accurate dental information from an intraoral scan might, for example, be useful to create a dental splint for navigation guidance during surgery. After the creation of the virtual patient model, advanced diagnostics and VSP can be performed.

Advanced diagnostics

In a dedicated software environment, further manipulation and analysis of the patient model can be performed. Advanced diagnostics is the expansion of the information that is readily available in the image data. This additional information can be obtained through image manipulation. Segmentation, mentioned earlier in relation to the generation of a surface model, is such a technique: voxels belonging to the same tissue type or anatomical structure are annotated within the image volume. This process may be done manually (coloring of the image set) or through thresholding, in which voxels greater than a certain gray-scale value (HU) are selected. This thresholding is, for instance, used in differentiating the bony structures from the soft tissues before a surface model of these bony structures is generated.

The paper-thin orbital floor and medial wall hamper the accuracy of threshold segmentation: more elaborate segmentation algorithms may be used to acquire an accurate

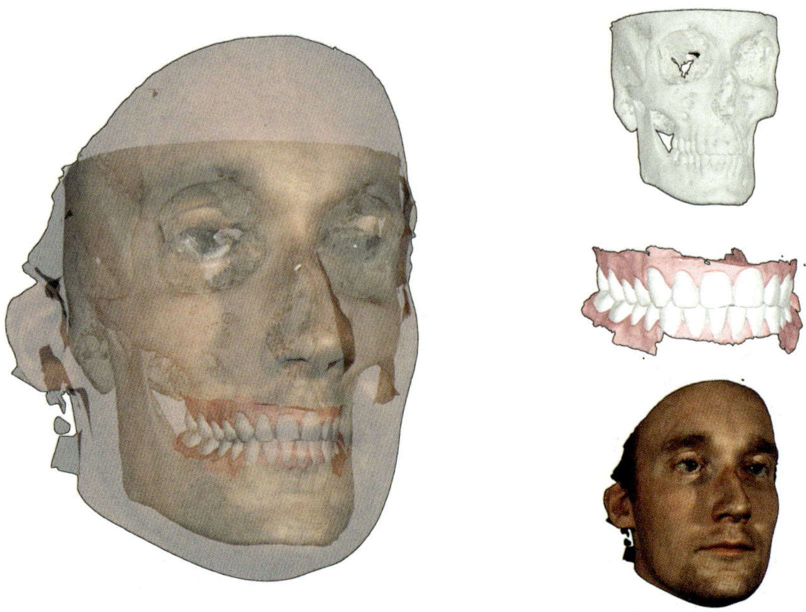

Fig. 2 Combining different imaging modalities to generate an extended virtual patient model. In this example, a cone-beam CT scan, intraoral scan and 3D stereophotograph are registered. (*Courtesy of* Ruud Schreurs, MSc, Cornelis Klop, MSc, and Thomas J. J. Maal, MSc, PhD.)

segmentation of the orbit and its contents (Fig. 3). One example of this is atlas-based segmentation, in which an atlas consisting of a patient model with presegmented anatomical structures is registered to the current patient scan (Fig. 4).[6,15,18] Atlas-based segmentation can provide reliable segmentation, even when CT image quality is suboptimal. Small manual adjustments might be needed to optimize the segmentation result (Fig. 5), especially in the case of deviating anatomy or disorder.[2,18] Because accurate segmentation of the orbit is a prerequisite for many advanced diagnostic and virtual planning processes, much research has been performed on improvement of accuracy or user-friendliness of segmentation techniques for orbital anatomy.[15,22–24]

A virtual 3D model of the segmented structures can be reconstructed similar to the process which is used to generate a hard-tissue patient model from the bony tissue segmentation. Of particular interest are the bilateral orbits, orbital contents, and, for an orbitozygomatic complex fracture, the zygomatic complex. The 3D shape of an object may be analyzed, and the volume of the object can be measured within the software. This method enables comparison of the orbital content between affected and unaffected orbits and thus quantification of the enlargement of the affected orbit. The segmented structures can subsequently be manipulated in the virtual environment in the ongoing process of adding diagnostic information to the virtual patient model. In unilateral orbital fractures, mirroring provides exact insight into the displacement of the affected orbital walls (Fig. 6).[3,5–7] In orbitozygomatic fractures (Fig. 7), segmented anatomical structures, obtained through different segmentation workflows, may be combined to obtain a complete template of the unaffected side before mirroring (Fig. 8). This way, the displacement of the orbital floor, zygomatic arch, and prominence (relative to the unaffected contralateral side) can be seen from 1 mirrored object (Fig. 9).[6,18,25,26]

Virtual surgical planning

The indication for surgery is established on clinical findings, possibly supported by findings in the advanced diagnostics process. The goal of VSP is to reconstruct the pretraumatized anatomy as closely as possible.[27–29] The VSP continues on information acquired from the advanced diagnostics process. This information in itself may comprise the surgical planning: the mirroring of the zygomatic complex provides a reconstruction of the premorbid anatomy of the affected structure. The mirrored orbit provides an adequate reconstruction for the affected orbit as well, but reduction of the dislocated bony parts is infeasible: alloplastic materials are frequently necessary to reconstruct the orbital floor and/or medial wall. The surgical planning is therefore more elaborate than mirroring alone: the optimal position of the reconstruction material (eg, a preformed titanium orbital implant) is also planned.

If a preformed titanium orbital implant is used, a virtual stereolithographic model (STL) of the implant is imported in the planning environment. The position of the implant can be manipulated in the virtual patient to find an optimal position for the implant in the current patient (Figs. 10 and 11).[6,30,31] Several parameters are taken into account in the positioning process: covering of the defect, support on the dorsal ledge, fixation possibility on the orbital rim, prevention of interference with existing bony structures, reconstructing the contour as closely as possible to the mirrored orbit, and bony support at the medial tip of the implant (Fig. 12). The virtual patient offers the possibility to perform virtual surgery and evaluate the outcome within the patient model. Multiple possible implant positions for the imported implant can be evaluated before coming to a decision on the desired position. If necessary, additional implants, with different sizes or from other manufacturers, may be imported to compare their fit and find the implant with the optimal size and shape for the individual reconstruction (Fig. 13).[6,10,28]

A suboptimal virtual implant fit of a preformed implant and clinical indication (and/or the surgeon's preference) may lead to the decision to perform the reconstruction with a premolded or patient-specific implant (PSI) (Fig. 14; see Fig. 18). The basis for the design of the implant is, again, the extended virtual patient model with all information that has been added in the advanced diagnostics and preliminary planning phase (Fig. 15; see Fig. 19). Information can be extracted from the virtual patient model for additive manufacturing (eg, 3D printing)

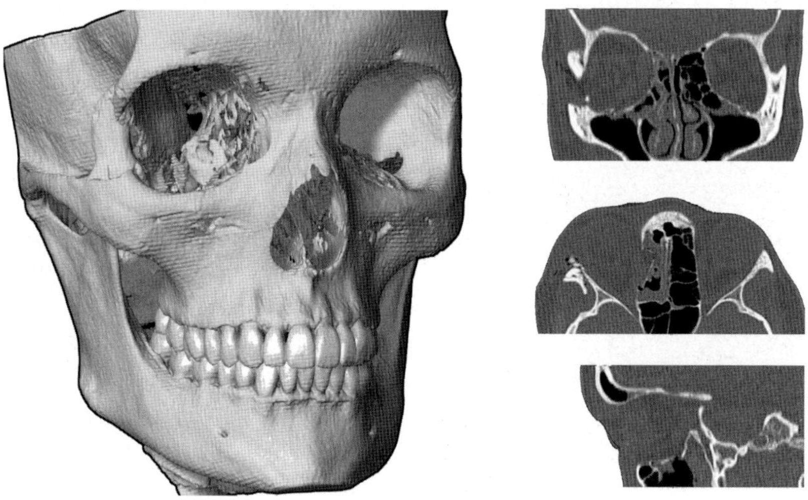

Fig. 3 Hard-tissue model and multiplanar views of patient 1. The 3D surface model is acquired from a threshold segmentation process. The orbital contents are not segmented accurately enough for further analysis. (*Courtesy of* Ruud Schreurs, MSc, Cornelis Klop, MSc, and Thomas J. J. Maal, MSc, PhD.)

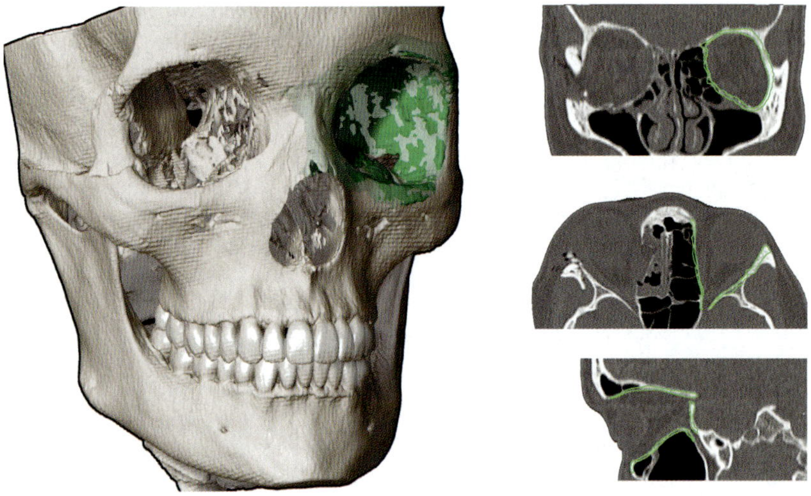

Fig. 4 Atlas-based segmentation of the unaffected contralateral orbit (patient 1). The atlas-based segmentation was performed in Brainlab iPlan Cranial (Brainlab AG, Munich, Germany). (*Courtesy of* Ruud Schreurs, MSc, Cornelis Klop, MSc, and Thomas J. J. Maal, MSc, PhD.)

(Figs. 16 and 17).[3,30,32–34] In the case of premolding an implant, a template of the mirrored, unaffected orbit may be printed to mold an implant before, or during, surgery. Additional information may be embedded in the 3D print, or in separate 3D prints; for instance, the defect itself or desired boundaries of the implant. Generation of a PSI is also based on exported virtual models from the patient model. In this case, the process of generating the implant's shape is virtual rather than physical: the exported information serves as a digital template for the virtual design of the PSI. The exported models may be manipulated beforehand; for instance, to create an overcorrection of the orbital volume in a designated area (see Fig. 20).[5] An STL of the PSI, or a preliminary design, can be imported in the software to check that it meets all parameters on implant shape and positioning, and to see whether the design will provide a unique fit to the designated position (see Fig. 21). Possible screw-hole positions for implant fixation can be evaluated in the virtual planning environment as well. In a secondary reconstruction, the position of existing osteosynthesis fixation can be indicated in the virtual patient model

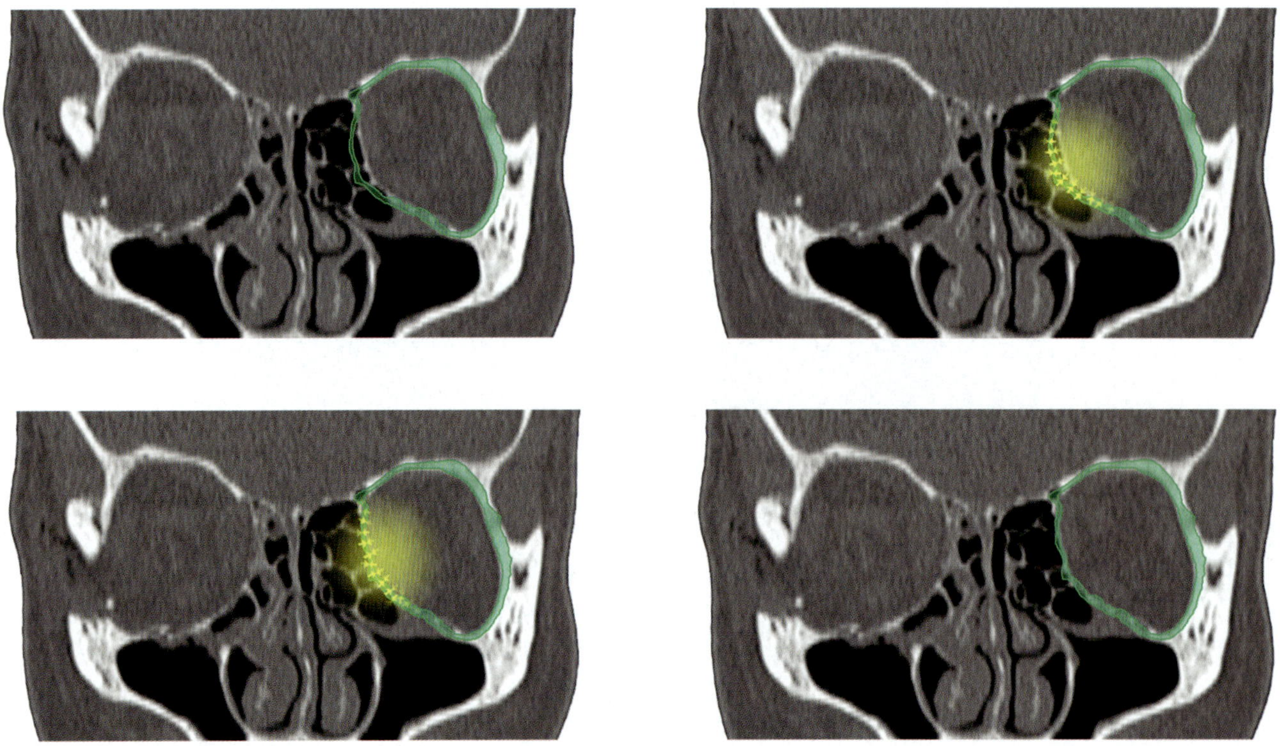

Fig. 5 Small manual adjustments of the resulting atlas-based segmentation. These small adjustments might be necessary in a small number of cases, especially if the anatomy differs greatly from the anatomy in the template. (*Courtesy of* Ruud Schreurs, MSc, Cornelis Klop, MSc, and Thomas J. J. Maal, MSc, PhD.)

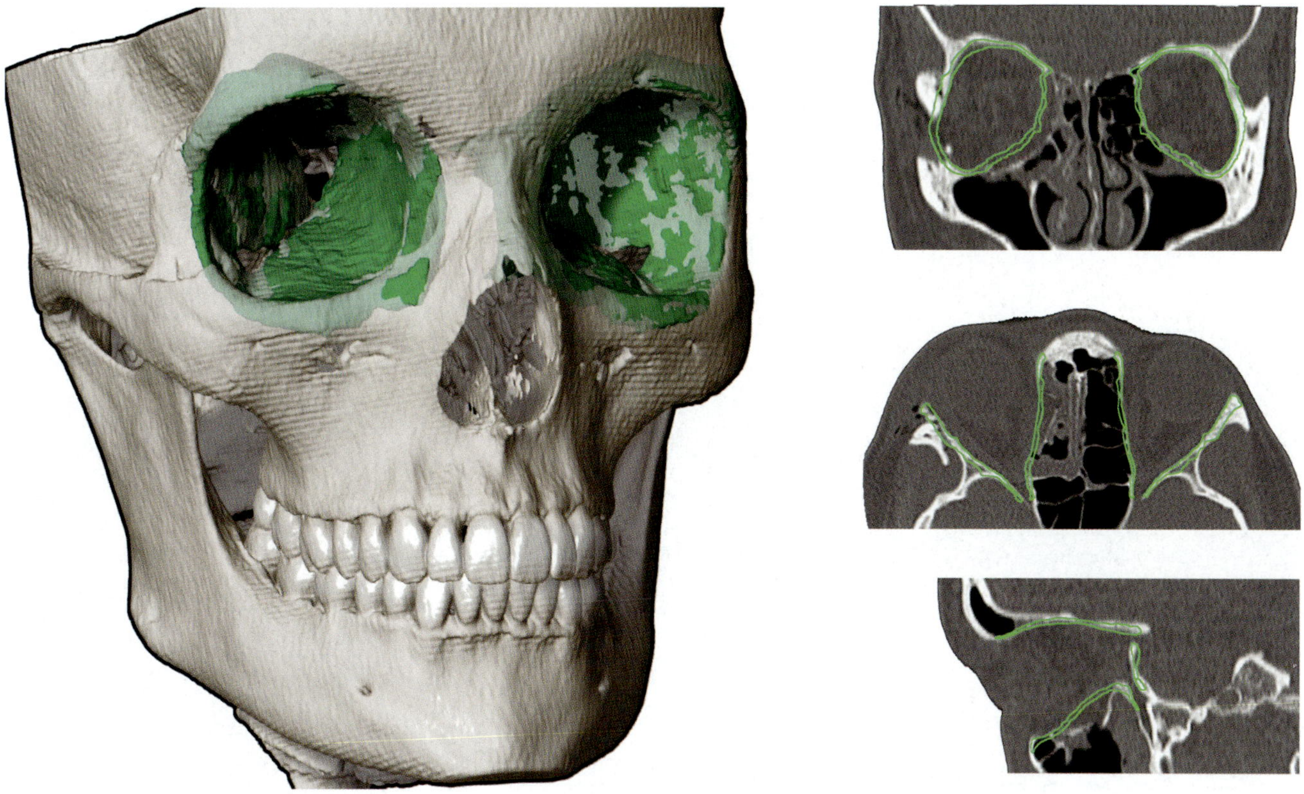

Fig. 6 Mirroring of the unaffected orbit, to obtain additional diagnostic information about the affected orbit (patient 1). (*Courtesy of* Ruud Schreurs, MSc, Cornelis Klop, MSc, and Thomas J. J. Maal, MSc, PhD.)

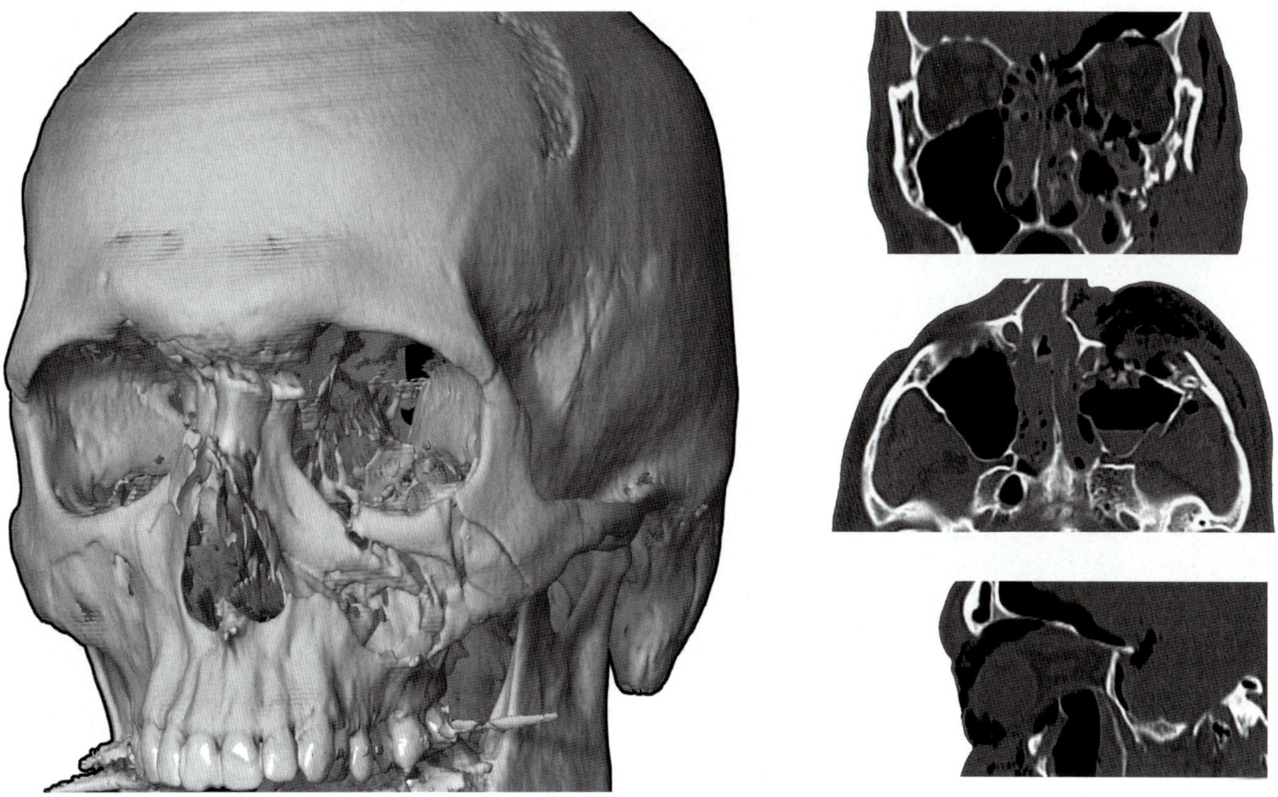

Fig. 7 Hard-tissue model and multiplanar views of patient 2. A naso-orbitoethmoid type I fracture and comminuted orbitozygomatic complex fracture can be seen. (*Courtesy of* Ruud Schreurs, MSc, Cornelis Klop, MSc, and Thomas J. J. Maal, MSc, PhD.)

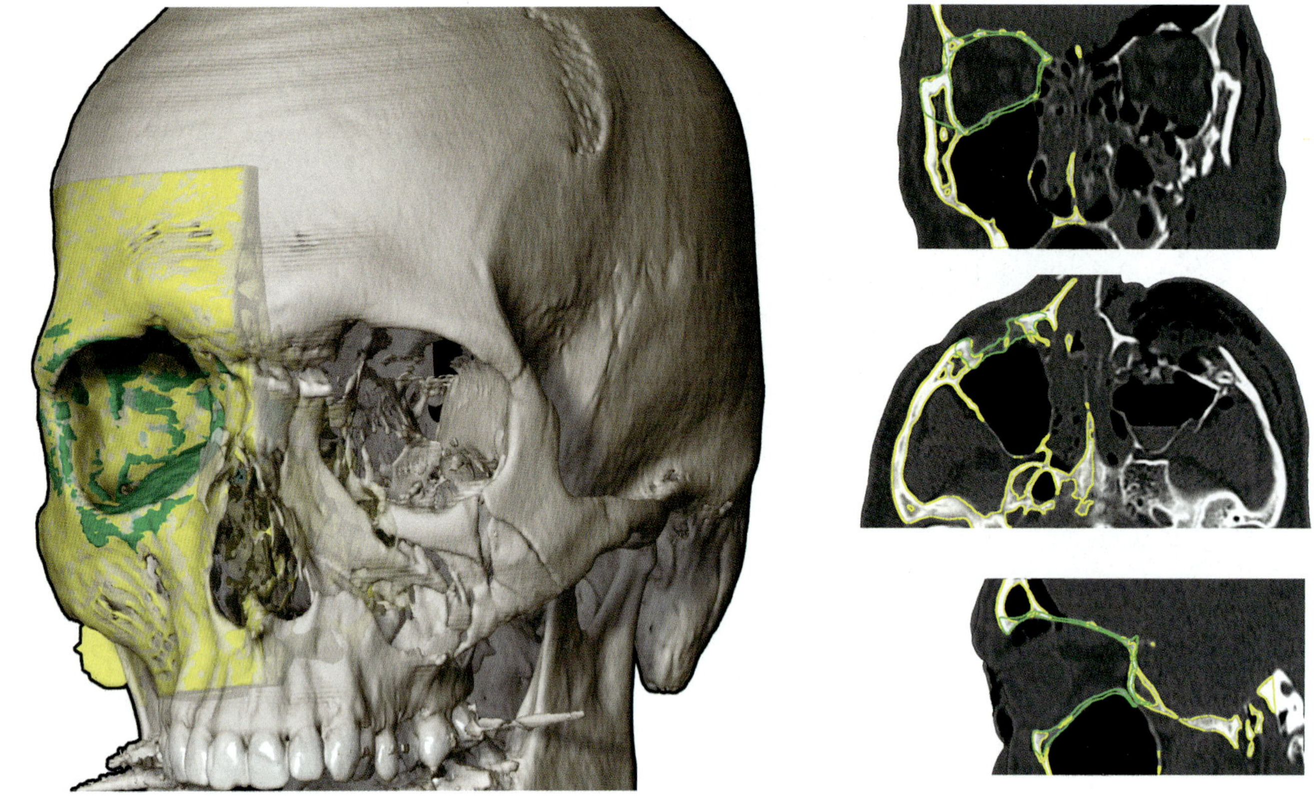

Fig. 8 Threshold segmentation of bone (*yellow*) and atlas-based segmentation of orbit (*green*), to be combined into 1 template (patient 2). (*Courtesy of* Ruud Schreurs, MSc, Cornelis Klop, MSc, and Thomas J. J. Maal, MSc, PhD.)

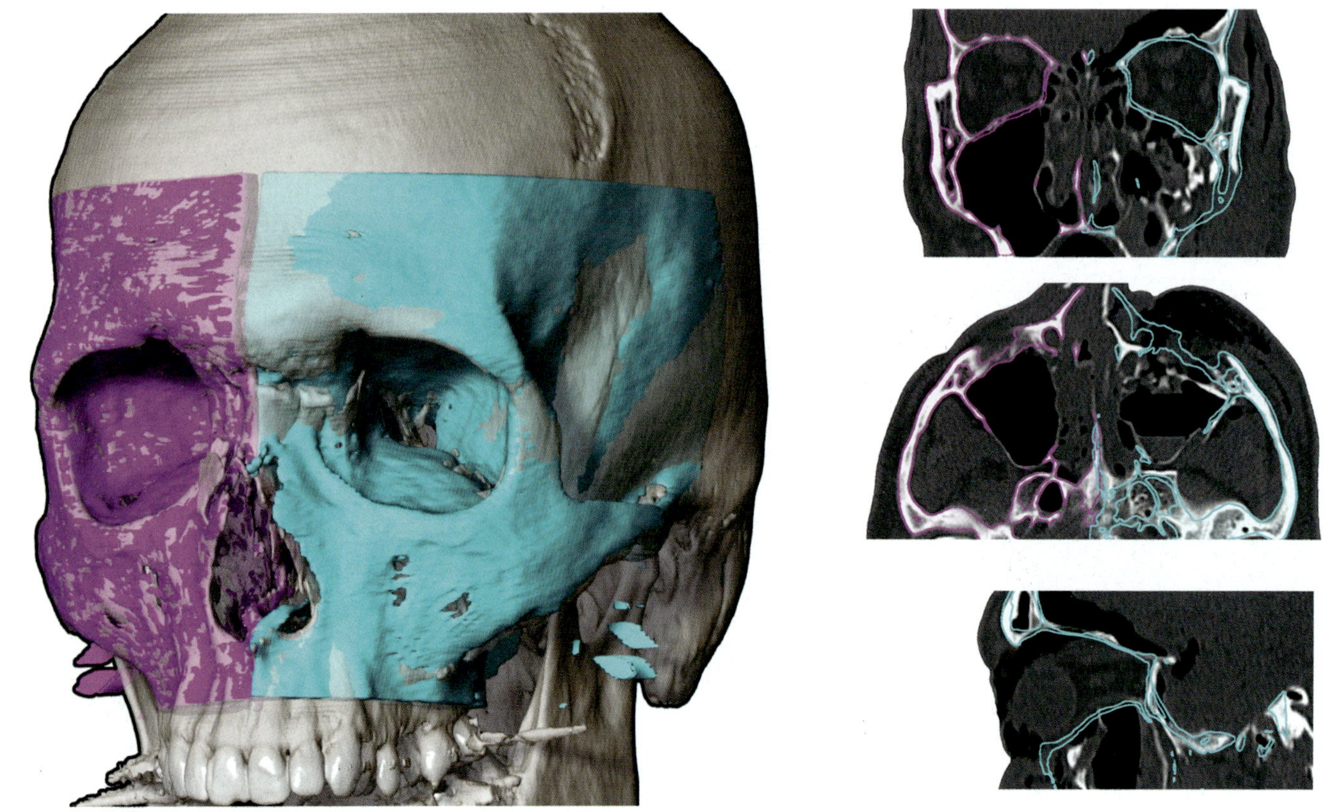

Fig. 9 Template consisting of segmentations from Fig. 8 are combined in the purple template, and mirrored to the contralateral side (*cyan*) to obtain information about the zygomatic displacement and the orbital fracture (patient 2). (*Courtesy of* Ruud Schreurs, MSc, Cornelis Klop, MSc, and Thomas J. J. Maal, MSc, PhD.)

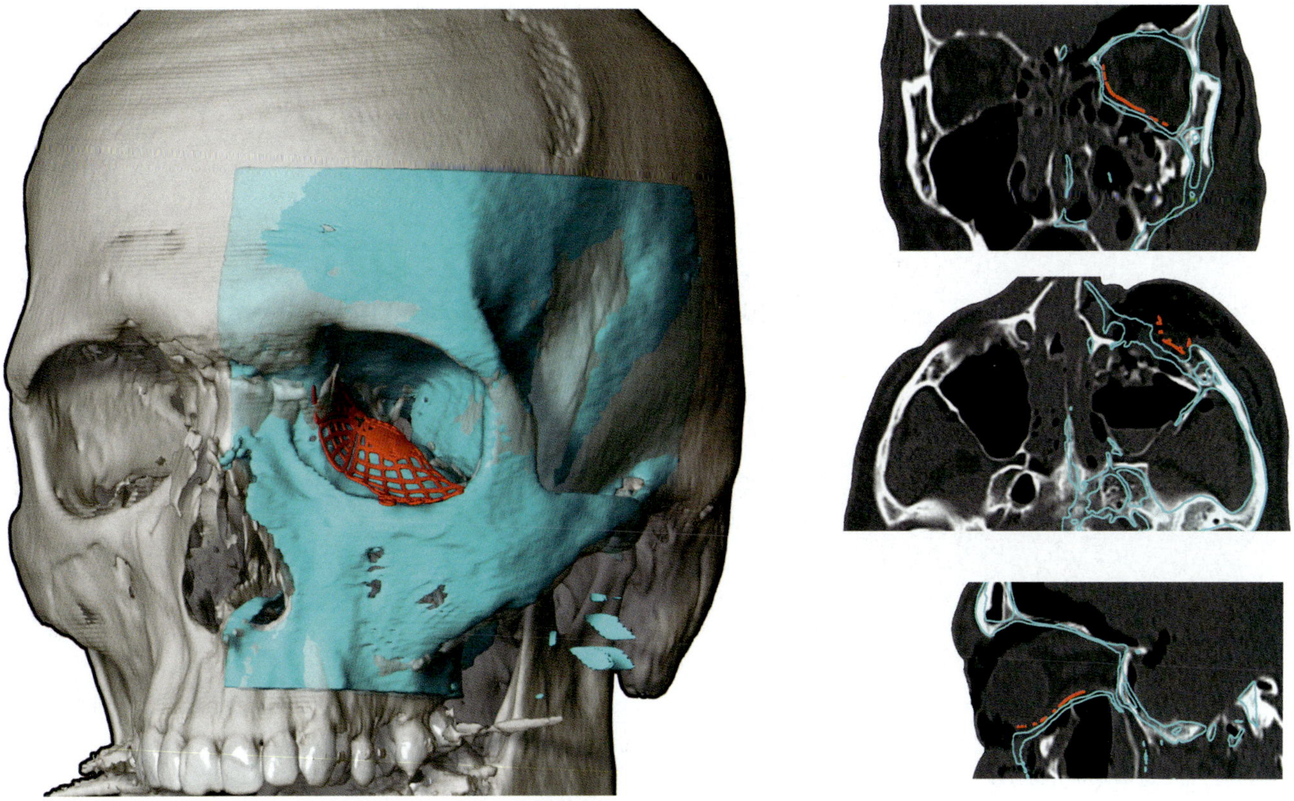

Fig. 10 VSP (patient 2). A preformed implant has been virtually positioned to reconstruct the orbit as closely as possible to the template obtained in Fig. 9. (*Courtesy of* Ruud Schreurs, MSc, Cornelis Klop, MSc, and Thomas J. J. Maal, MSc, PhD.)

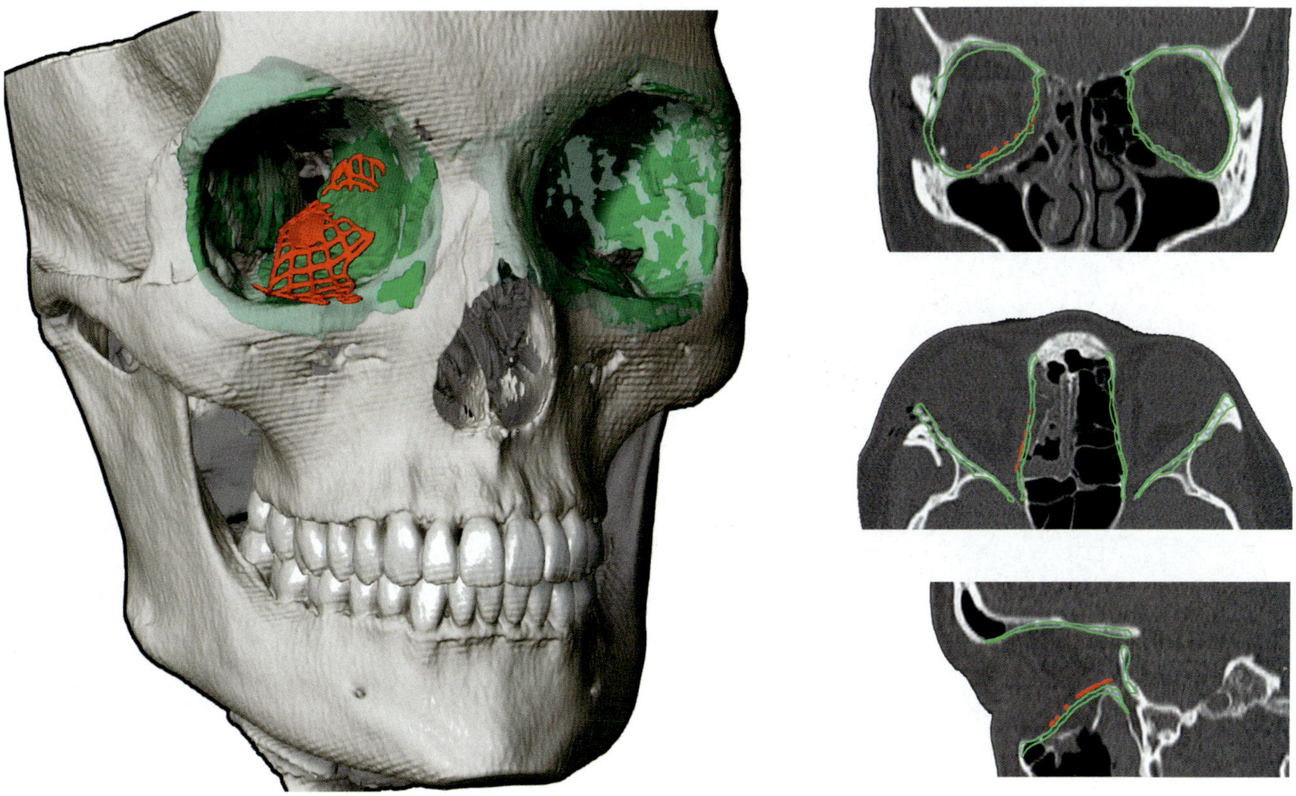

Fig. 11 VSP (patient 1). A preformed implant has been virtually positioned to reconstruct the orbit as closely as possible to the template obtained in Fig. 6 keeping the details in Fig. 12 in mind. (*Courtesy of* Ruud Schreurs, MSc, Cornelis Klop, MSc, and Thomas J. J. Maal, MSc, PhD.)

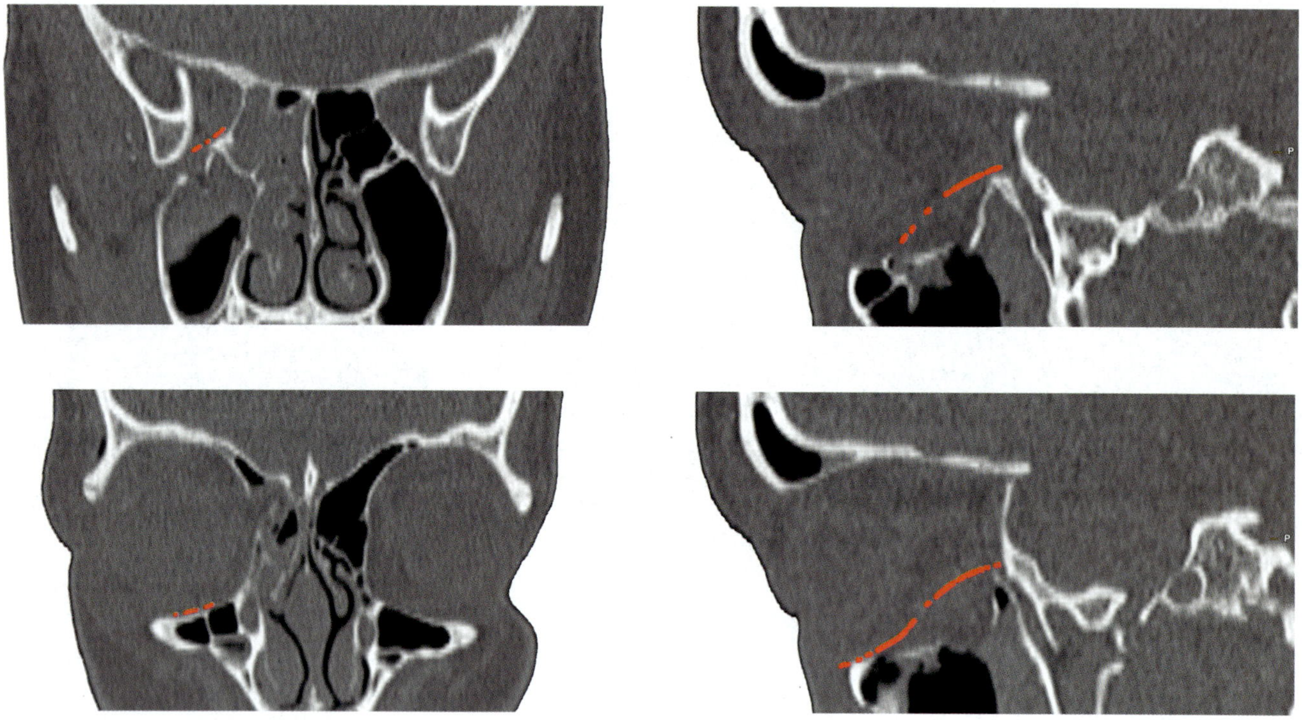

Fig. 12 Positioning parameters (patient 1). Support on the ledge (*top*) and fixation possibility on the orbital rim (*bottom*) is seen in the coronal and sagittal views. (*Courtesy of* Ruud Schreurs, MSc, Cornelis Klop, MSc, and Thomas J. J. Maal, MSc, PhD.)

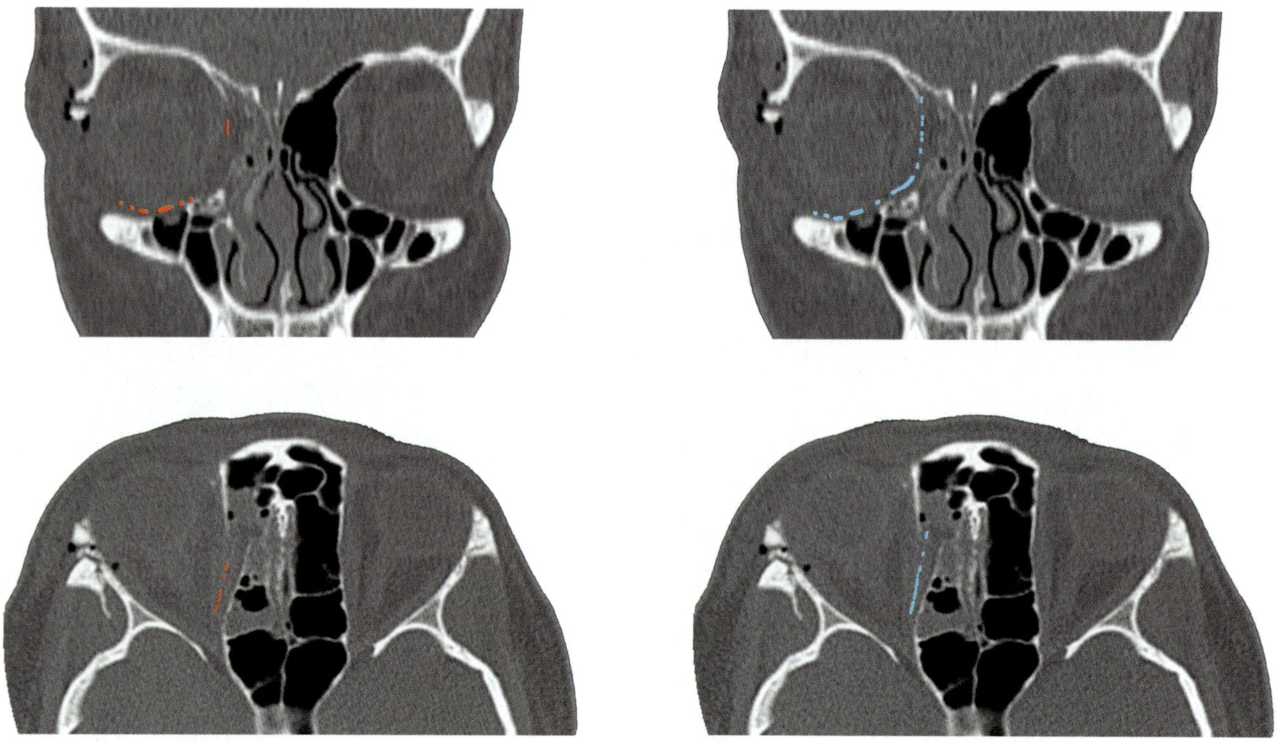

Fig. 13 Small implant (*red*) versus large implant (*blue*) (patient 1). The medial wall extension of the large implant interferes with the unaffected bony structures of the medial wall, and cannot be positioned without cutting the implant. Because the small implant follows the contour of the mirrored orbit adequately (Fig. 11) and does not interfere with existing bony structures, the small implant was selected in this case. (*Courtesy of* Ruud Schreurs, MSc, Cornelis Klop, MSc, and Thomas J. J. Maal, MSc, PhD.)

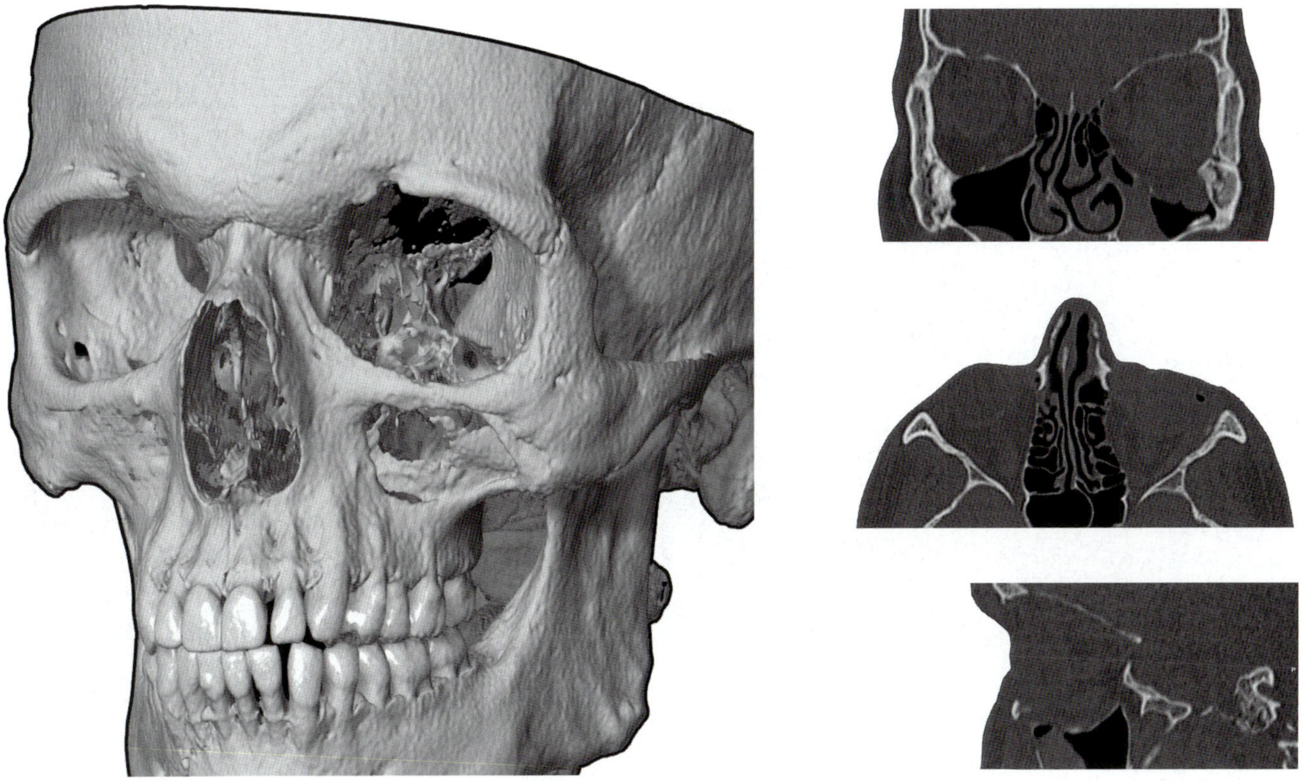

Fig. 14 Hard-tissue model and multiplanar views of patient 3. (*Courtesy of* Ruud Schreurs, MSc, Cornelis Klop, MSc, and Thomas J. J. Maal, MSc, PhD.)

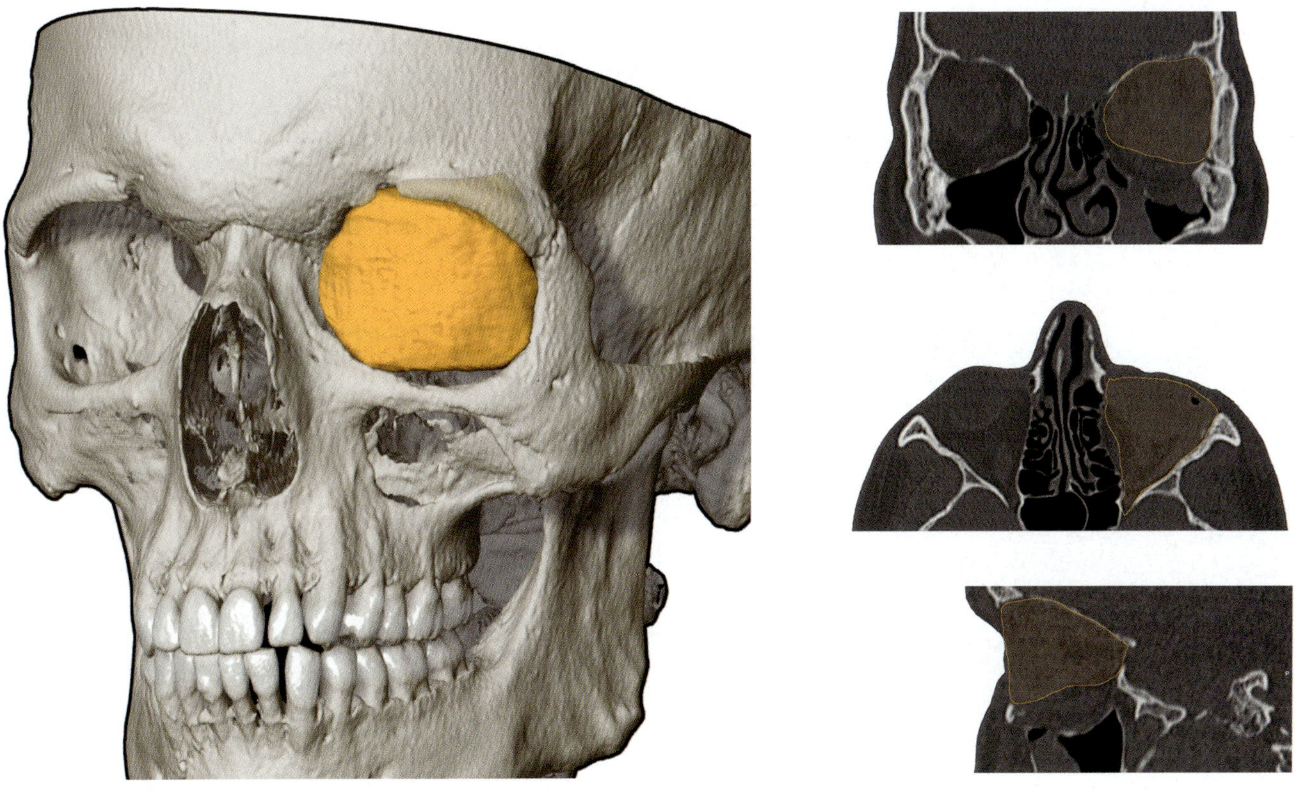

Fig. 15 Desired shape of the orbit after reconstruction (patient 3). (*Courtesy of* Ruud Schreurs, MSc, Cornelis Klop, MSc, and Thomas J. J. Maal, MSc, PhD.)

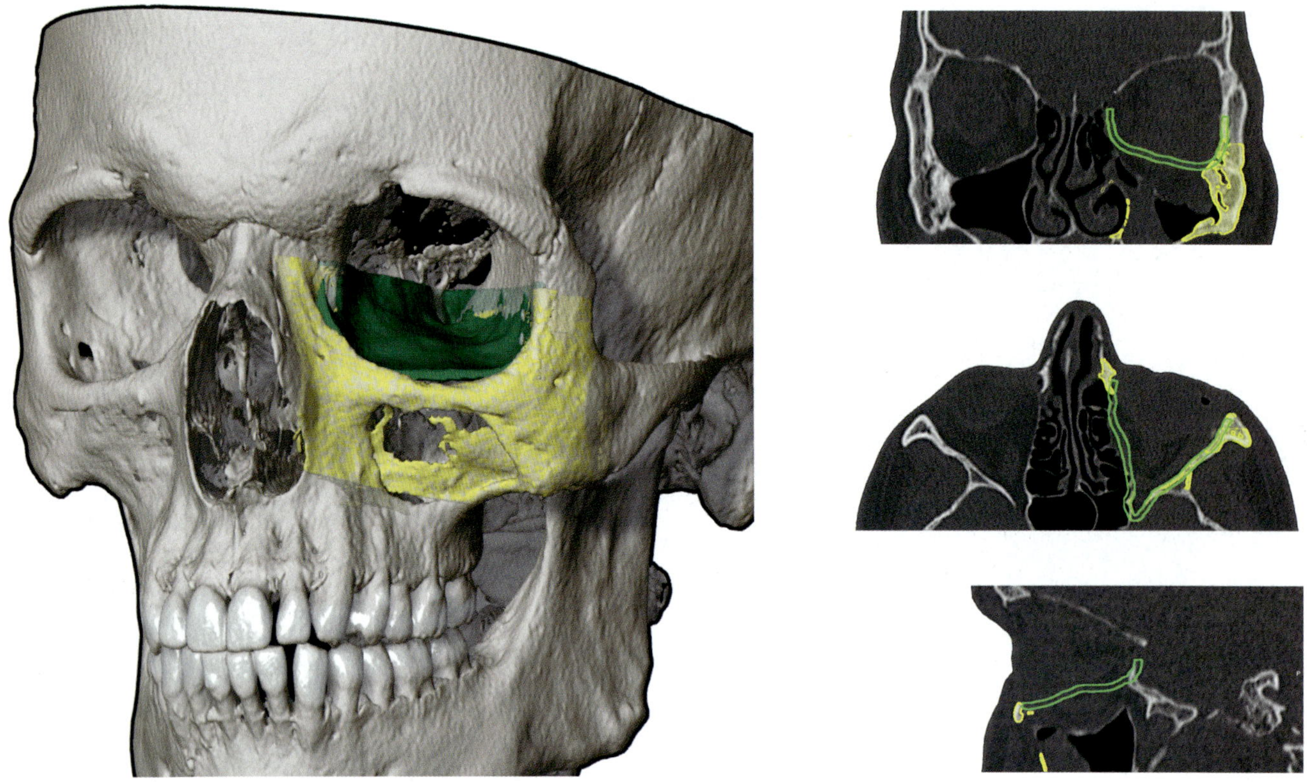

Fig. 16 Orbital floor corresponding with the shape in Fig. 15 (*green*), and existing bony structures (*yellow*) (patient 3). (*Courtesy of* Ruud Schreurs, MSc, Cornelis Klop, MSc, and Thomas J. J. Maal, MSc, PhD.)

(see Fig. 22). This way, the fixation of the PSI can be designed to overlap with the existing screw positions from the primary reconstruction, for additional feedback during positioning.[33]

Evaluation

Advanced diagnostics and VSP are the first, and arguably most important, steps in a CAS workflow for orbital reconstruction. The advanced diagnostics stage ensures that all available information is used in the decision-making process. The feasibility of the surgical intervention is assessed beforehand through the VSP, which rules out preventable surgical mismanagement such as the use of an unsuited implant for reconstruction, which was the case in the primary reconstruction of the patient in Figs. 18–22 (Fig. 23). The surgery may be simulated as many times as necessary to obtain the desired reconstruction of premorbid anatomy. An additional advantage of these simulations is that the surgeon is familiarized with the patient's specific anatomy and disorder. For training surgeons, this provides an enhanced learning experience,

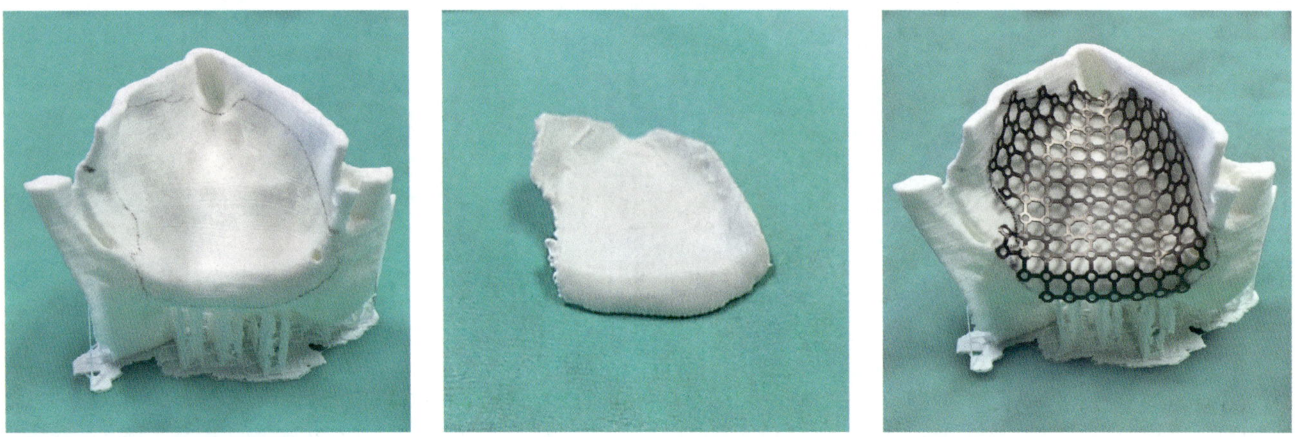

Fig. 17 3D printed template for bending the implant (patient 3), consisting of the structures visualized in Fig. 16 (*left*). An additional template extracted from the patient model, indicating the desired implant's contour, was 3D printed (*middle*). Based on these templates, an implant was premolded (*right*). (*Courtesy of* Ruud Schreurs, MSc, Cornelis Klop, MSc, and Thomas J. J. Maal, MSc, PhD.)

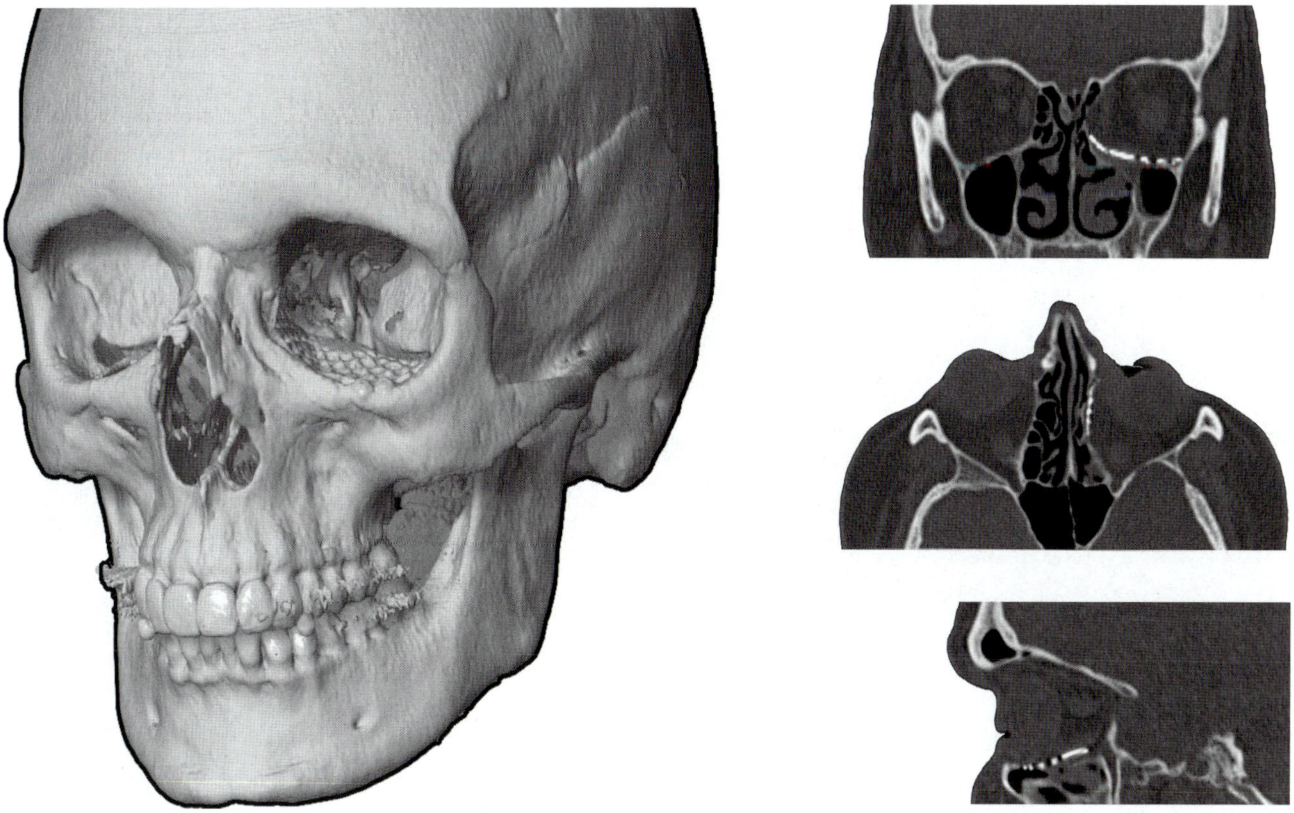

Fig. 18 Hard-tissue model and multiplanar views of patient 4. (*Courtesy of* Ruud Schreurs, MSc, Cornelis Klop, MSc, and Thomas J. J. Maal, MSc, PhD.)

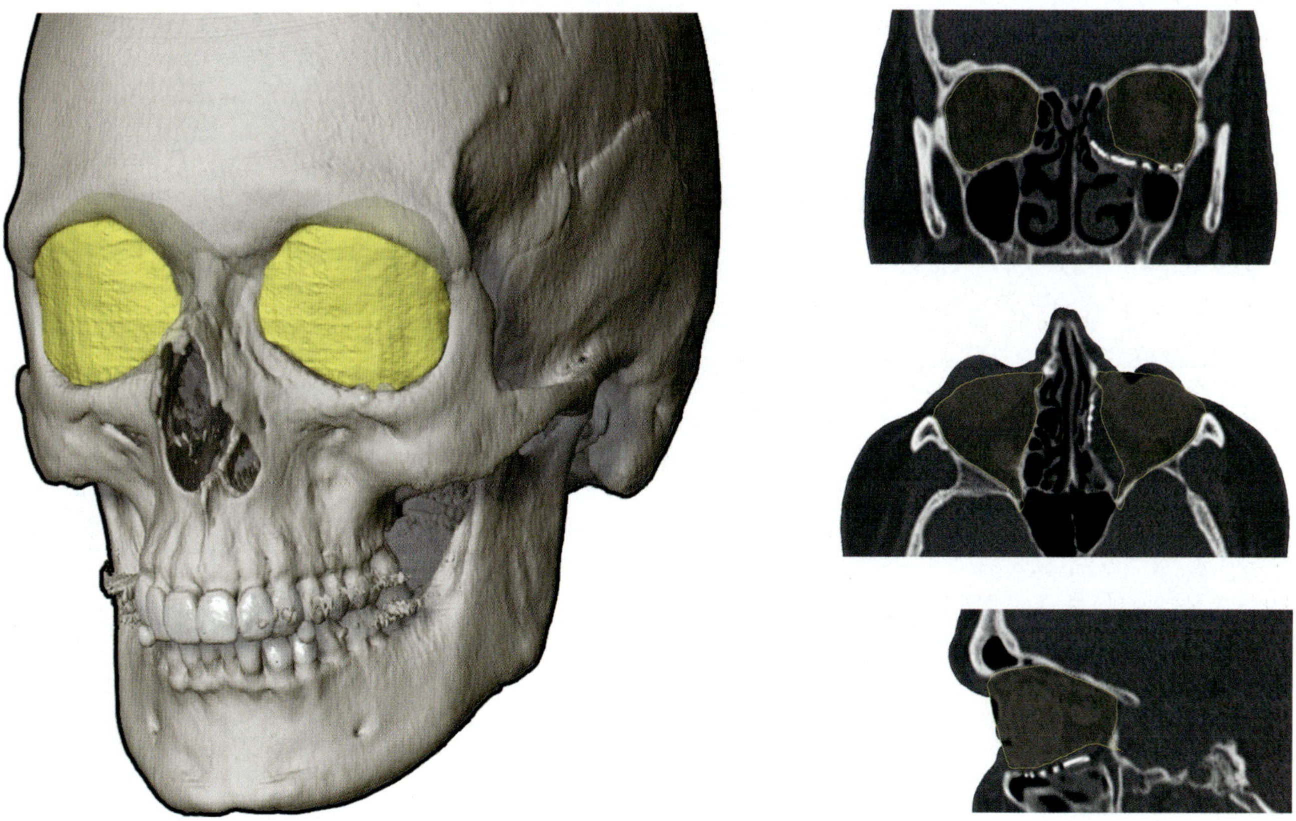

Fig. 19 Unaffected orbit and mirrored orbit, which serves as the basis for the PSI design (patient 4). (*Courtesy of* Ruud Schreurs, MSc, Cornelis Klop, MSc, and Thomas J. J. Maal, MSc, PhD.)

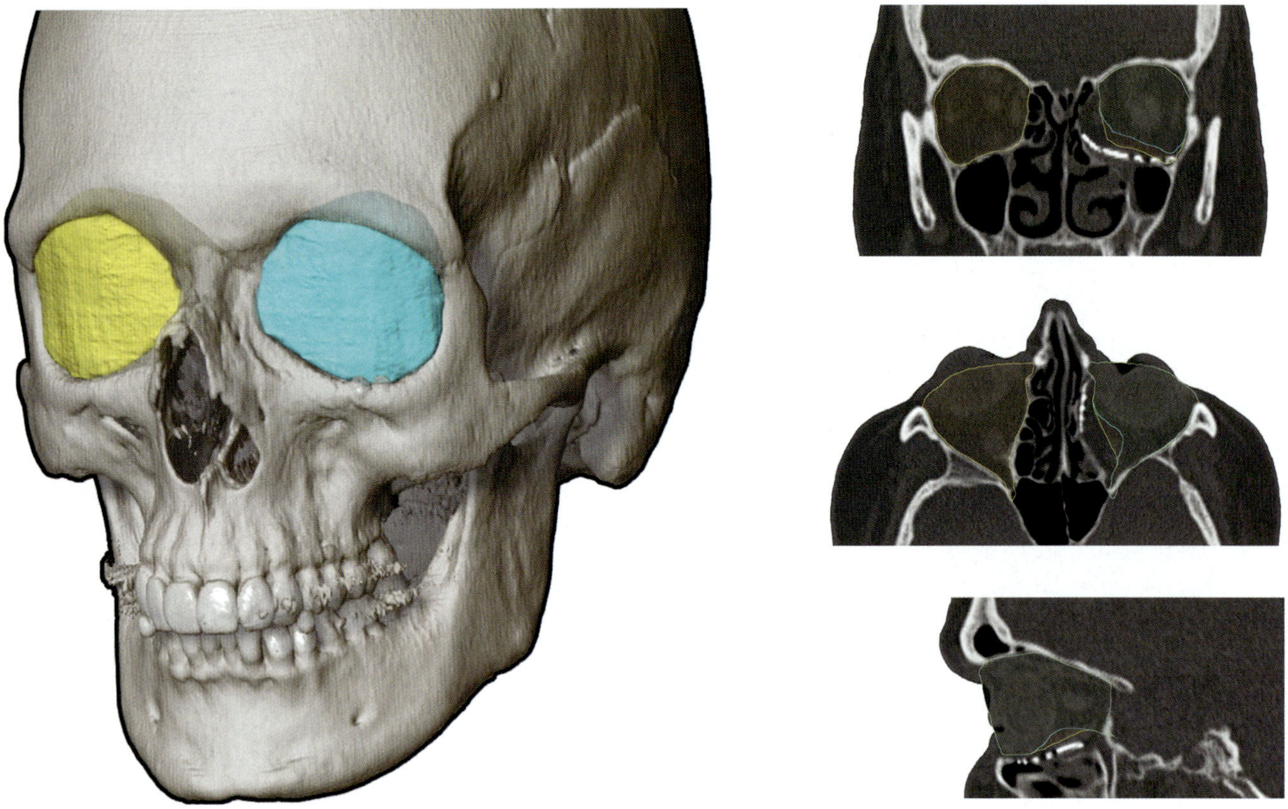

Fig. 20 Possibility of overcorrection (patient 4). The cyan model is a 1 cm^3 overcorrected model of the mirrored orbit. (*Courtesy of* Ruud Schreurs, MSc, Cornelis Klop, MSc, and Thomas J. J. Maal, MSc, PhD.)

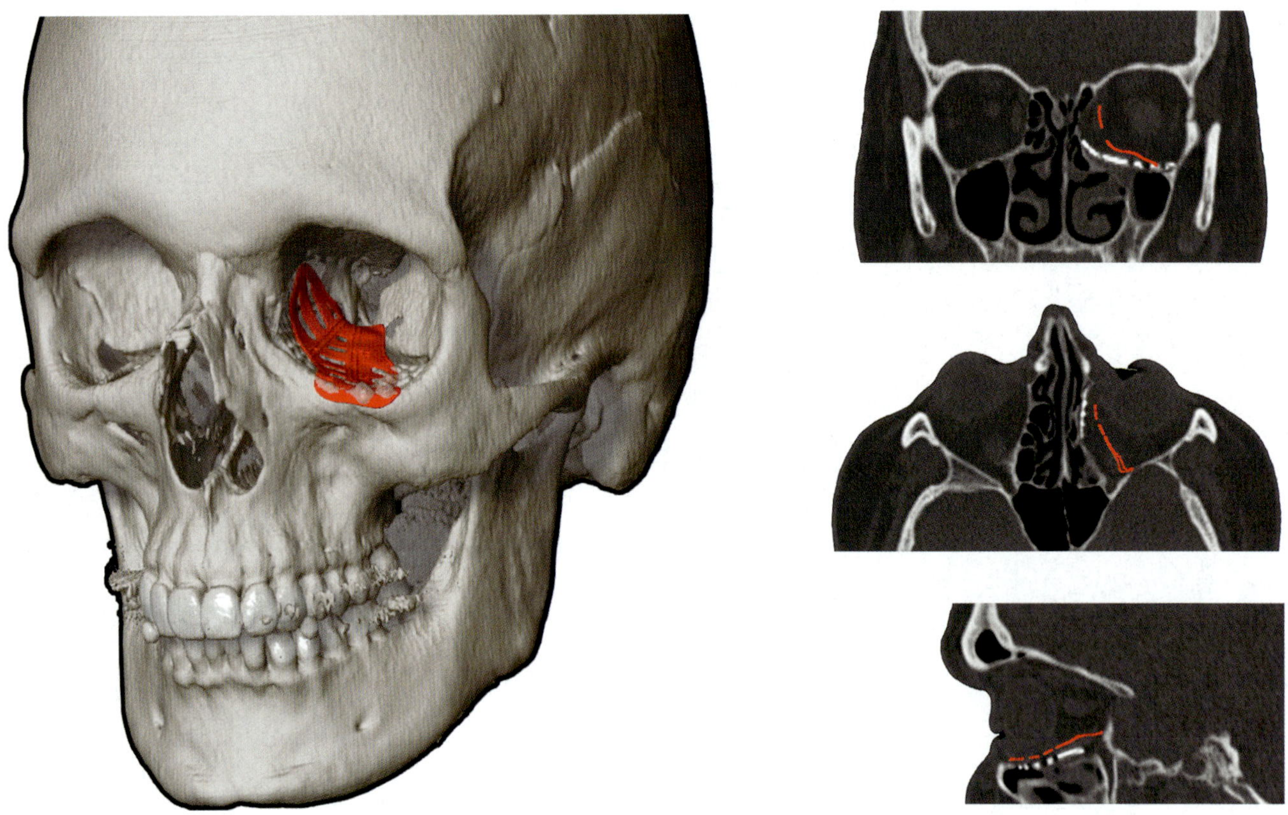

Fig. 21 Design of a PSI (patient 4). (*Courtesy of* Ruud Schreurs, MSc, Cornelis Klop, MSc, and Thomas J. J. Maal, MSc, PhD.)

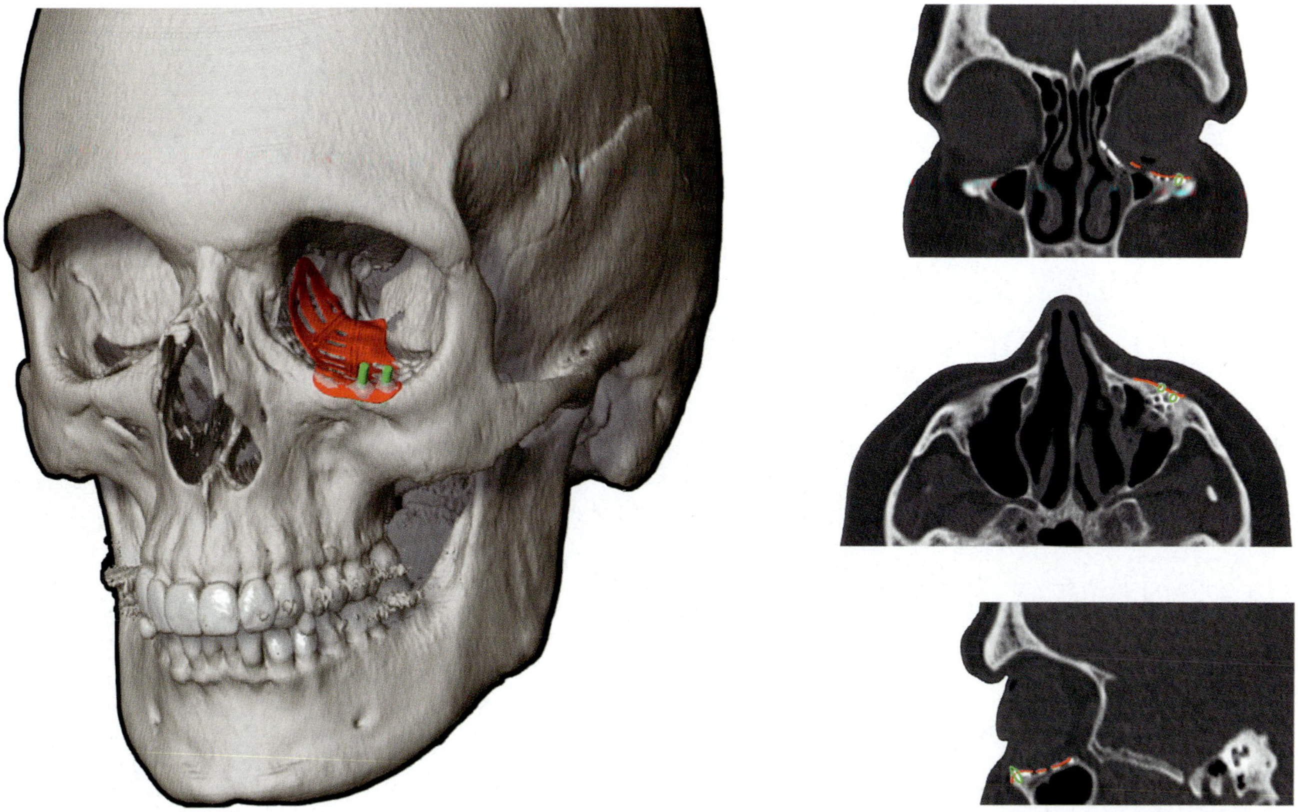

Fig. 22 Segmentation of existing osteosynthesis fixation (patient 4). The screw positions of the primary reconstruction are incorporated in the PSI design, to provide feedback on positioning. (*Courtesy of* Ruud Schreurs, MSc, Cornelis Klop, MSc, and Thomas J. J. Maal, MSc, PhD.)

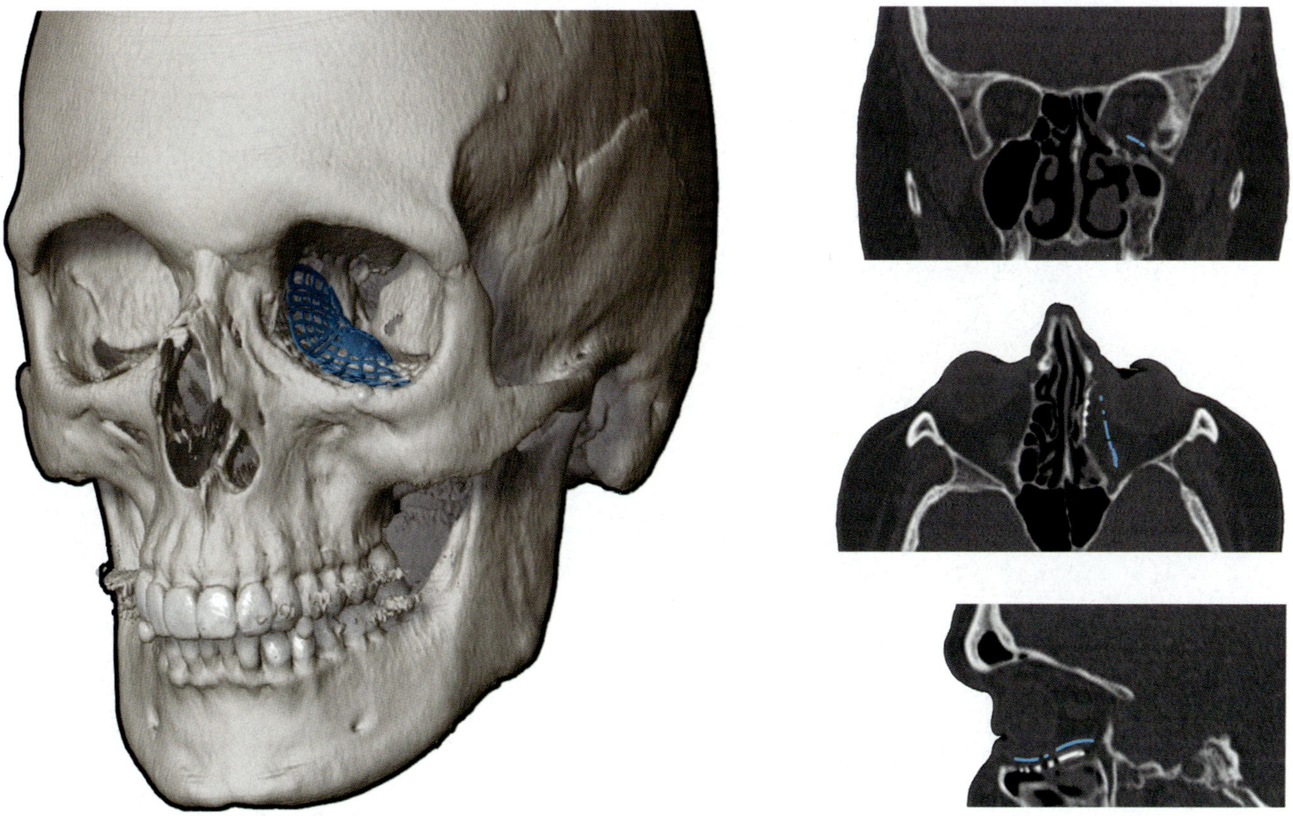

Fig. 23 Feasibility assessment of implant chosen for reconstruction (patient 4). If the contour of the mirrored orbit is followed, the implant has no support on the dorsal ledge. If support on the ledge were sought, the enlarged volume of the orbit would not be corrected properly. (*Courtesy of* Ruud Schreurs, MSc, Cornelis Klop, MSc, and Thomas J. J. Maal, MSc, PhD.)

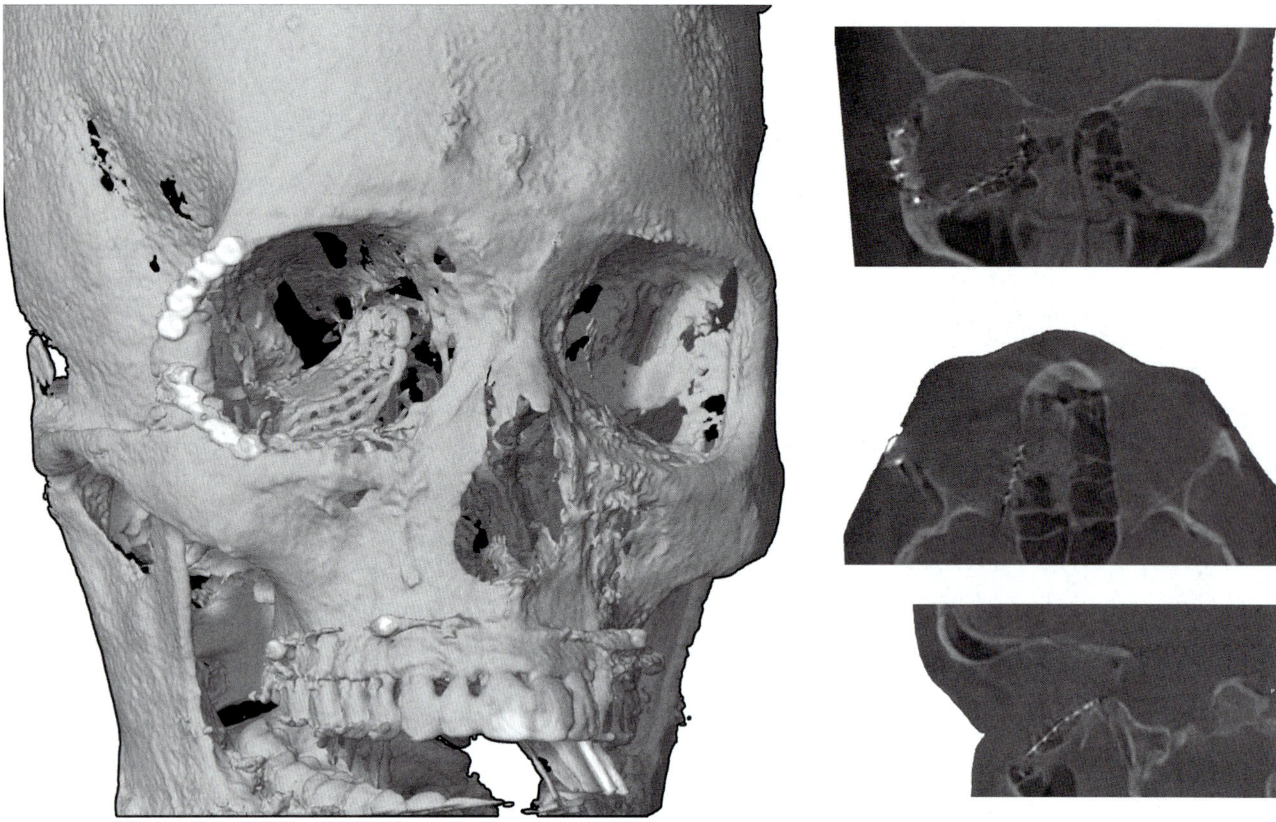

Fig. 24 Intraoperative imaging of patient 1. (*Courtesy of* Ruud Schreurs, MSc, Cornelis Klop, MSc, and Thomas J. J. Maal, MSc, PhD.)

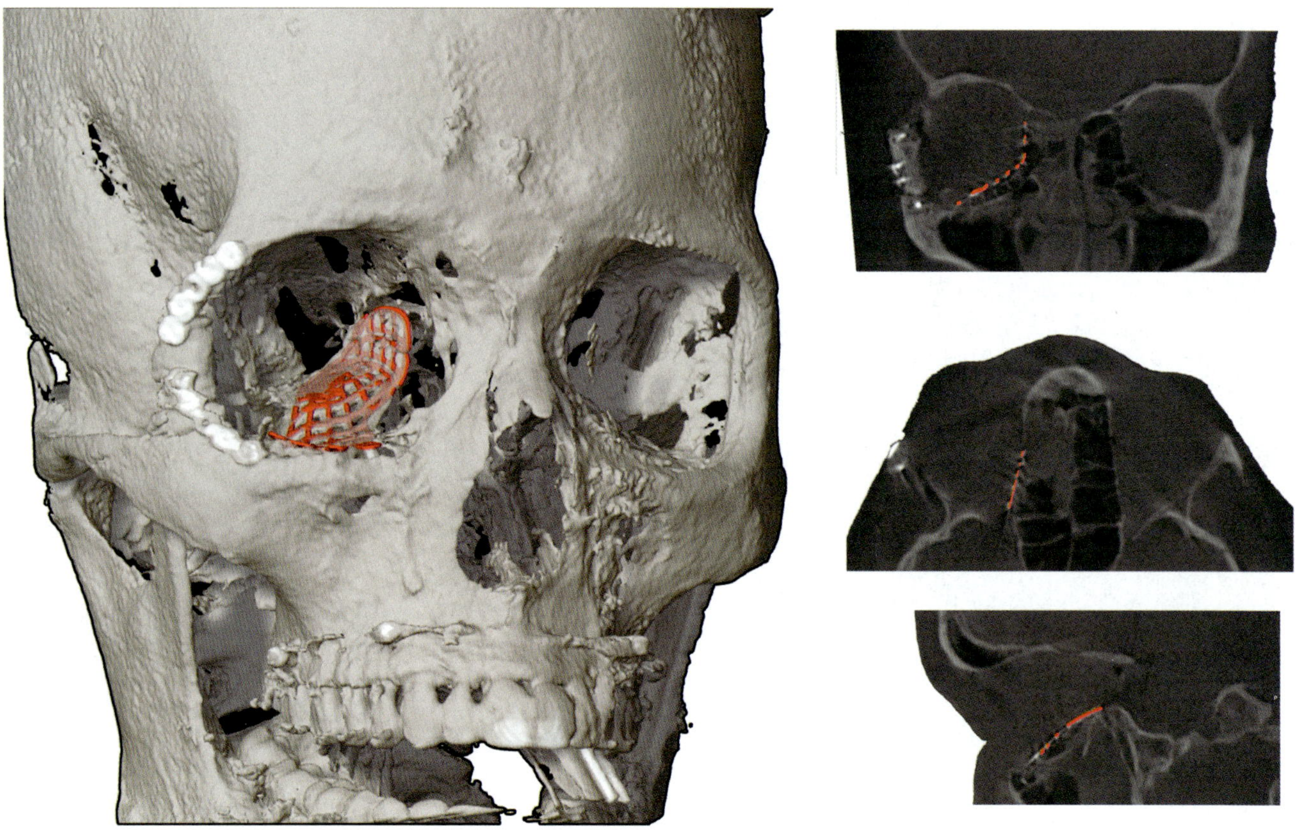

Fig. 25 Computer-assisted evaluation of surgical result (patient 1). The planned implant position was obtained and no adjustments are necessary. (*Courtesy of* Ruud Schreurs, MSc, Cornelis Klop, MSc, and Thomas J. J. Maal, MSc, PhD.)

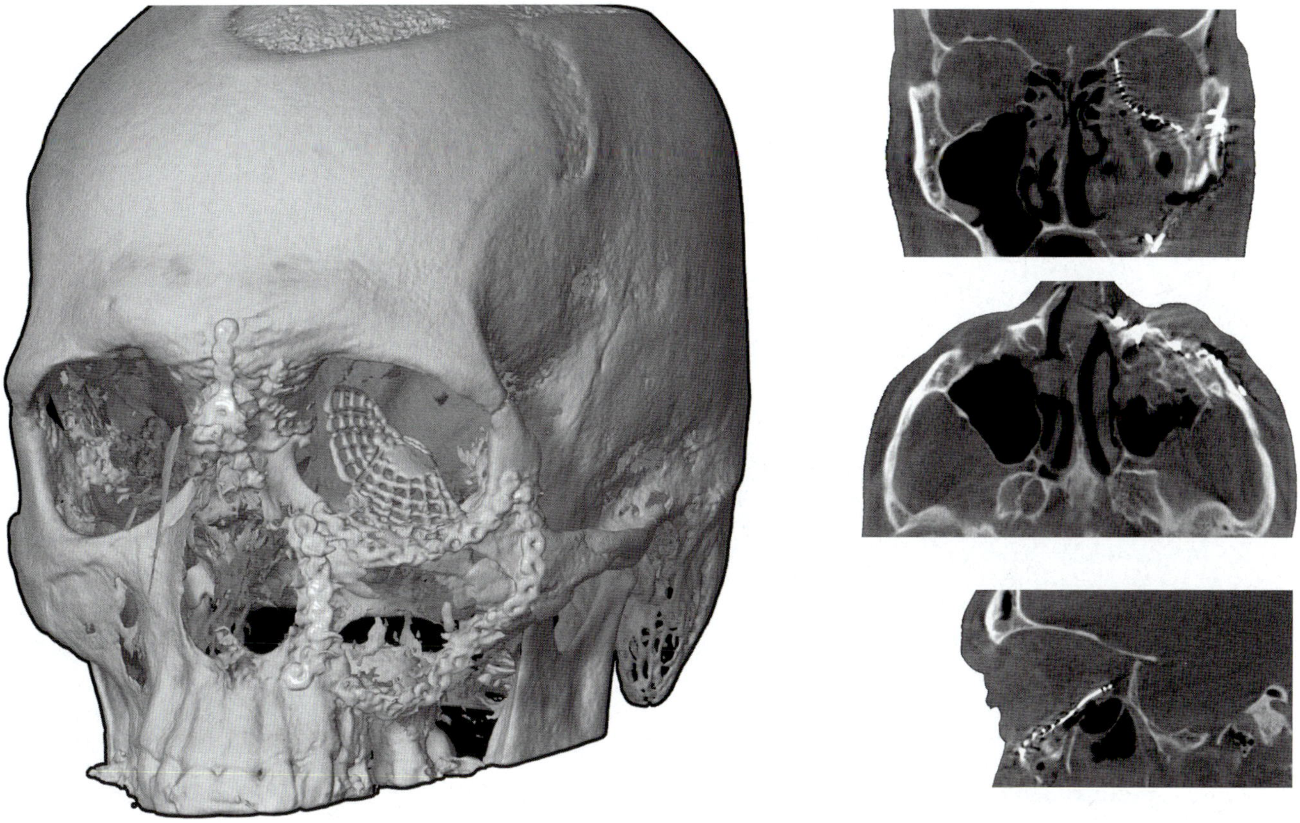

Fig. 26 Postoperative imaging of patient 2. (*Courtesy of* Ruud Schreurs, MSc, Cornelis Klop, MSc, and Thomas J. J. Maal, MSc, PhD.)

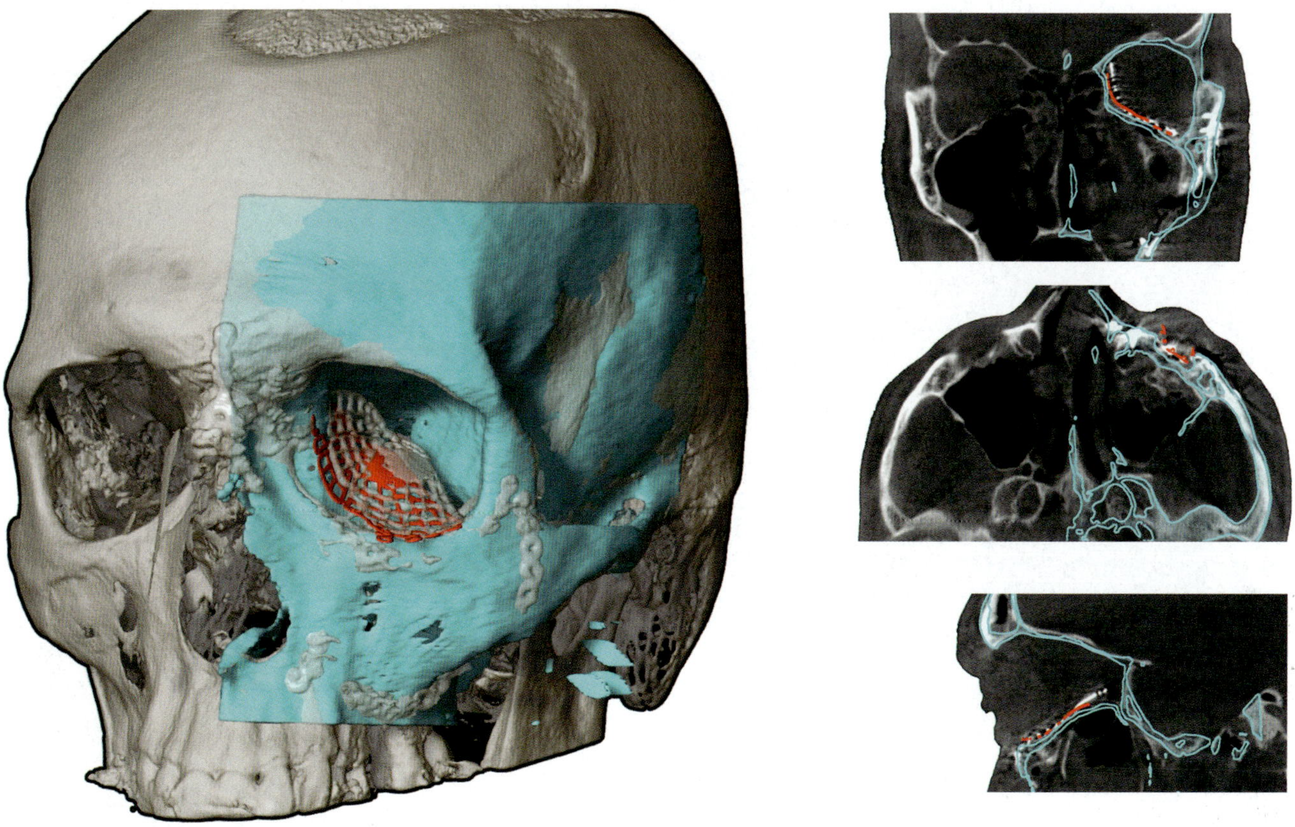

Fig. 27 Computer-assisted evaluation of surgical result (patient 2). The zygomatic complex is repositioned according to the virtual surgical plan, but the acquired implant position deviates from the planned position. (*Courtesy of* Ruud Schreurs, MSc, Cornelis Klop, MSc, and Thomas J. J. Maal, MSc, PhD.)

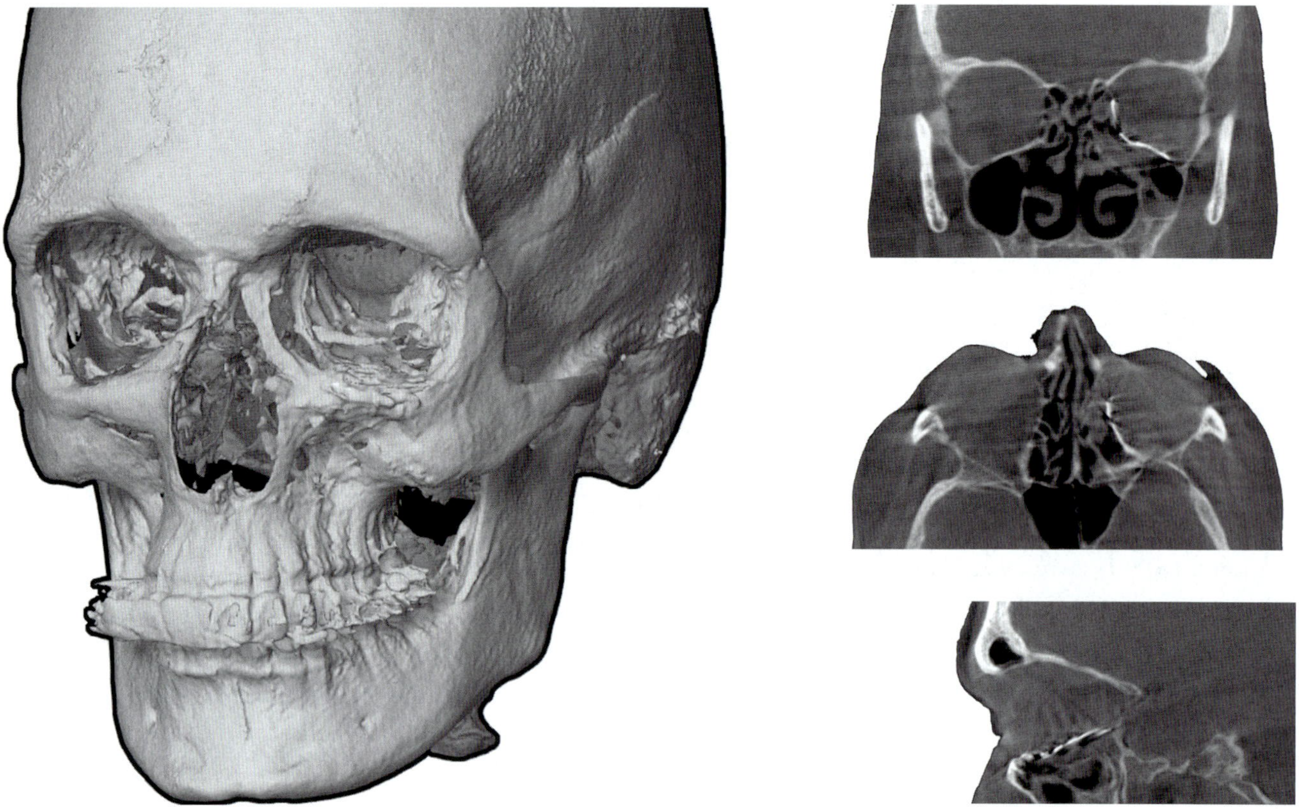

Fig. 28 Postoperative imaging of patient 4. (*Courtesy of* Ruud Schreurs, MSc, Cornelis Klop, MSc, and Thomas J. J. Maal, MSc, PhD.)

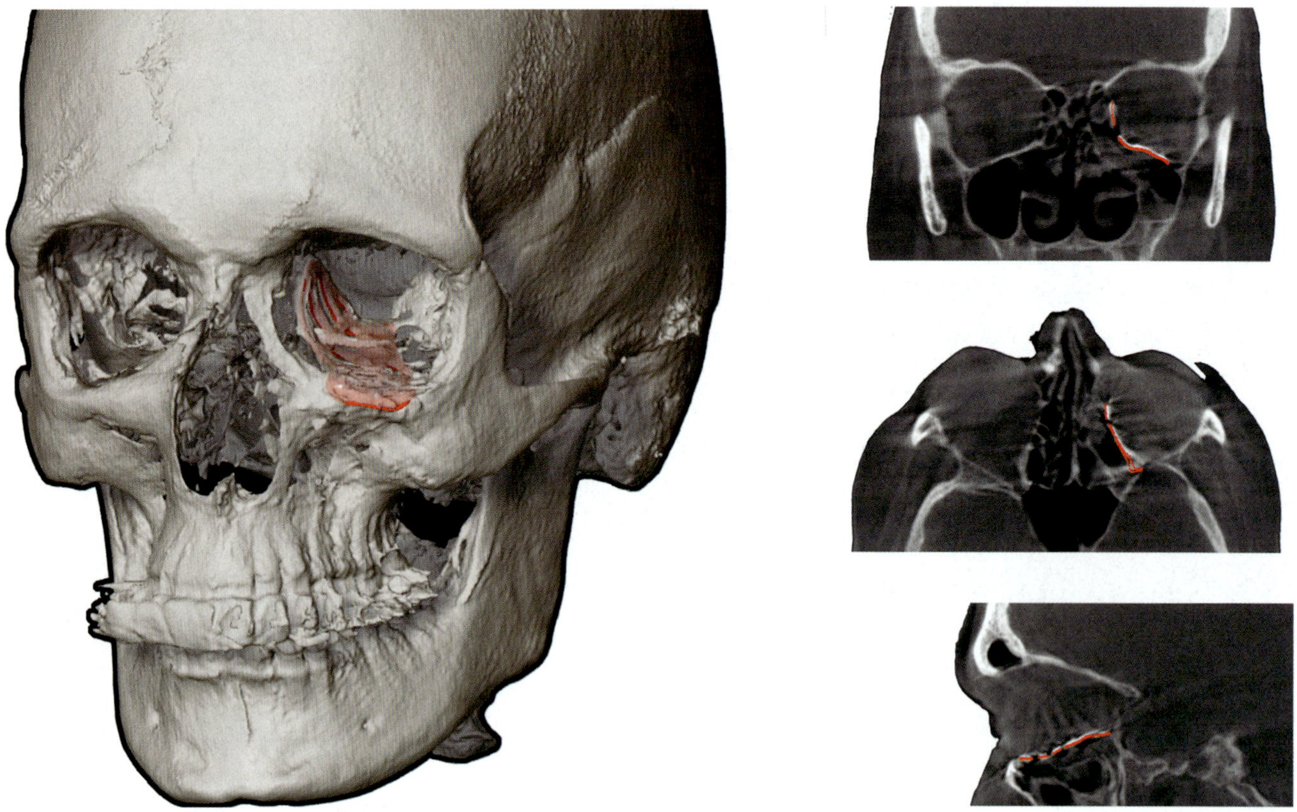

Fig. 29 Computer-assisted evaluation of surgical result (patient 4). The planned implant position was obtained. (*Courtesy of* Ruud Schreurs, MSc, Cornelis Klop, MSc, and Thomas J. J. Maal, MSc, PhD.)

whereas experienced surgeons are able to anticipate intraoperative difficulties from the information in the virtual surgical plan.

The CAS workflow entails intraoperative feedback and postoperative evaluation after advanced diagnostics and VSP. The virtual surgical plan sets a target for the surgeon, but the feedback during the operation can be extended beyond just visualization in the CAS workflow. The shape of a premolded implant or PSI can guide the surgeon to the planned implant position. The planning may be imported in a surgical navigation system, which can provide dynamic feedback on implant position during surgery. These feedback mechanisms may aid surgeons in achieving the desired reconstruction result.[8,10,17,27,35–37] Both feedback mechanisms are discussed in greater detail in Schreurs and colleagues' article, "Intraoperative Feedback and Quality Control in Orbital Reconstruction: The Past, the Present and the Future," in this issue. Image fusion of the intraoperative or postoperative imaging to the virtual surgical plan enables detailed comparison between planned and acquired implant position.[2,9,19] This evaluation of the final surgical result (Figs. 24–29), combined with clinical outcome and difficulties encountered during surgery, yield feedback and possible improvements in any of the stages for the next patient who is treated using the CAS workflow.

Clinics care points

- An important preparation step for computer-assisted surgery in orbital reconstruction is to create a virtual 3D model from the CT data. This model can be augmented with additional 3D information to generate an accurate virtual patient model.
- The virtual patient model enables advanced diagnostics and 3D virtual surgical planning, which ensure a better inspection of the problem and the possible solutions during the preoperative phase.
- Virtual surgical planning is a valuable tool in orbital reconstruction in the preoperative setting, but it can also be utilized intraoperatively for feedback, and postoperatively for evaluation.
- Postoperative evaluation within the computer-assisted surgery workflow provides meaningful feedback for future cases.

Disclosure

The authors have nothing to disclose.

References

1. Baumann A, Sinko K, Dorner G. Late reconstruction of the orbit with patient-specific implants using computer-aided planning and navigation. J Oral Maxillofac Surg 2015;73(12):S101–6.
2. Gander T, Essig H, Metzler P, et al. Patient specific implants (PSI) in reconstruction of orbital floor and wall fractures. J Cranio-Maxillofacial Surg 2015;43(1):126–30.
3. Rana M, Chui CHK, Wagner M, et al. Increasing the accuracy of orbital reconstruction with selective laser-melted patient-specific implants combined with intraoperative navigation. J Oral Maxillofac Surg 2015;73(6):1113–8.
4. Cha JH, Lee YH, Ruy WC, et al. Application of rapid prototyping technique and intraoperative navigation system for the repair and reconstruction of orbital wall fractures. Arch Craniofac Surg 2016;17(3):146.
5. Kärkkäinen M, Wilkman T, Mesimäki K, et al. Primary reconstruction of orbital fractures using patient-specific titanium milled implants: the Helsinki protocol. Br J Oral Maxillofac Surg 2018;56(9):791–6.
6. Mahoney NR, Peng MY, Merbs SL, et al. Virtual fitting, selection, and cutting of preformed anatomic orbital implants. Ophthal Plast Reconstr Surg 2017;33(3):196–201.
7. Scolozzi P. Applications of 3D orbital computer-assisted surgery (CAS). J Stomatol Oral Maxillofac Surg 2017;118(4):217–23.
8. Azarmehr I, Stokbro K, Bell RB, et al. Contemporary techniques in orbital reconstruction: a review of the literature and report of a case combining surgical navigation, computer-aided surgical simulation, and a patient-specific implant. J Oral Maxillofac Surg 2020;78(4):594–609.
9. Schreurs R, Dubois L, Becking AG, et al. Quantitative assessment of orbital implant position-a proof of concept. PLoS One 2016;11(3). https://doi.org/10.1371/journal.pone.0150162.
10. Jansen J, Schreurs R, Dubois L, et al. The advantages of advanced computer-assisted diagnostics and three-dimensional preoperative planning on implant position in orbital reconstruction. J Craniomaxillofac Surg. 2018. https://doi.org/10.1016/j.jcms.2018.02.010.
11. Kubal WS. Imaging of orbital trauma. Radiographics 2008;28(6):1729–39.
12. Lin KY, Ngai P, Echegoyen JC, et al. Imaging in orbital trauma. Saudi J Ophthalmol 2012;26(4):427–32.
13. Chazen JL, Lantos J, Gupta A, et al. Orbital soft-tissue trauma. Neuroimaging Clin N Am 2014;24(3):425–37.
14. Boyette JR, Pemberton JD, Bonilla-Velez J. Management of orbital fractures: challenges and solutions. Clin Ophthalmol 2015;9:2127.
15. Jansen J, Schreurs R, Dubois L, et al. Orbital volume analysis: validation of a semi-automatic software segmentation method. Int J Comput Assist Radiol Surg 2016;11(1). https://doi.org/10.1007/s11548-015-1254-6.
16. Grob S, Yonkers M, Tao J. Orbital fracture repair. In: Seminars in plastic surgery, vol. 31. New York: Thieme Medical Publishers; 2017. p. 31–9.
17. Cai EZ, Koh YP, Hing ECH, et al. Computer-assisted navigational surgery improves outcomes in orbital reconstructive surgery. J Craniofac Surg 2012;23(5):1567–73.
18. Wagner MEH, Lichtenstein JT, Winkelmann M, et al. Development and first clinical application of automated virtual reconstruction of unilateral midface defects. J Craniomaxillofac Surg. 2015;43(8):1340–7.
19. He Y, Zhang Y, Yu GY, et al. Expert consensus on navigation-guided unilateral orbital fracture and orbital floor reconstruction techniques. Chin J Dent Res 2020;23(1):51–5.
20. TJJ Maal, Plooij JM, Rangel FA, et al. The accuracy of matching three-dimensional photographs with skin surfaces derived from cone-beam computed tomography. Int J Oral Maxillofac Surg 2008;37(7):641–6.
21. Baan F, Bruggink R, Nijsink J, et al. Fusion of intra-oral scans in cone-beam computed tomography scans. Clin Oral Investig 2020. https://doi.org/10.1007/s00784-020-03336-y.
22. Wagner MEH, Gellrich N-C, Friese K-I, et al. Model-based segmentation in orbital volume measurement with cone beam computed tomography and evaluation against current concepts. Int J Comput Assist Radiol Surg 2016;11(1):1–9.
23. Hsung T-C, Lo J, Chong M-M, et al. Orbit segmentation by surface reconstruction with automatic sliced vertex screening. IEEE Trans Biomed Eng 2017;65(4):828–38.
24. Kim H, Son T, Lee J, et al. Three-dimensional orbital wall modeling using paranasal sinus segmentation. J Craniomaxillofac Surg 2019;47(6):959–67.
25. Susarla SM, Duncan K, Mahoney NR, et al. Virtual surgical planning for orbital reconstruction. Middle East Afr J Ophthalmol 2015;22(4):442.

26. Ho J-PTF, Schreurs R, Milstein DMJ, et al. Measuring zygomaticomaxillary complex symmetry three-dimensionally with the use of mirroring and surface based matching techniques. J Craniomaxillofac Surg. 2016;44(10). https://doi.org/10.1016/j.jcms.2016.07.034.
27. Wilde F, Schramm A. Intraoperative imaging in orbital and midface reconstruction. Facial Plast Surg 2014;30(05):545–53.
28. Bittermann G, Metzger MC, Schlager S, et al. Orbital reconstruction: prefabricated implants, data transfer, and revision surgery. Facial Plast Surg 2014;30(05):554–60.
29. Rana M, Holtmann H, Kanatas AN, et al. Primary orbital reconstruction with selective laser melted core patient-specific implants: overview of 100 patients. Br J Oral Maxillofac Surg 2019; 57(8):782–7.
30. Doerfler H-M, Huempfner-Hierl H, Kruber D, et al. Template-based orbital wall fracture treatment using statistical shape analysis. J Oral Maxillofac Surg 2017;75(7):1475-e1.
31. Hierl T, Kruber D, Doerfler H-M, et al. Computer-aided versus conventional planning in orbital traumatology using preformed meshes: development of a new workflow. J Oral Maxillofac Surg 2019;77(8):1663–72.
32. Kim YC, Jeong WS, Park T, et al. The accuracy of patient specific implant prebented with 3D-printed rapid prototype model for orbital wall reconstruction. J Craniomaxillofac Surg. 2017;45(6):928–36.
33. Schreurs R, Dubois L, Becking AG, et al. The orbit first! A novel surgical treatment protocol for secondary orbitozygomatic reconstruction. J Craniomaxillofac Surg 2017;45(7). https://doi.org/10.1016/j.jcms.2017.03.026.
34. Kang S, Kwon J, Ahn CJ, et al. Generation of customized orbital implant templates using 3-dimensional printing for orbital wall reconstruction. Eye 2018;32(12):1864–70.
35. Hsieh T-Y, Vong S, Strong EB. Orbital reconstruction. Curr Opin Otolaryngol Head Neck Surg 2015;23(5):388–92.
36. Dubois L, Schreurs R, Jansen J, et al. Predictability in orbital reconstruction: a human cadaver study. Part II: navigation-assisted orbital reconstruction. J Craniomaxillofac Surg 2015;43(10): 2042–9.
37. Dubois L, Essig H, Schreurs R, et al. Predictability in orbital reconstruction. A human cadaver study, part III: implant-oriented navigation for optimized reconstruction. J Craniomaxillofac Surg 2015;43(10):2050–6.

Intraoperative Feedback and Quality Control in Orbital Reconstruction

The Past, the Present, and the Future

Ruud Schreurs, MSc [a,b,*], Frank Wilde, MD, DDS [c,d], Alexander Schramm, MD, DDS [c,d], Nils-Claudius Gellrich, MD, DDS [e]

KEYWORDS

• Computer-assisted surgery • Orbit • Orbital reconstruction • Surgical navigation • Intraoperative imaging • Patient-specific implants • Intraoperative feedback • Quality control

KEY POINTS

- The development and implementation of medical technology in orbital reconstructive surgery is a logical consequence of the philosophy to optimize the treatment procedure before, during, and after surgery in terms of maximum control for the surgeon and the aim for optimal outcome for the individual patient.
- During the surgical procedure, the optimal virtual surgical planning must be transferred to the surgical site as accurately as possible; for this purpose, a variety of different methods and devices may be used and even combined, depending on the complexity of the task.
- The adage that "the best way to predict the future is to invent it" (Alan Kay) has proved true for orbital reconstruction in the past and will be the key to future innovations.

Introduction: the rationale of technology in orbital surgery

Over the last 20 years, rapid changes in digital medical technology have occurred if it comes to "making the invisible visible." Especially in craniomaxillofacial surgery, complex reconstructive procedures in primary or secondary cases have always been a challenge in the past and will remain as such in the future. Patients have a different view on their pathology than the surgeon has: the patient has an outside-oriented perspective, which relates to outer appearance and appropriate function. The surgeon has to take the outer tissue envelope into consideration to focus on the inside-oriented perspective, which is the craniofacial skeleton, and the associated soft tissues to analyze the amount of individual deformity, to modify these, and to finally achieve an appropriate esthetic result for that patient combined with adequate function.

Detailed knowledge of the anatomic structures is fundamental for orbital surgery: inadequate reconstructions potentially lead to unsatisfactory results.[1] For this reason, clinical assessment, combined with imaging techniques used for diagnosis and treatment planning, must meet the highest standards. It is only then possible to answer the most important question in orbital fracture management: do we have to explore an orbital defect? This ongoing debate is further discussed in Leander Dubois and colleagues' article,"Ongoing Debate in Clinical Decision Making in Orbital Fractures: Indications, Timing, and Biomaterials," in this issue. If surgery is indicated, it is the task of the surgeon to minimize the risk for the patient and achieve the adequate result, which brings the following questions: do we have a plan for our intended result? Is this plan achievable? Is the plan adequate? Is the plan available during surgery? Can feedback on the plan be obtained intraoperatively? Did we achieve the intended result?

These questions led to the introduction and implementation of computer-assisted surgery. From this perspective, all phases of treatment (before, during, and after the surgical procedure) should be optimized for the individual patient. Medical technology turned out to be the cornerstone to take this idea to reality: with technological developments, the limitations in orbital reconstruction could be overcome and the predictability of the results improved. This article covers the intraoperative phase of computer-assisted surgery; with the "why" provided, focus is on the past developments that led to

[a] Department of Oral and Maxillofacial Surgery, Amsterdam UMC Location AMC and Academic Center for Dentistry Amsterdam (ACTA), Meibergdreef 9, 1105 AZ Amsterdam, the Netherlands
[b] Department of Oral and Maxillofacial Surgery, Radboud University Medical Centre Nijmegen, Geert Grooteplein Zuid 10, Nijmegen 6525 GA, the Netherlands
[c] Department of Oral, Maxillofacial and Plastic Surgery, German Armed Forces Hospital of Ulm, Oberer Eselsberg 40, Ulm 89081, Germany
[d] Department of Oral and Maxillofacial Surgery, University Hospital, Ulm University, Albert-Einstein-Allee 23, Ulm 89081, Germany
[e] Department of Oral and Maxillofacial Surgery, Hannover Medical School, Carl-Neuberg-Str. 1, Hannover 30625, Germany
* Corresponding author.
E-mail address: r.schreurs@amsterdamumc.nl

Atlas Oral Maxillofacial Surg Clin N Am 29 (2021) 97-108

https://doi.org/10.1016/j.cxom.2020.11.006

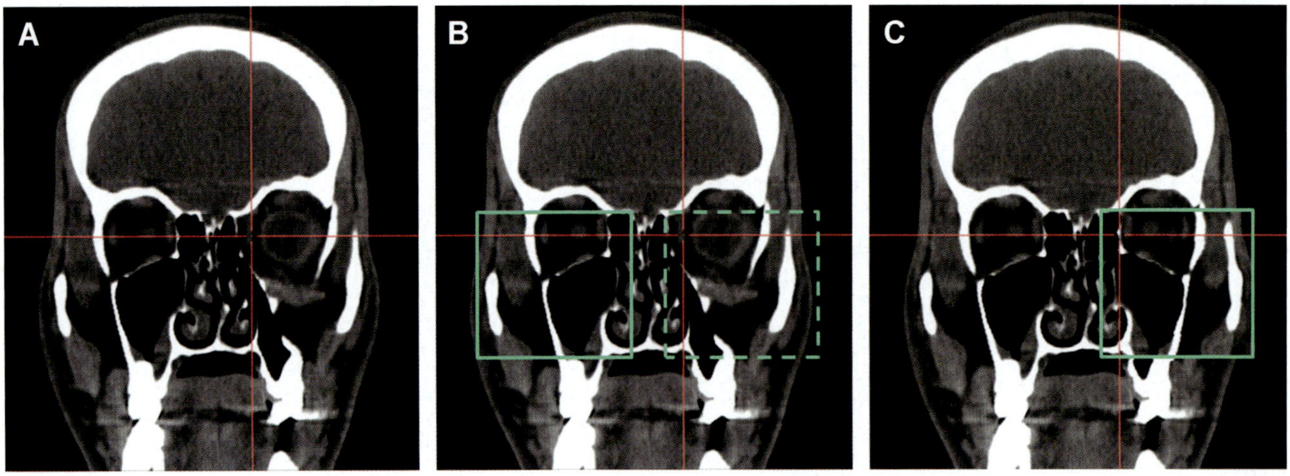

Fig. 1 Visualization of an early virtual surgical planning for an orbitozygomatic complex fracture. A volume of interest is indicated on the unaffected side (*A*) and mirrored to the affected side (*B*), effectively generating a secondary DICOM dataset with the desired reconstruction (*C*). Only the coronal view is shown here for simplification, but all multiplanar directions are available to the surgeon. (*Courtesy of* Ruud Schreurs, MSc, Frank Wilde, MD, DDS, Alexander Schramm, MD, DDS, and Nils-Claudius Gellrich, MD, DDS.)

intraoperative control, the current state of the art, and the possible future of feedback and quality control in orbital surgery: the how, the now, and the wow.

How: the history of intraoperative feedback

Historically, several 2-dimensional (2D) radiographs had been used to approach orbital deformity correction. Today none of these have any impact anymore, and—by the way—there never could be a plan nor a control to what was loaded in and on the orbit. Surgery of the orbit based on 2D radiographs must have been a walk in the mist and darkness. The headway to 3D imaging, in case of orbital reconstruction helical and cone-beam computed tomography (CBCT) (only in selected cases combined with MRI), meets the requirement to treat a 3D defect with the aid of a 3D data set. However, in the eighties of the last decade these data were only used to look at, which meant that trying to understand the individual patient's deformity depended on the views selected by the radiologist. From the nineties onwards, computer technology allowed the surgeon to interactively use the volume data sets on independent analyzing platforms. Clinicians became able to modify the individual volume data set to the intended result.

Mirroring the unaffected side onto the deformed side was the first attempt to virtually correct the bony framework and create a digital blueprint for the reconstruction in unilateral craniofacial defects (Fig. 1). This technique was developed and taken into routine by the Freiburg group of Rainer Schmelzeisen, Alexander Schramm, and Nils-Claudius Gellrich, in cooperation with the former Leibinger Company, trying to make the STN Zeiss/Leibinger navigation system applicable for craniomaxillofacial surgery in those days.[2] All planning had to be performed on the navigation machine itself; it was only in the early 2000s that medical industry was able to serve the demands of the surgeon, and virtual planning became feasible with software on stand-alone machines, independent of the navigation system. It was the cooperation with Brainlab that

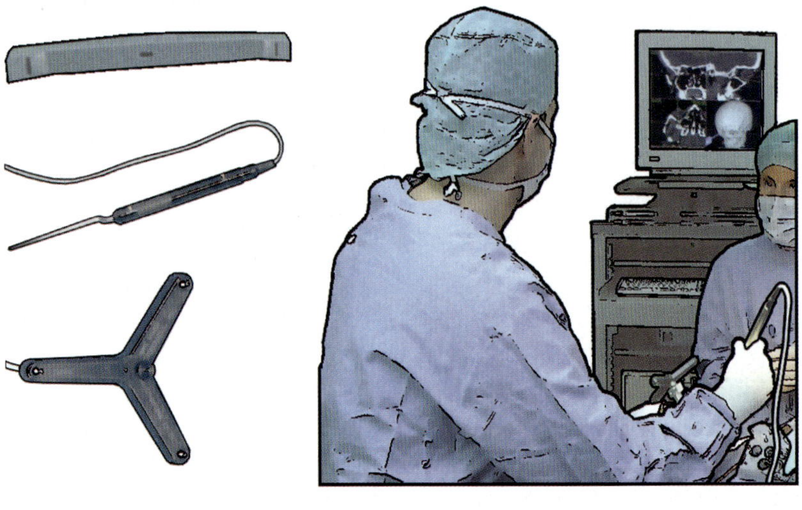

Fig. 2 Instruments of an early navigation system (*left*) and the use of the navigation system (*right*). This system was an optical tracking system with active light-emitting diodes (LEDs) on the instrument and reference array, whose signal was captured by the camera in the top left. Currently, passive and wireless optical systems (see Fig. 8) are most frequently used. (*Courtesy of* Ruud Schreurs, MSc, Frank Wilde, MD, DDS, Alexander Schramm, MD, DDS, and Nils-Claudius Gellrich, MD, DDS.)

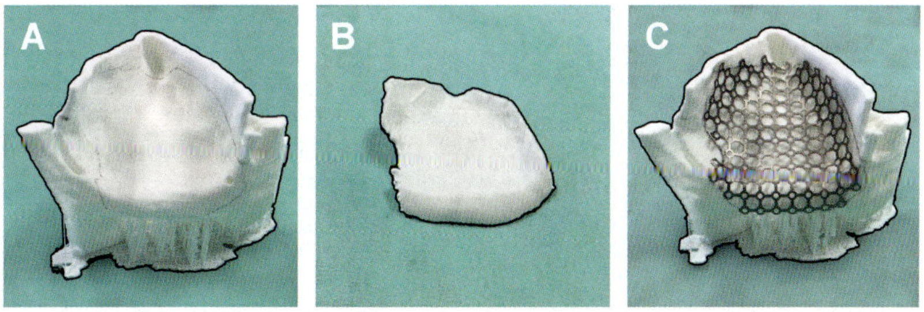

Fig. 3 Prebent implant on an individualized biomodel. In (*A*), the individualized biomodel is shown, whereas (*B*) shows the desired shape of the implant, as constructed in the virtual planning software. The result of the prebent implant is shown in (*C*). (*Courtesy of* Ruud Schreurs, MSc, Frank Wilde, MD, DDS, Alexander Schramm, MD, DDS, and Nils-Claudius Gellrich, MD, DDS.)

resulted in this advancement in planning logistics and the availability of advanced software tools for virtual planning.[3]

The navigation technology may be viewed as the offspring of frame-based stereotaxy, introduced by Horsley and Clarke in 1908.[4–7] Their Horsley-Clarke apparatus, of which the first was produced at a cost of £300, included the use of geometric measurements in a Cartesian coordinate frame.[5,6] An atlas of the position of brain structures within the coordinate frame was generated for cats and monkeys, and the frame and atlas could even be compensated for different head sizes.[5] It was not until 1947 that a modified version of the apparatus, proposed by Spiegel and Wycis, was used in human brain surgery.[8] The link with the preoperative imaging was made with the introduction of frameless stereotaxy in 1987: the position of the pointer tip of an articulating mechanical arm was related to the image data acquired before the operation.[7,9] Optical tracking of the instrument and patient meant increased freedom of movement and easier use of the navigation system.[7] The use of navigation in orbital surgery, almost a decade after Horsley and Clarke laid the groundwork, was kick-started with an article describing the use in a group of 18 patients by the Freiburg group.[2] An image of one of the navigation systems used in these days is provided in Fig. 2.

Developments in 3D imaging have had another effect next to the development of surgical planning and the utilization during surgical navigation: 3D imaging technology became available in the OR itself. Already in the early 1980s applications of imaging during neurosurgery were described, but the fixed position of the scanner and limited image quality hampered it widespread use.[10–13] Advances in image quality, image equipment, and mobility of intraoperative CT or CBCT scanners over the years paved the way for utilization within oral and maxillofacial surgery: it is not surprising that reconstruction of orbital defects was among the first applications.[14]

In the meantime, the gap had to be closed between virtual planning, navigation, and intraoperative imaging on one side and the implant to achieve the desired result on the other. Individualization of orbital implants was historically achieved by preshaping whatever biomaterial during surgery and was thereby depending on the experience and skills of the individual surgeon. Deeply respected colleagues such as Beat Hammer, Joe Gruss, Paul Manson, and others had their own way to prebend, or mold on a nonindividual reference model, with outstanding results. But even at that time they already included some kind of reference, whether it was schematic drawings only or the aforementioned reference skull draped with a sterile foil to serve as an aid for molding the reconstruction material. With further development of 3D printing technologies more and more individualized biomodels of the given (deformed) patient's anatomy or the virtually corrected anatomy became available to shape a nonpreformed biomaterial toward an individual implant, either preoperatively or intraoperatively (Fig. 3).[15,16] This technique still is a valid and an adequate method, which helps to master nearly all kind of craniofacial deformity correction. Latest technology allows to even provide 3D-printed patient-specific biomodels, which are autoclavable.

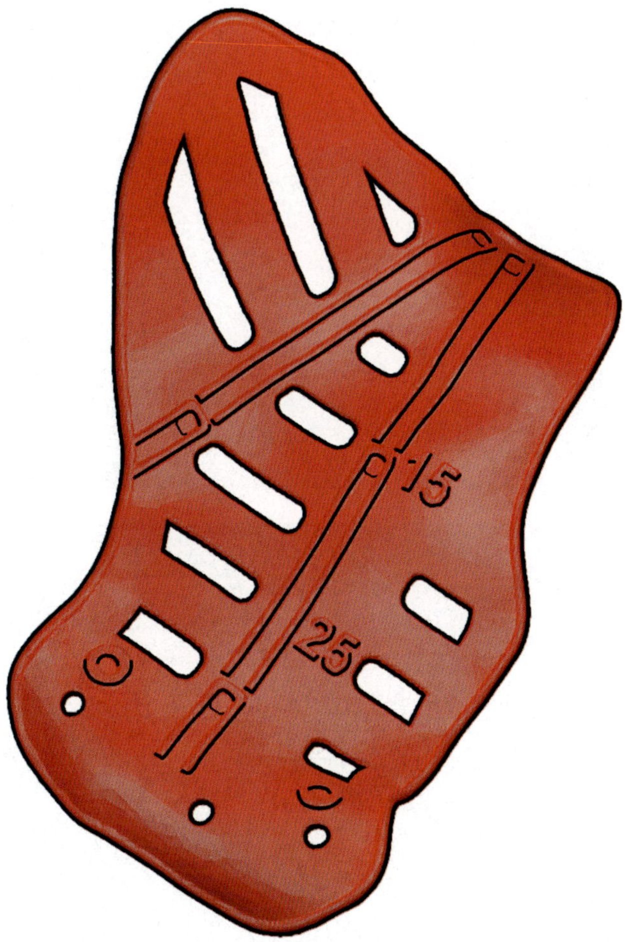

Fig. 4 Patient-specific implant with functionalization and preventive design parameters. The different thickness, cord-style outer boundary, and navigation markers and rulers can be distinguished. (*Courtesy of* Ruud Schreurs, MSc, Frank Wilde, MD, DDS, Alexander Schramm, MD, DDS, and Nils-Claudius Gellrich, MD, DDS.)

A different approach to shaping an implant was developed in parallel. Research on the average shape of the orbit performed by Marc Metzger's group (Freiburg) was a preface for the development of a preformed orbital implant based on the average shape of the orbit and possible defects encountered.[17–19] In theory, the use of such an implant prevents the necessity of preoperative or intraoperative bending altogether, thus saving time and being less dependent on the molding skills of the surgeon.[19,20] Another advantage lies in the possibility to import a virtual model of the preformed implant in the virtual surgical planning. The optimal position of the implant can be determined based on characteristics of patient and defect; it is even possible to evaluate preformed implants of several sizes or different manufacturers (see also article,"Advanced Diagnostics and Three-dimensional Virtual Surgical Planning in Orbital Reconstruction", in this issue).[20–22]

With emerging skills of analyzing patient's volume data sets, the view of taking an individual virtual plan toward an adequate individual anatomic shaped implant changed the requirements of what an implant should be able to provide and represent: above the effect of an anatomic replacement the terms "functionalization" and "preventive design" of an implant came up. Functionalization implies that functions were added to the implant, for example, position control information was added for navigation purposes. Furthermore, anatomic extensions or flings can be added to an implant, so that the implant properly leavers on reliable structures in the defect site. Preventive design implies that typical mistakes that might occur with specific procedures can be diminished: in reconstructive orbital surgery this refers to change of implant shape, sharp edges, and possible interference with the optic nerve or eye muscles especially in the orbital cone area. This is why the Hannover Group with Majeed Rana and Nils-Claudius Gellrich developed a patient-specific orbital implant with a distinct topography of different thickness, a slightly thickened circular outer rounded cord-style implant border, an inverted snow-shovel design in the area of the posterior ledge, and multiple linear openings perpendicular to the transition zone for the medial orbital wall and perpendicular to the parasagittal oblique vector for the orbital floor.[23] These implementations can be seen in Figs. 4.

Now: current concepts in state-of-the-art quality control

Diagnosis precedes the computer-assisted reconstruction of the orbit and is based on clinical findings and 3D imaging.[24–28]

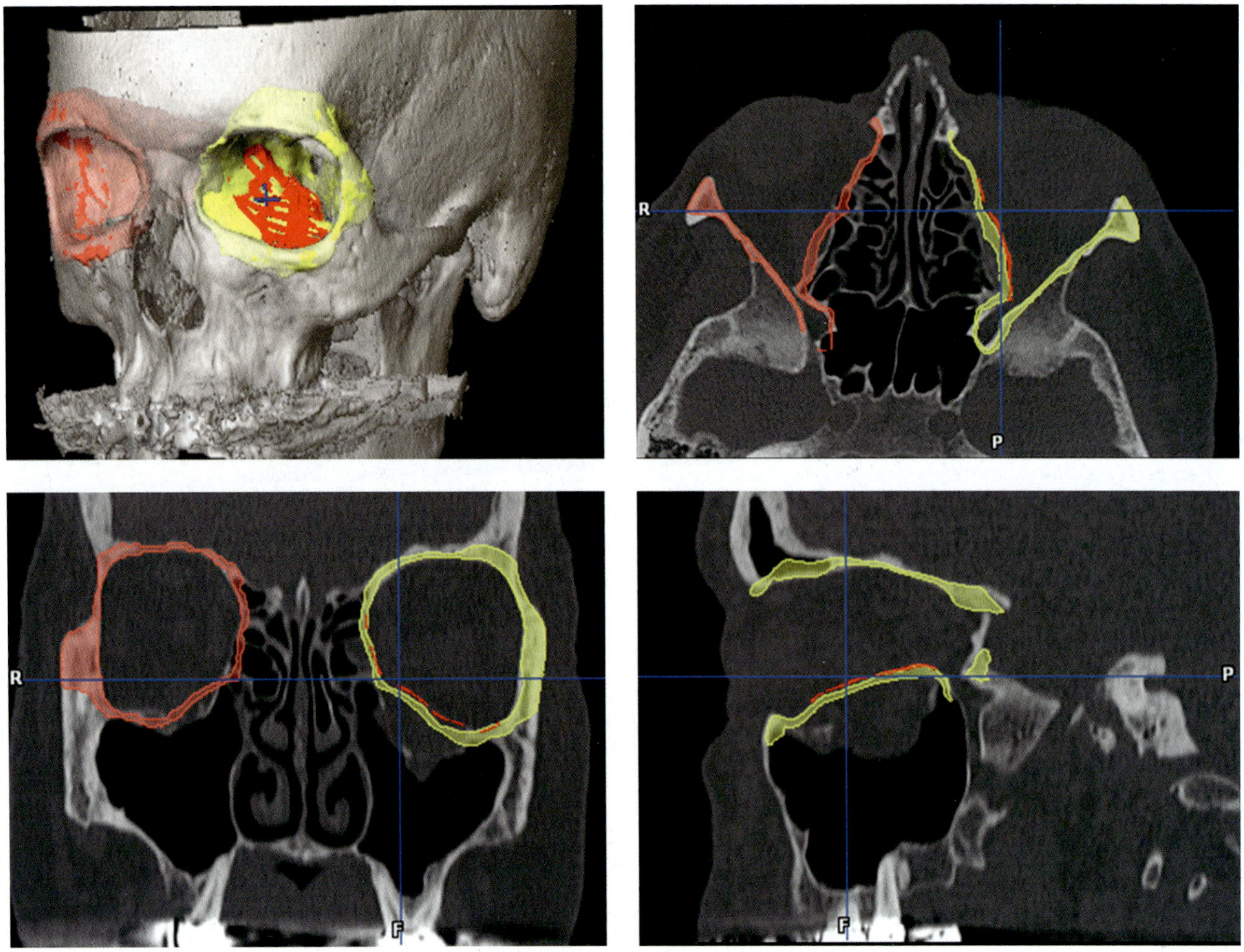

Fig. 5 Multiplanar view of the virtual reconstruction with a virtually placed patient-specific implant that was imported into the left orbit as an STL data set after industrial planning (*red contour line*). Virtual implant placement allows the accuracy of fit to be verified before the implant is manufactured. (*Courtesy of* Ruud Schreurs, MSc, Frank Wilde, MD, DDS, Alexander Schramm, MD, DDS, and Nils-Claudius Gellrich, MD, DDS.)

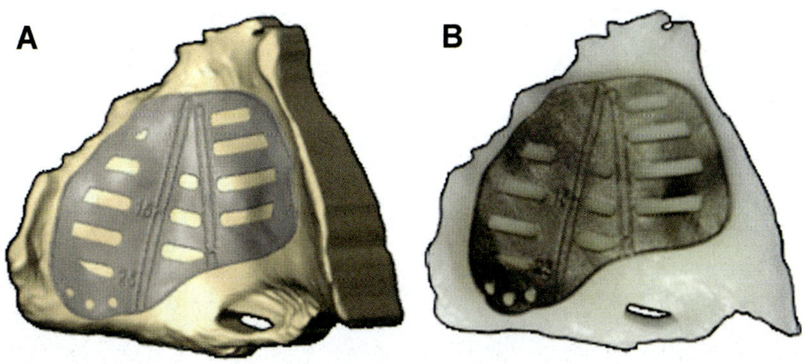

Fig. 6 Computer-aided design of the patient-specific implant (*A*) and the selective laser-melted patient-specific implant corresponding to the design (*B*). (*Courtesy of* Ruud Schreurs, MSc, Frank Wilde, MD, DDS, Alexander Schramm, MD, DDS, and Nils-Claudius Gellrich, MD, DDS.)

As discussed in article,"Advanced Diagnostics and Three-dimensional Virtual Surgical Planning in Orbital Reconstruction", in this issue CT must be regarded as the gold standard for primary diagnosis preceding orbital reconstruction and should be preferred. It provides not only excellent resolution of bone structures but, unlike CBCT, also allows soft-tissue structures to be evaluated, especially with the use of contrast agent.[28] In current concepts of intraoperative feedback workflows, virtual surgical planning and simulation of the reconstruction serves as the reference of the feedback obtained. The objective of surgical planning is to perform an ideal reconstruction based on a virtual model that matches the desired outcome of surgery.[1,7,29,30]

Although discussed in greater detail in article,"Advanced Diagnostics and Three-dimensional Virtual Surgical Planning in Orbital Reconstruction", in this issue several important factors include that many different types of simulations may be performed without a loss of information, 2D and 3D images may be displayed in any plane before and during surgery, and virtual models (STL data) may be imported.[1,31–33] These factors allow that standard implants, anatomically preformed implants, and patient-specific implants can be virtually positioned in the patient data set preoperatively and their shape, size, and fit can be assessed (Fig. 5).[26,30,32] If a patient-specific implant is indicated for the orbital reconstruction, the next step on the ladder is to process virtual reconstruction STL data sets using computer-aided design (CAD) software for planning patient-specific implants (Fig. 6A) and to directly produce these implants using computer-aided manufacturing (CAM) techniques such

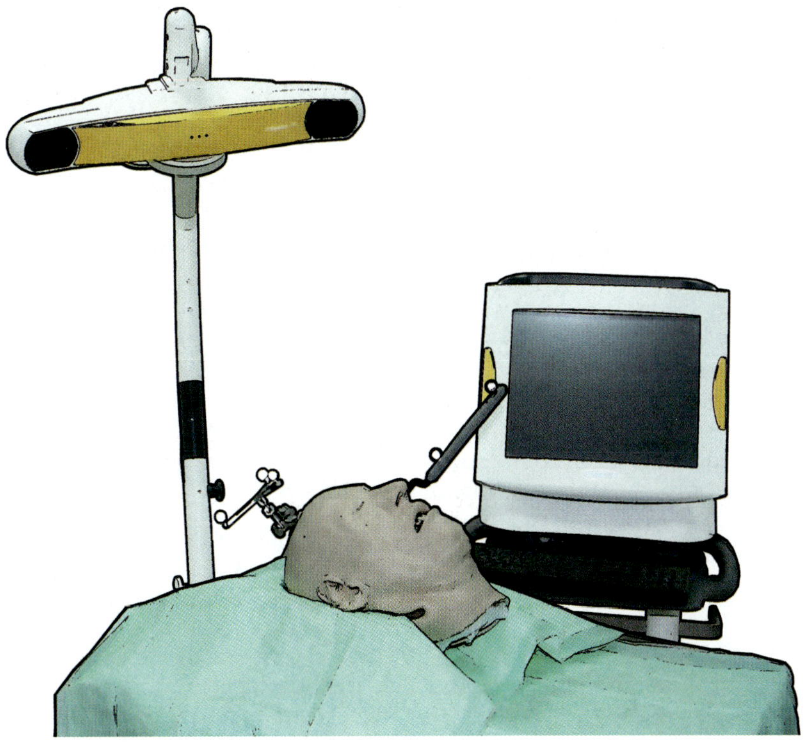

Fig. 7 Intraoperative setup of an indirect navigation system: camera with integrated LEDs, pointer with 2 reflective spheres, reference array with 3 reflective spheres attached to the calvaria, touch screen. (*Courtesy of* Ruud Schreurs, MSc, Frank Wilde, MD, DDS, Alexander Schramm, MD, DDS, and Nils-Claudius Gellrich, MD, DDS.)

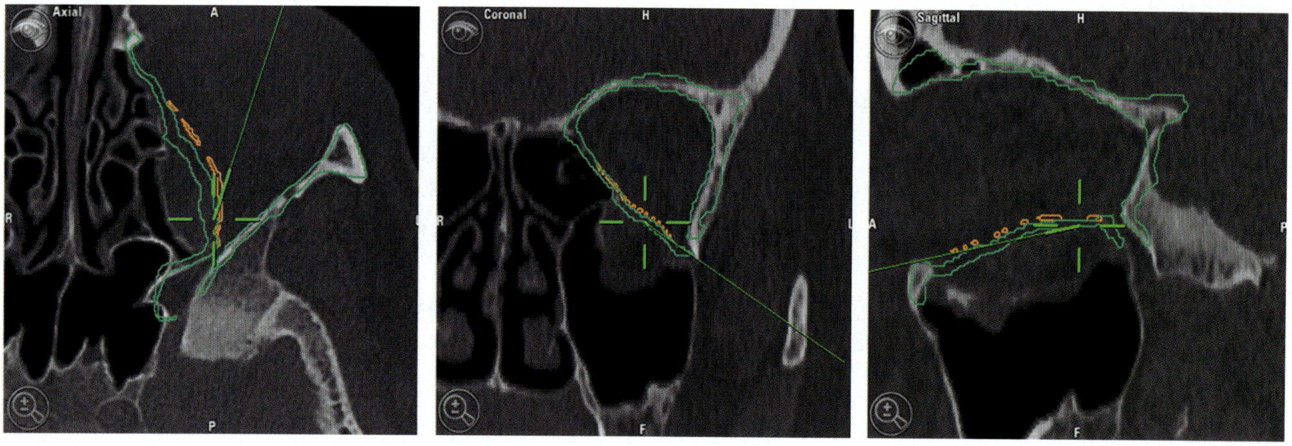

Fig. 8 Screenshots from multiplanar views on the navigation screen during surgery. The green line with the green cross represents the pointer in the orbit to control the position and fit of inserted implants during surgery. (*Courtesy of* Ruud Schreurs, MSc, Frank Wilde, MD, DDS, Alexander Schramm, MD, DDS, and Nils-Claudius Gellrich, MD, DDS.)

as selective laser melting (Fig. 6B). During the surgical procedure, surgeons have the difficult task of transferring the result of virtual computer-assisted planning to the surgical site as accurately as possible. For this purpose, they can use and combine a variety of different methods and devices, depending on the complexity of the task.

Patient-specific implants

Customized CAD-/CAM-fabricated implants are increasingly used for orbital reconstructions. Titanium mesh structures have proved their favorable material characteristics for orbital reconstructions. Selective laser melting of titanium powder allows high-precision titanium mesh structures of any complexity and geometry to be manufactured. Because it is now possible to obtain such patient-specific implants within 5 working days from planning to delivery, it has become possible to use such implants even for primary and not exclusively for secondary reconstructions. The aforementioned functionalization and preventive design parameters are incorporated as much as possible in the implant's design, so that not only "the perfect lid could be manufactured for an individual pot" but also "the perfect lid could sit in the perfect position." The exact fit of the implant, the use of surgical guides, the incorporation of "old" screw hole positions from the primary reconstruction (in secondary cases), and the use of navigation markers or rulers all aid in achieving this goal.[23,34] The challenge to obtain a correct postoperative result without the use of these implants is definitely higher. Apart from the orbit—which pioneered these implant developments with much higher demands and clinical relevance—any other implant used in craniomaxillofacial surgery or even the human body profits from these advances in orbital surgery.

Intraoperative navigation

Nowadays, intraoperative navigation with modern infrared-based navigation systems has become an integral part of computer-assisted maxillofacial reconstruction.[1,7] Before the start of the surgical procedure, the patient in the operation room must be "fused" with the image data set that is displayed on the screen. This process is known as registration and is based on reference points that must be clearly identifiable and reproducible both on the patient and in the image data set. Because the patient's position must be permanently tracked because patient movements during surgery cannot be prevented or may even be necessary during the procedure, a reference array is attached to the patient's head, which allows the navigation system to register all patient movements without limiting head mobility (see Fig. 7).[1,7,32]

Once the patient is registered with the DICOM set, the tip of the pointer can be visualized in the image volume on the screen of the navigation system, which enables surgeons to verify the realignment of bone fragments and the position and fit of inserted implants during surgery and to make any necessary changes without patient exposure to ionizing radiation. In this process, the virtual reconstruction that has been made during the planning phase serves as an intraoperative template that helps surgeons align bone fragments and/or place implants (Fig. 8).[1,7,29,30] The direction of the navigation rulers, or the position of navigation markers, allows easier interpretation of the acquired implant position by the surgeon.[23,35]

Intraoperative imaging

Although functionalized implants and intraoperative navigation can provide usable information during reconstruction, the surgical outcome in orbital surgery should always be validated and documented in 3D by the use of CT or CBCT. Although intraoperative navigation can already provide relatively precise information about the position of osteosynthesis material and the repositioning of bone fragments, it cannot completely replace a radiological examination, because navigation can never visualize the entire surgical site. It is recommendable that such a radiological validation should be performed during the surgical procedure immediately after reconstruction, which allows necessary modifications such as incorrect positions of bone fragments and implants to be made during the surgical procedure.[27,30,32] CBCT technology offers several advantages that make this modality superior. CBCT systems are available as mobile, ceiling-suspended, or floor-mounted 3D C-arm systems for use in the operating room or as small compact CBCT systems for intraoperative use (Fig. 9).[32] The systems produce image series for multiplanar visualization in the axial,

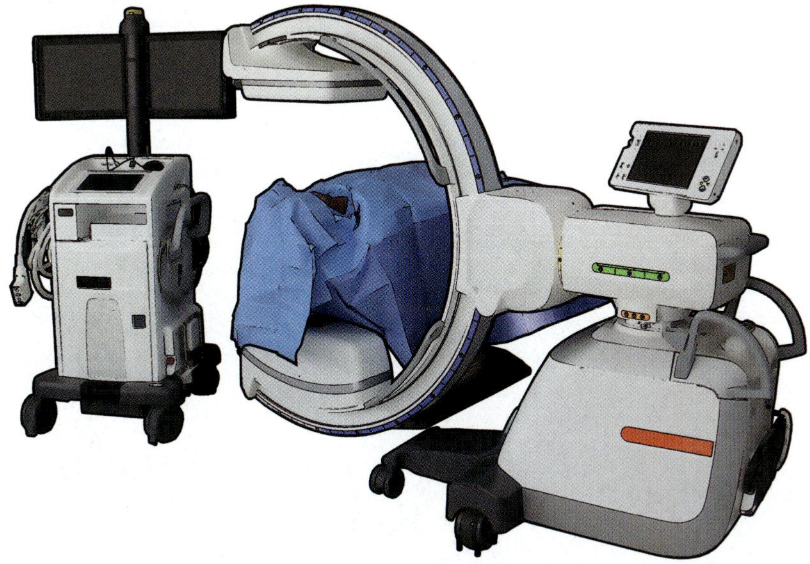

Fig. 9 Mobile 3D C-arm device for intraoperative imaging in action. (*Courtesy of* Ruud Schreurs, MSc, Frank Wilde, MD, DDS, Alexander Schramm, MD, DDS, and Nils-Claudius Gellrich, MD, DDS.)

coronal, and sagittal planes and thus allow hard tissues to be imaged during surgery. Images that are produced by these systems are nowadays of such good quality that additional postoperative imaging is usually not required anymore.[27]

The purpose of intraoperative and postoperative 3D imaging is not only to perform a surgical procedure under radiological control but also to provide data sets for computer-assisted fusion with preoperative image data sets and especially with preoperative computer planning. Image fusion allows differences between preoperative planning and surgical outcome to be visualized and, if required, to be quantitatively evaluated within the scope of quality assurance (Fig. 10).

Wow: the future of orbital reconstruction

Technological innovation will affect the utilization of all of the abovementioned technologies for intraoperative feedback and even add novel methods of obtaining feedback during surgery. Separate feedback modalities are already combined into a symbiotic feedback system: the aforementioned functionalization of a patient-specific implant design allows it to be equipped with navigation rulers and markers to optimize navigation feedback (see Fig. 4).[23,36] The unique fit and addition of rulers and markers in the design is an example of 2 combined feedback mechanisms that allow improved feedback

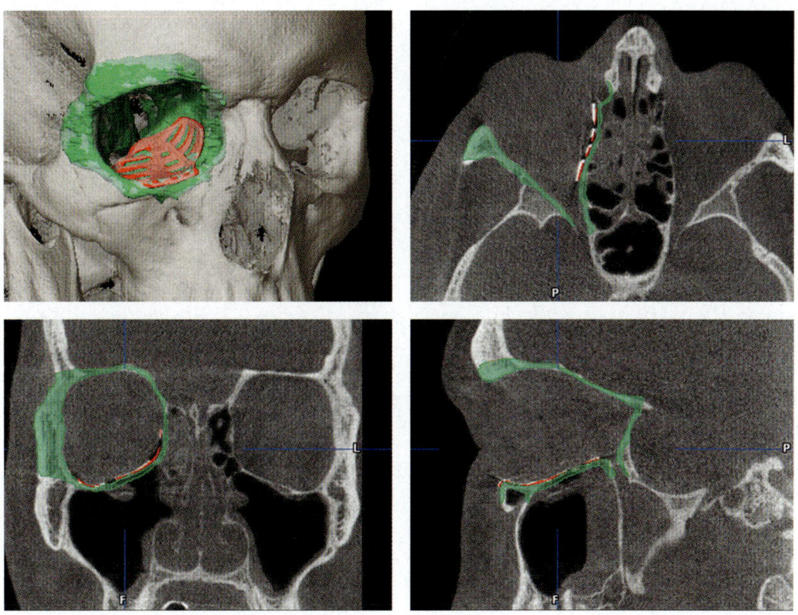

Fig. 10 Multiplanar view of intraoperative 3D imaging with superimposition of virtual planning. The green contour line shows the virtual reconstruction of the orbit and the red contour the planned implant. The image shows good fit of the radio-opaque implant in accordance with virtual planning. (*Courtesy of* Ruud Schreurs, MSc, Frank Wilde, MD, DDS, Alexander Schramm, MD, DDS, and Nils-Claudius Gellrich, MD, DDS.)

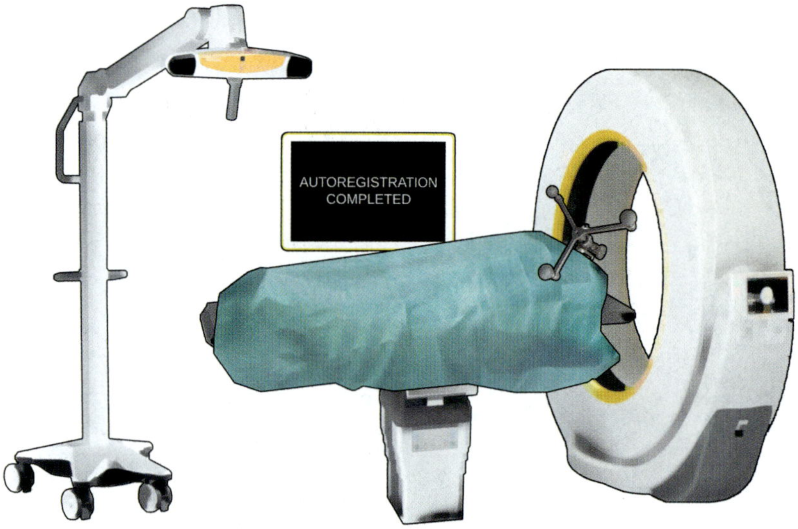

Fig. 11 Autoregistration setup. Intraoperative imaging is combined with the registration procedure for navigation, allowing (re-) registration in the operation room without the need for user intervention. (*Courtesy of* Ruud Schreurs, MSc, Frank Wilde, MD, DDS, Alexander Schramm, MD, DDS, and Nils-Claudius Gellrich, MD, DDS.)

intraoperatively. Another example is the fact that intraoperative imaging can be transferred to the preoperative planning modality automatically to generate instant feedback on the reconstruction result[37–39] and may even provide (re-) registration if used in combination with intraoperative navigation (Fig. 11). Registration of the patient to the virtual surgical plan can now be performed without the need for user intervention. Still, improvements to the already comprehensive feedback are possible in several areas, such as preoperative design, preoperative simulation, intraoperative visualization, and intraoperative control.

The design of a patient-specific implant is nowadays performed largely manually: a designer from a third-party company designs the implant in consultation with the surgeon, or in specific cases the design is performed in-house by a clinical technician or the surgeon. In every scenario, the design is based on the individual patient's characteristics but influenced by experience and preference of designer and surgeon. Design considerations such as implant's size, compelling fit, and feedback mechanisms incorporated are operator dependent, and the quality of intraoperative feedback obtained from the shape and fit of the patient-specific implant is affected by previous experience in patient-specific implant design. An overview of the design workflow is provided in Fig. 12A. The use of artificial intelligence in the preoperative planning process could induce automation in the patient-specific implant design process, while bearing optimal intra-operative feedback in mind (Fig. 12B), and this could save time in the planning process, perfect the compelling fit, and make individualized treatment more accessible to surgeons without previous experience in patient-specific implant design.

Obtaining experience in orbital reconstruction is difficult in general, because of the keyhole access and limited exposure of the surgical field. The intraoperative feedback modalities may aid in the understanding of the procedure, but they are no substitute for hands-on learning experience. Preoperative surgical simulation could provide a possible solution.[40] In current state-of-the-art simulation, a walk-through of the complete surgery is performed on a 3D-printed model consisting of several components, which simulate the tactile feedback of anatomic structures encountered.[41] The virtual model is seen in Fig. 13A, and the physical components are seen in Fig. 13B. Intraoperative navigation for quality control in the simulation setting makes the training surgeon familiar with its use and interpretation (Fig. 13C). Simulation could also benefit experienced surgeons, for complex conditions or procedures. Currently, physical models are used, because virtual simulation is associated with high cost and difficulty to simulate invasive procedures. If these drawbacks are overcome, virtual simulation obviates production time and cost and has the potential to simulate patient-specific surgeries (repetitively) and be incorporated in the computer-assisted surgery workflow.

Visualization during surgery could also benefit from further developments. Although frequently compared with car navigation, intraoperative navigation is not nearly as intuitive. Feedback is provided to review the acquired position, rather than real-time during positioning, and interpretation of implant position from the navigation pointer's position is left to the surgeon. Real-time, intuitive feedback during positioning (similar to car navigation) requires the implant to be tracked at all times and its position expressed relative to the target position. A navigation-compatible positioning instrument for orbital reconstruction has been proposed that meets these requirements (Fig. 14), and software has been developed to provide real-time instructions on positioning, both visually and quantitatively.[42] Positioning with the instrument and the real-time navigation feedback obtained are visualized in Fig. 15. The effect on implant position has been established in preclinical testing (see article, "Advanced Concepts of Orbital Reconstruction: A Unique Attempt to Scientifically Evaluate Individual Techniques in Reconstruction of Large Orbital Defects," in this issue.).[43]

Current methods using visual feedback require the surgeon to evaluate 3D information on a 2D screen and switch focus between surgical site and monitor. Augmented reality possesses the possibility to tackle both problems by enhancing the surgeon's view of the surgical site with a virtual overlay.[44–47] The information presented in this overlay could be the virtual planning: in Fig. 16A, the surgeon's view of the real world is seen; the virtual layer in Fig. 16B contains objects from the

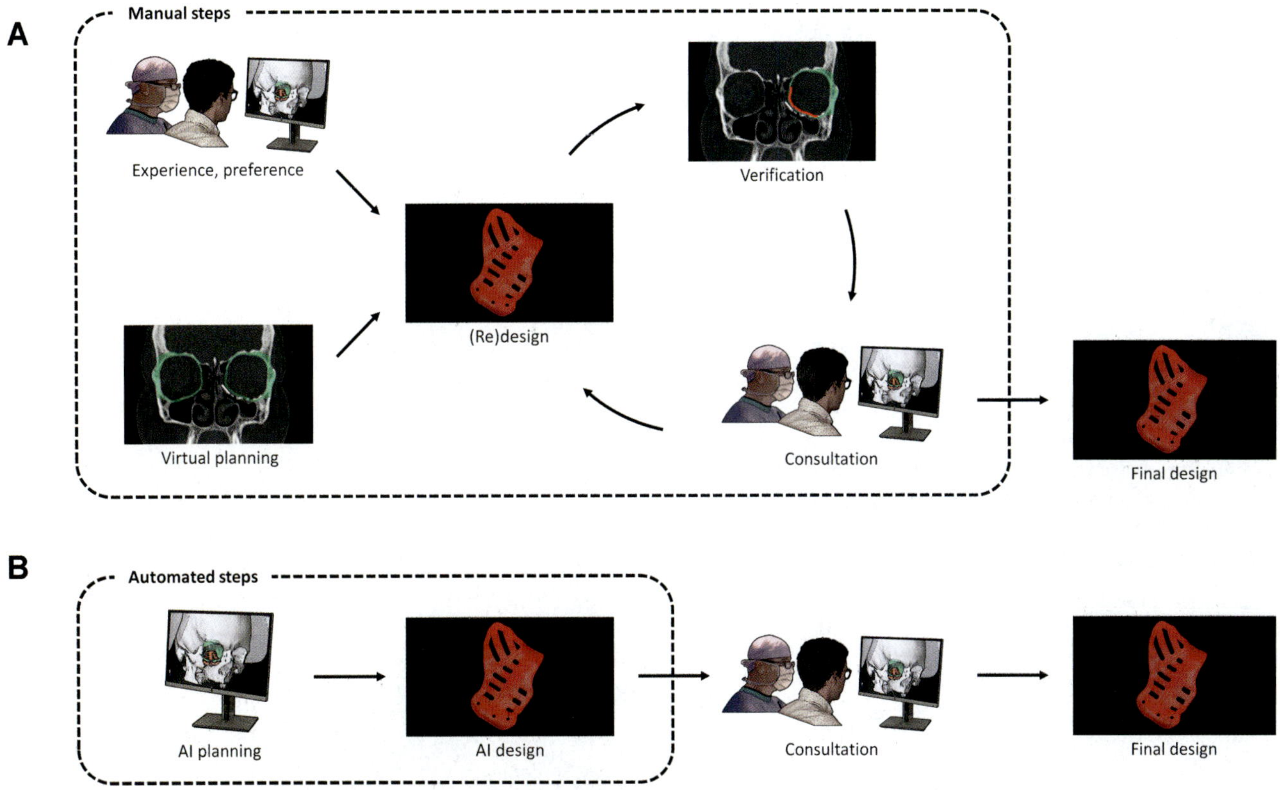

Fig. 12 Visualization of current PSI design workflow (*A*), with much of the design choices based on experience and preference of the surgeon and designer. Many manual steps need to be completed in order to obtain the final PSI design. In (*B*), a proposed AI-supported workflow is visualized. The planning and preliminary design is performed largely automatically, saving time and making PSI design more accessible to surgeons without previous experience in PSI treatment. AI, artificial intelligence; PSI, patient-specific implant. (*Courtesy of* Ruud Schreurs, MSc, Frank Wilde, MD, DDS, Alexander Schramm, MD, DDS, and Nils-Claudius Gellrich, MD, DDS.)

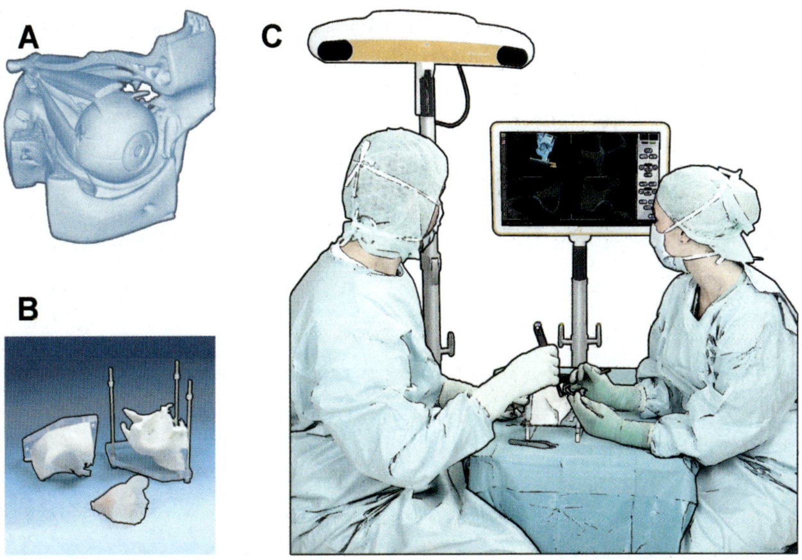

Fig. 13 Surgical simulation of orbital reconstruction. The virtual model of the orbit and orbital contents is visualized in (*A*). Physical models based on the virtual model are generated through 3D printing; the individual components consist of different materials to simulate tactile feedback during surgery (*B*). The simulation is compatible with intraoperative navigation, which allows the surgeon to get familiar with the interpretation of the feedback the system provides. The complete setup is seen in (*C*). (*Courtesy of* Ruud Schreurs, MSc, Frank Wilde, MD, DDS, Alexander Schramm, MD, DDS, and Nils-Claudius Gellrich, MD, DDS.)

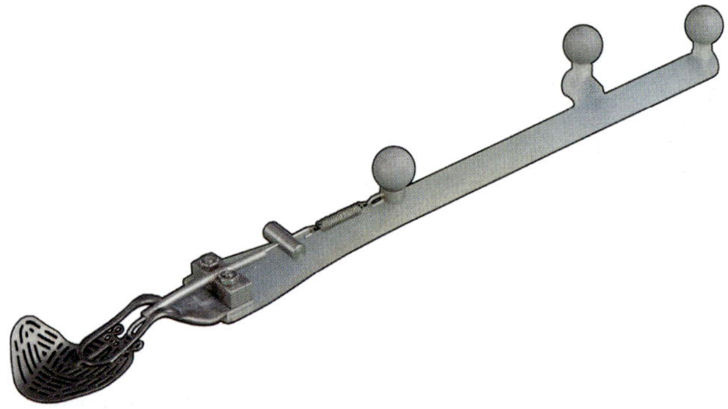

Fig. 14 Navigation-compatible positioning instrument. The orbital implant can be attached to the instrument in a unique way (and detached after fixation); the position of the orbital implant can be calculated from the position of the navigation feedback the instrument generates. (*Courtesy of* Ruud Schreurs, MSc, Frank Wilde, MD, DDS, Alexander Schramm, MD, DDS, and Nils-Claudius Gellrich, MD, DDS.)

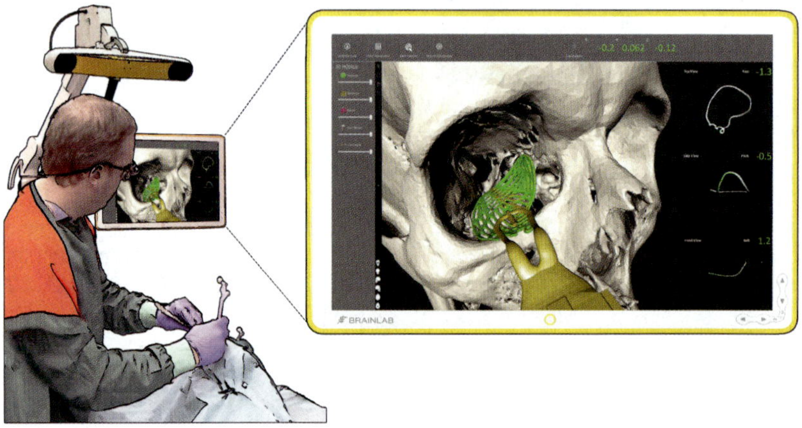

Fig. 15 Real-time navigation setup and feedback. The orbital implant is tracked through the instrument, which the surgeon uses to position the orbital implant. Real-time feedback consists of a 3D view of the planned and current position of the implant; the color changes according to the current deviation. Separate views representing a top view, side view, and frontal view of the implant outline are added for detailed positioning information. Quantitative feedback on rotation and translation is provided next to the separate views and top, respectively. (*Courtesy of* Ruud Schreurs, MSc, Frank Wilde, MD, DDS, Alexander Schramm, MD, DDS, and Nils-Claudius Gellrich, MD, DDS.)

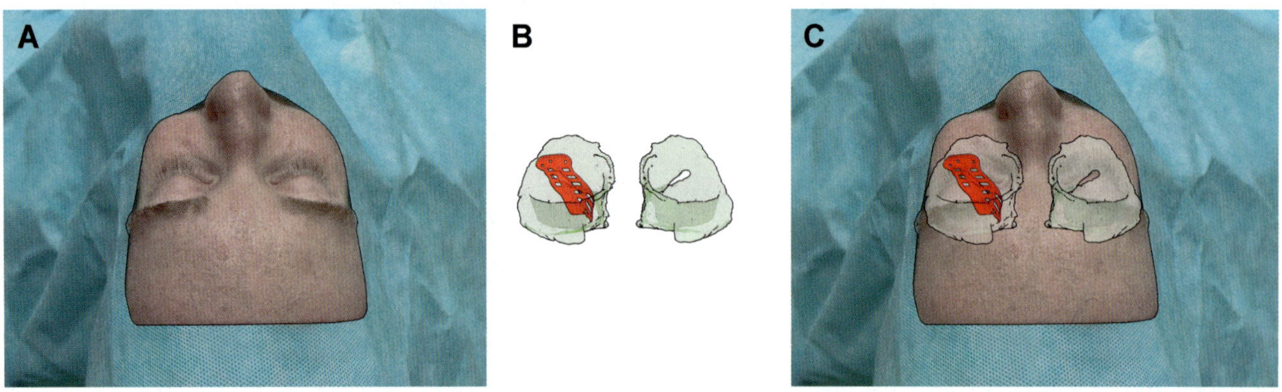

Fig. 16 Principle of augmented reality. The real world, as seen by the surgeon, is seen in (*A*). In (*B*), the virtual layer to be augmented on the real-world view is shown, which corresponds to the planned objects in the virtual surgical planning. In (*C*), the augmented reality view is shown: the virtual layer is added to the real world for a combined view. (*Courtesy of* Ruud Schreurs, MSc, Frank Wilde, MD, DDS, Alexander Schramm, MD, DDS, and Nils-Claudius Gellrich, MD, DDS.)

planning. In Fig. 16C, the augmented view of the surgeon is seen. Even more valuable feedback may become available through combination with real-time navigation: a see-through view of the orbit with the planned and current implant position could be added to the operator's view.

In a more distant future, robotic-assisted orbital reconstruction may become available. Several approaches could be imagined, ranging from simple tasks such as aiding in fixation by stabilizing the acquired implant position to more complex methods, such as movement constraints for the surgeon to keep clear of vital anatomic structures and minimize the amount of iatrogenic damage.[48,49] Fully autonomous implant insertion may even be feasible from a technical point of view, but this may be constrained by medicolegal issues. The key to successful implementation of any of these futuristic technologies in orbital reconstruction may be the same as the strategy seen in current intraoperative feedback methods: combining techniques to use their respective strengths and cover the individual frailties.

CLINICS CARE POINTS

- Patient-specific implants hold the highest potential for optimal reconstruction of an orbital defect. A design tailored to the defect and surrounding anatomy, and functionalization of the implant for combination with other feedback techniques, ensure an optimal implant that leads to an optimal reconstruction.
- Intraoperative navigation has become an integral part of computer-assisted maxillofacial reconstruction. It is able to provide feedback to improve predictability during orbital reconstruction.
- The surgical outcome in orbital reconstruction should always be validated and documented. If imaging is performed intraoperatively, necessary modifications may be made during the surgical procedure and revision surgeries may be prevented.

Disclosure

The authors have nothing to disclose.

References

1. Schramm A, Gellrich NC. Intraoperative navigation und computerassistierte Chirurgie. Schwenzer N Und Ehrenfeld M Zahn-Mund-Kieferheilkunde. Mund Kiefer Gesichtschir 2011;4:479–99.
2. Gellrich N-C, Schramm A, Hammer B, et al. Computer-assisted secondary reconstruction of unilateral posttraumatic orbital deformity. Plast Reconstr Surg 2002;110(6):1417–29.
3. Metzger MC, Bittermann G, Dannenberg L, et al. Design and development of a virtual anatomic atlas of the human skull for automatic segmentation in computer-assisted surgery, preoperative planning, and navigation. Int J Comput Assist Radiol Surg 2013; 8(5):691–702.
4. Horsley V, Clarke RH. The structure and functions of the cerebellum examined by a new method. Brain 1908;31(1):45–124.
5. Schurr PH, Merrington WR. The Horsley–Clarke stereotaxic apparatus. Br J Surg 1978;65(1):33–6.
6. Jensen RL, Stone JL, Hayne RA. Introduction of the human Horsley-Clarke stereotactic frame. Neurosurgery 1996;38(3):563–7.
7. Schramm A, Gellrich N-C, Schmelzeisen R. Navigational surgery of the facial skeleton. Springer Science & Business Media; 2007.
8. Spiegel EA, Wycis HT, Marks M, et al. Stereotaxic apparatus for operations on the human brain. Science 1947;106(2754): 349–50.
9. Watanabe E, Watanabe T, Manaka S, et al. Three-dimensional digitizer (neuronavigator): new equipment for computed tomography-guided stereotaxic surgery. Surg Neurol 1987;27(6):543–7.
10. Shalit MN, Israeli Y, Matz S, et al. Intra-operative computerized axial tomography. Surg Neurol 1979;11(5):382–4.
11. Lunsford LD, Parrish R, Albright L. Intraoperative imaging with a therapeutic computed tomographic scanner. Neurosurgery 1984; 15(4):559–61.
12. Schichor C, Terpolilli N, Thorsteinsdottir J, et al. Intraoperative computed tomography in cranial neurosurgery. Neurosurg Clin N Am 2017;28(4):595–602.
13. Nimsky C, Carl B. Historical, current, and future intraoperative imaging modalities. Neurosurg Clin N Am 2017;28(4):453–64.
14. Stanley RB. Use of intraoperative computed tomography during repair of orbitozygomatic fractures. Arch Facial Plast Surg 1999; 1(1):19–24.
15. Doerfler H-M, Huempfner-Hierl H, Kruber D, et al. Template-based orbital wall fracture treatment using statistical shape analysis. J Oral Maxillofac Surg 2017;75(7):1475-e1.
16. Kim YC, Jeong WS, Park T, et al. The accuracy of patient specific implant prebented with 3D-printed rapid prototype model for orbital wall reconstruction. J Craniomaxillofac Surg 2017;45(6):928–36.
17. Metzger MC, Schön R, Tetzlaf R, et al. Topographical CT-data analysis of the human orbital floor. Int J Oral Maxillofac Surg 2007; 36(1):45–53.
18. Bell RB. Computer planning and intraoperative navigation in cranio-maxillofacial surgery. Oral Maxillofac Surg Clin North Am 2010; 22(1):135–56.
19. Metzger MC, Schmelzeisen R. Craniomaxillofacial Implants Based on 3D Modeling. Digital Technologies in Craniomaxillofacial Surgery. Springer; 2018. p. 167–73.
20. Strong EB, Fuller SC, Wiley DF, et al. Preformed vs intraoperative bending of titanium mesh for orbital reconstruction. Otolaryngol Head Neck Surg 2013;149(1):60–6.
21. Bittermann G, Metzger MC, Schlager S, et al. Orbital reconstruction: prefabricated implants, data transfer, and revision surgery. Facial Plast Surg 2014;30(05):554–60.
22. Hierl T, Kruber D, Doerfler H-M, et al. Computer-aided versus conventional planning in orbital traumatology using preformed meshes: development of a new workflow. J Oral Maxillofac Surg 2019;77(8):1663–72.
23. Rana M, Chui CHK, Wagner M, et al. Increasing the accuracy of orbital reconstruction with selective laser-melted patient-specific implants combined with intraoperative navigation. J Oral Maxillofac Surg 2015;73(6):1113–8.
24. Manson PN, Markowitz B, Mirvis S, et al. Toward CT-based facial fracture treatment. Plast Reconstr Surg 1990;85(2):202–12.
25. Tanrikulu R, Erol B. Comparison of computed tomography with conventional radiography for midfacial fractures. Dentomaxillofac Radiol 2001;30(3):141–6.
26. Wilde F, Hilbert J, Kamer L, et al. The combination of automatic segmentation, preformed implants, intraoperative navigation and intraoperative imaging in primary orbital wall reconstruction: description of a new method. Int J Comput Assist Radiol Surg 2009;4:134.
27. Wilde F, Lorenz K, Ebner A-K, et al. Intraoperative imaging with a 3D C-arm system after zygomatico-orbital complex fracture reduction. J Oral Maxillofac Surg 2013;71(5):894–910.
28. Wikner J, Riecke B, Gröbe A, et al. Imaging of the midfacial and orbital trauma. Facial Plast Surg 2014;30(05):528–36.
29. Hohlweg-Majert B, Schön R, Schmelzeisen R, et al. Navigational maxillofacial surgery using virtual models. World J Surg 2005; 29(12):1530–8.
30. Schramm A, Wilde F. Die computergestützte Gesichtsschädelrekonstruktion. HNO 2011;59(8):800.
31. Markiewicz MR, Bell RB. Modern concepts in computer-assisted craniomaxillofacial reconstruction. Curr Opin Otolaryngol Head Neck Surg 2011;19(4):295–301.

32. Wilde F, Schramm A. Intraoperative imaging in orbital and midface reconstruction. Facial Plast Surg 2014;30(05):545–53.
33. Parthasarathy J. 3D modeling, custom implants and its future perspectives in craniofacial surgery. Ann Maxillofac Surg 2014; 4(1):9.
34. Schreurs R, Dubois L, Becking AG, et al. The orbit first! A novel surgical treatment protocol for secondary orbitozygomatic reconstruction. J Craniomaxillofac Surg 2017;45(7). https://doi.org/10.1016/j.jcms.2017.03.026.
35. Dubois L, Essig H, Schreurs R, et al. Predictability in orbital reconstruction. A human cadaver study, part III: implant-oriented navigation for optimized reconstruction. J Craniomaxillofac Surg 2015;43(10):2050–6.
36. Gander T, Essig H, Metzler P, et al. Patient specific implants (PSI) in reconstruction of orbital floor and wall fractures. J Craniomaxillofac Surg 2015;43(1):126–30.
37. Grauvogel TD, Becker C, Hassepass F, et al. Comparison of 3D C-arm–based registration to conventional pair-point registration regarding navigation accuracy in ENT surgery. Otolaryngol Head Neck Surg 2015;152(2):266–71.
38. Carl B, Bopp M, Saß B, et al. Intraoperative computed tomography as reliable navigation registration device in 200 cranial procedures. Acta Neurochir (Wien) 2018;160(9):1681–9.
39. Carl B, Bopp M, Saß B, et al. Reliable navigation registration in cranial and spine surgery based on intraoperative computed tomography. Neurosurg Focus 2019;47(6):E11.
40. Selzer DJ. Overview of Simulation in Surgery. Comprehensive Healthcare Simulation: Surgery and Surgical Subspecialties. Springer; 2019. p. 13–23.
41. Lichtenstein JT, Zeller AN, Lemound J, et al. 3D-printed simulation device for orbital surgery. J Surg Educ 2017;74(1):2–8.
42. Schreurs R, Dubois L, Becking AG, et al. Implant-oriented navigation in orbital reconstruction. Part 1: technique and accuracy study. Int J Oral Maxillofac Surg 2017;47(3):395–402.
43. Schreurs R, Dubois L, Ho J, et al. Implant-oriented navigation in orbital reconstruction part II: preclinical cadaver study. Int J Oral Maxillofac Surg 2019;49(5):678–85.
44. Vigh B, Müller S, Ristow O, et al. The use of a head-mounted display in oral implantology: a feasibility study. Int J Comput Assist Radiol Surg 2014;9(1):71–8.
45. Wang J, Suenaga H, Yang L, et al. Video see-through augmented reality for oral and maxillofacial surgery. Int J Med Robot 2017; 13(2):e1754.
46. Meulstee JW, Nijsink J, Schreurs R, et al. Toward holographic-guided surgery. Surg Innov 2018;26(1). 1553350618799552.
47. Wang J, Shen Y, Yang S. A practical marker-less image registration method for augmented reality oral and maxillofacial surgery. Int J Comput Assist Radiol Surg 2019;14(5):763–73.
48. Davies B. A review of robotics in surgery. Proc Inst Mech Eng H. 2000;214(1):129–40.
49. Camarillo DB, Krummel TM, Salisbury JK Jr. Robotic technology in surgery: past, present, and future. Am J Surg 2004;188(4):2–15.

Evidence-Based Decision Making in Orbital Fractures

Implementation of a Clinical Protocol

Peter J.J. Gooris, MD, DMD, PhD, FEBOMFS [a,b,c,*], Jesper Jansen, MD, DMD, PhD [d], J. Eelco Bergsma, MD, DMD, PhD [c], Leander Dubois, DDS, MD, DMD, PhD [d]

KEYWORDS

• Orbital fracture • Clinical treatment protocol • Functional guideline • Sequential orthoptic evaluation

KEY POINTS

- An evidence-based clinical protocol for orbital fractures will facilitate in the decision making of which type of treatment is most beneficial.
- Limited enophthalmos and diplopia without muscle entrapment: a wait-and-see policy is justified when adequate consecutive orthoptic evaluation can be carried out and sufficient recovery of eye motility is demonstrated.
- If there is an indication for surgical intervention with computer-assisted surgery, including virtual surgical planning, the use of a patient-specific implant and intraoperative navigation will increase the predictability of the orbital reconstruction.
- If correct criteria are met, a nonsurgical approach toward orbital wall fractures shows promising results and functional outcome.

Introduction

In 1957, Smith and Reagan[1] described the mechanism of internal orbit correction after a blow-out fracture. The investigators advocated early intervention by exploration and reconstruction of the orbital defect. Ten years later, Converse and colleagues[2] published a 10-year survey on orbital fractures and recommended a more conservative approach. In the 1970s, Putterman, an ophthalmologist, identified contusion and edema of the extraocular muscles as the main cause of diplopia and advocated a nonsurgical approach to prevent surgical-related problems, such as scarring and atrophy.[3]

Koornneef,[4] in his thesis in 1976 described the specific histologic spatial aspects of the orbital musculo-fibrous tissue of the internal orbit. If the damage to this framework is limited in case of trauma, the intrinsic capacity of these orbital tissues keeps the globe in position even in case of a large orbital wall fracture (1982).[4]

The introduction of computed tomography (CT) for facial trauma in the mid-1980s resulted in better assessment and subsequently enabled three-dimensional (3D) visualization of the orbital content. This led to a more aggressive surgical approach; in time, the clinical symptoms and CT data were found to correlate, precipitating in new CT driven protocols with fewer surgical interventions. In 2002, Burnstine[5] published his landmark paper on the clinical recommendations for repair of isolated orbital floor fractures and reviewed evidence-based approaches. The implementation of computer-assisted surgery with advanced diagnostics and preoperative virtual planning, navigation guidance, and intraoperative imaging in the mid-2000s further improved the predictability in the outcome of a reconstruction.

Despite all the new developments and insight information, management of orbital wall fractures is still subject to ongoing debate. The complex soft tissue architecture of the periorbit and its response to trauma and surgery makes the causes of diplopia multifactorial and difficult to address. In this article, the focus lies on the clinical decisions, which can be made based on the true indications, as discussed in the Leander Dubois and colleagues' article, "Ongoing Debate in Clinical Decision Making in Orbital Fractures: Indications, Timing, and Biomaterials," in this issue.

Patient presentation on admission

A multidisciplinary approach is necessary. At first presentation, standardized oral and maxillofacial (OMF) and ophthalmologic examination, including orthoptic investigation, is performed. CT scans are made according to midfacial trauma protocol:

[a] Department of Oral and Maxillofacial Surgery, University of Washington Seattle, WA, USA
[b] Department of Oral and Maxillofacial Surgery, University Medical Centre Amsterdam, the Netherlands
[c] Department of Oral and Maxillofacial Surgery, Amphia Hospital Breda, Molengracht 21, Breda 4818 CK, the Netherlands
[d] Department of Oral and Maxillofacial Surgery, University Medical Centre Amsterdam, Meibergdreef 9, Amsterdam 1105 AZ, the Netherlands
* Corresponding author. Department of Oral and Maxillofacial Surgery, Amphia Hospital Breda, Molengracht 21, Breda 4818 CK, the Netherlands.
E-mail address: p.gooris@gmail.com

Atlas Oral Maxillofacial Surg Clin N Am 29 (2021) 109-127

https://doi.org/10.1016/j.cxom.2020.11.005

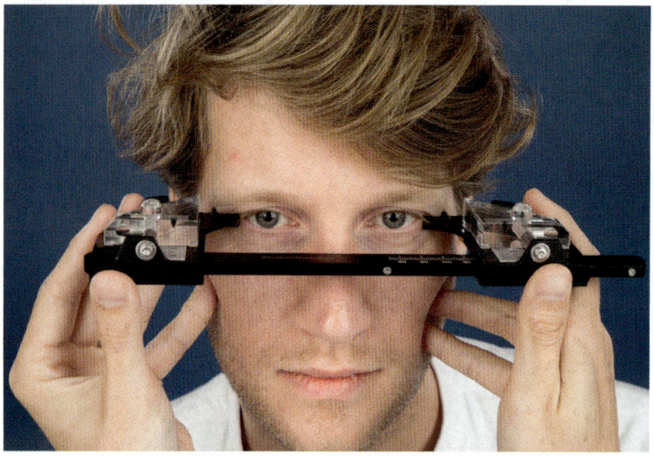

Fig. 1 Hertel exophthalmometer in use. (*Courtesy of* Leander Dubois, MD, DMD, PhD)

using a Siemens (Munich, Germany) Somatom Volume Zoom, equal exposure was used; 1-mm slice thickness, 1-mm increments, 120 kV, 30 mAs. Settings at window of 2000, a level of 400, field of view of 140 mm and a matrix size of 512 × 512.

Urgent indications for emergency orbital intervention are singled out: disturbed vision due to compression on the optic nerve in the case of a retrobulbar hematoma, globe perforation, severe globe dislocation, entrapped extraocular muscle, especially in case of a white-eyed blow-out fracture, and the occurrence of an oculo-cardiac reflex, were already discussed in the Gijsbert J. Hötte and Ronald O. B. De Keizer's article, "Ocular Injury and Emergencies Around the Globe," in this issue. In most of these indications, close collaboration with an ophthalmologist is mandatory.

After thorough examination by the OMF surgeon, ophthalmologic examination is required to assess vision of both eyes, assess ophthalmologic history (pretraumatic pathology, such as amblyopia or squint), and inspection of the globe and contents. Hertel measurement may be carried out by either the OMF surgeon or ophthalmologist (Fig. 1).

Orthoptic tests are required to objectivate existing diplopia and motility disturbances.

Final clinical decision making is based on the clinical findings, subjective and objective measurements, and CT imaging results.

The role of orthoptic evaluation

Objective and repeated measurements should be performed by the orthoptist. In the orthoptic examination, among other measurements, the following items are measured: prism cover test, ductions, and the field of binocular single vision (BSV).

Measuring the ductions and BSV is done with the Goldmann perimeter, with the patient sitting in front of the device (Fig. 2A, B). In a trauma setting, the measurements can sometimes be

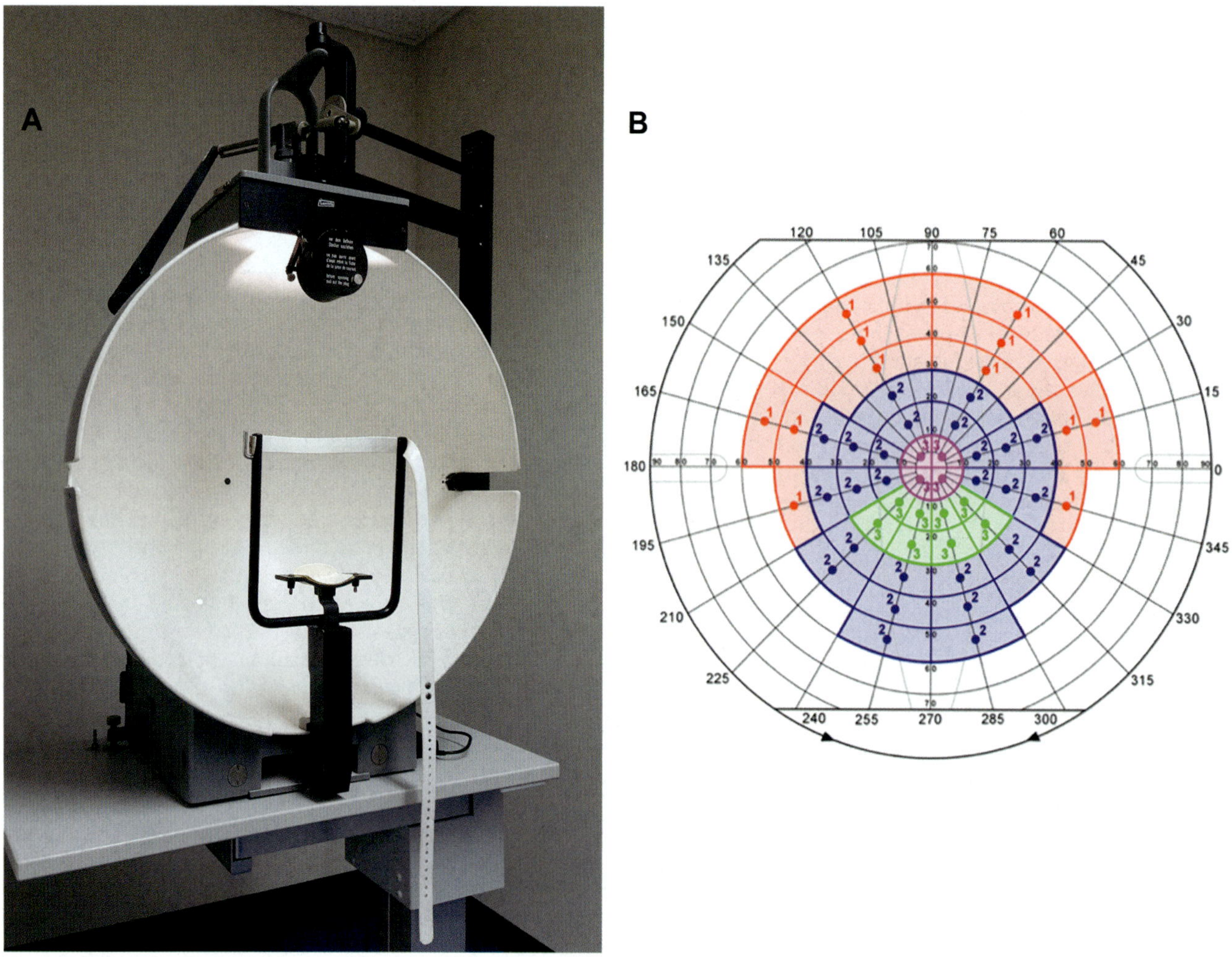

Fig. 2 (*A*) Goldmann perimeter. (*B*) BSV score chart. (*Courtesy of* Hinke Marijke Jellema, CO, MMedSci, PhD, Amsterdam, the Netherlands)

difficult to perform because of logistics, limited mobility of the patient, or considerable periorbital swelling. In that case, several attempts should be made in time to perform the measurements to gain information at the successive moments. Baseline measurements are important to assess the improvement of ductions and BSV within the first 10 to 14 days after the trauma. It is also known that patients with a BSV less than 60 or diplopia in the central gaze will benefit from surgery, although generally there is a high chance that diplopia will persist even after orbital reconstruction.[6] A limited motility of less than 15° (absolute restriction) is often the result of entrapment of incarcerated tissue. A relative motility disorder is often the result of swelling, protruding orbital content, and/or pain. Diplopia can occur as a result of the motility disorder, but it is also possible that there is no diplopia in a minimal motility disorder due to habituation and adjustment of the central nervous system. The Yvette Braaksma- Besselink and Hinke Marijke Jellema's article, "Orthoptic Evaluation and Treatment in Orbital Fractures," in this issue, can be consulted for a detailed explanation of the orthoptic examination.

Decision making

The indications for and timing of surgery are the main topics in the ongoing debate on the management of orbital wall fractures, as described in the Leander Dubois and colleagues' article, "Ongoing Debate in Clinical Decision Making in Orbital Fractures: Indications, Timing, and Biomaterials," in this issue. Generally, small asymptomatic fractures do not require surgery, whereas larger fractures with early enophthalmos do require orbital reconstruction. The indications for immediate reconstruction are clear to most clinicians. Controversy arises in cases with large orbital wall fractures without early enophthalmos. In some studies, surgery is indicated based on the size (>2 cm^2 or >50%) of the fracture, which is measured on a CT scan or in the case of severe diplopia and limited motility within several days after trauma.[5,7] The assumption is that early surgery (<2 weeks) results in a better clinical outcomes and causes less iatrogenic damage.[5] However, the size of the fracture as such does not necessarily correlate with the development of late enophthalmos, whereas moderate diplopia is demonstrated to resolve without intervention.[8] Early surgical treatment holds a risk for overtreatment in patients who may have recovered spontaneously over time. The indication debate has subsequently shifted to discussion on the type of fractures that may be eligible for late repair (>2 weeks). There are differing views in the literature; it has been shown that delayed reconstruction has no limiting effect on the clinical outcome; it allows time to tell you whether diplopia is slowly improving and whether enophthalmos will occur.[8–11]

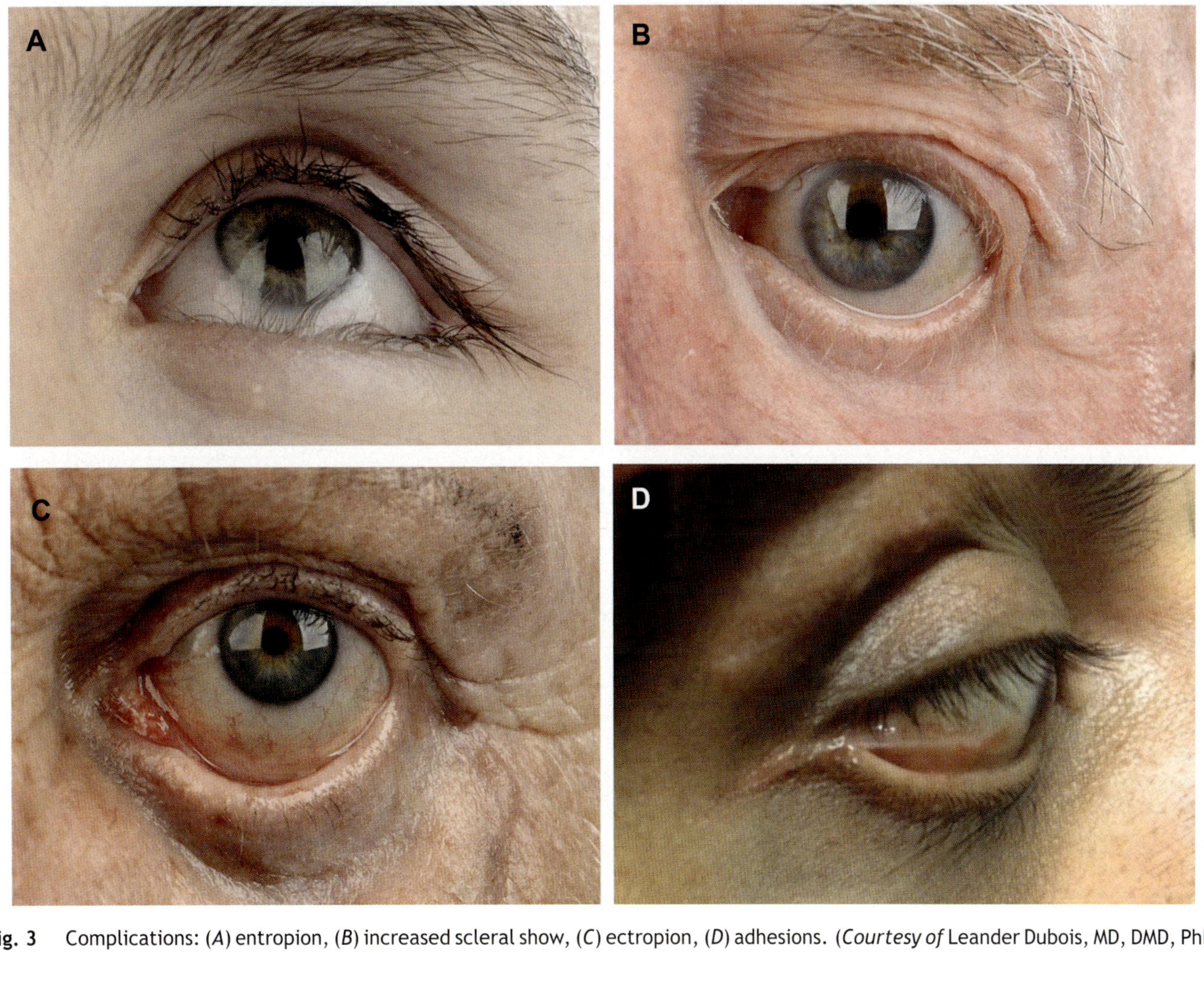

Fig. 3 Complications: (*A*) entropion, (*B*) increased scleral show, (*C*) ectropion, (*D*) adhesions. (*Courtesy of* Leander Dubois, MD, DMD, PhD)

When surgical intervention (orbital wall reconstruction) is indicated, several studies have demonstrated that virtual surgical planning (VSP) can assist the surgeon in achieving a better and more predictable treatment outcome.[12–14] Navigation-assisted surgery will further enhance the predictability of the orbital wall reconstruction.[15,16] The corresponding principles are explained in more detail in the Ruud Schreurs and colleagues' article, "Advanced Diagnostics and Three-dimensional Virtual Surgical Planning in Orbital Reconstruction"; and Ruud Schreurs and colleagues' article, "Advanced Concepts of Orbital Reconstruction: A Unique Attempt to Scientifically Evaluate Individual Techniques in Reconstruction of Large Orbital Defects," in this issue. Using the popular transconjunctival approach, adequate exposure of the medial and lateral wall and orbital floor is accomplished and access to the posterior ledge is provided.[17,18] A comprehensive overview of how primary orbital fractures should be treated is given in the Simon Holmes' article, "Primary Orbital Fracture Repair," in this issue.

Both the surgical and nonsurgical approach can result in complications. The most common nonsurgical complications are persisting motility restrictions/diplopia and early or late enophthalmos. Complications of the surgical treatment strategy must be differentiated in approach-related and those related to the surgical procedure. Relatively common approach-related complications are entropion (trans-conjunctival), increased scleral show, ectropion (subciliary) and adhesions (Fig. 3). Other complications include persistent motility restrictions or persistent enophthalmos, which may remain.[19]

If surgical intervention is waived, one should realize that it may take several weeks before clinical symptoms resolve; however, late surgical intervention is generally assumed to result in more negative sequelae.[10,11] Nevertheless, a systematic review of the literature shows no effect of delayed treatment and good clinical outcome can be seen after late reconstructions.[20] In the early stage, it is difficult to predict how the soft tissue will recuperate. Indications for surgery should be based on existing rather than expected problems. For that reason, a clinical protocol with special emphasis on nonsurgical treatment based on functional evaluation is suggested (Fig. 4).

The clinical protocol derived from Jansen and colleagues[8] is described as follows.

Clinical examination is performed:

- Examination by the OMF surgeon:
  - Subjective diplopia, enophthalmos, infraorbital hypesthesia, hypoglobus, pain, and other symptoms. A CT scan is obtained according to protocol when a fracture is suspected. Rule out indications for immediate surgery within 24 hours.
- Ophthalmic examination:
  - Exophthalmometry (enophthalmos of >2 mm at first presentation or after 2 weeks is an indication for early surgery with 2–3 weeks), vision, bulb pressure.
- Orthoptic examination:
  - Ductions: the motility perimeter (Goldmann) is used to measure the ductions in all 4 directions with the head accurately in primary position (see the Yvette Braaksma-Besselink and Hinke Marijke Jellema's article, "Orthoptic Evaluation and Treatment in Orbital Fractures," in this issue). Abduction or adduction of less than 25° and elevation or depression of less than 15° at first presentation are indications for early surgery within 2 weeks. If after 2 weeks of follow-up the ductions have improved less than 8°, there is an indication for delayed surgery between 2 and 3 weeks. Orthoptic evaluation is repeated after 3, 6, and 12 months if necessary.

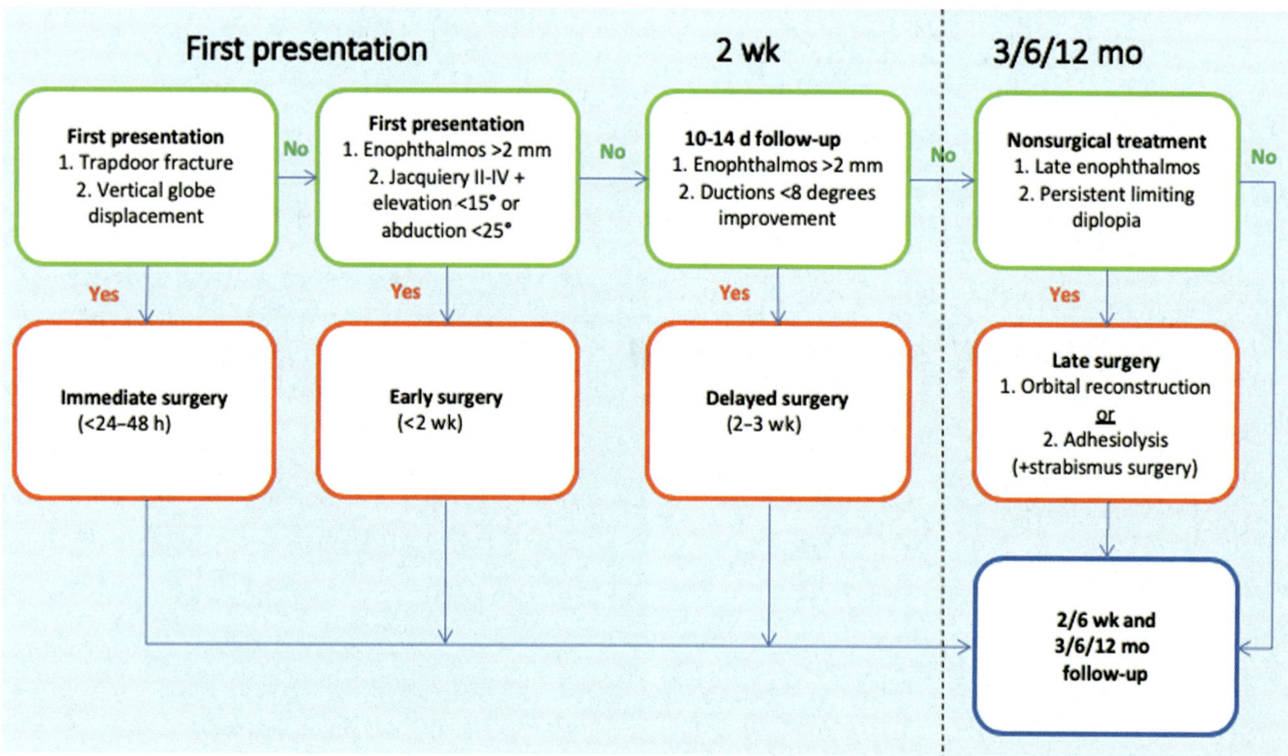

Fig. 4 Flow chart and timeline of the evidence-based clinical protocol for orbital fracture management.

- Field of binocular vision (BSV) is performed with the use of the motility perimeter (Goldmann); the BSV is scored at a score sheet from 0 to 100 points.

Recovery

It is important to closely monitor the patient immediately after surgery of the orbit.

Frequent vision control (once every 15 minutes for the initial 2 hours) is necessary, as loss of vision is an alarming symptom, which is most likely to be caused by increasing pressure on the optic nerve either as a result of progressive orbital soft tissue swelling or retrobulbar hematoma. Color vision diminishes first (color red first, followed by green) and is an early warning sign of compression of the optic nerve. The nursing staff in the recovery room should be informed and alerted of these signs. Decompression via a lateral canthotomy may be indicated, as an emergency procedure in such cases. When stable, the patient is brought back to the ward where frequent monitoring of vision control is still important; however, the frequency can be cut down to once every hour.

The patient will stay in the hospital for 24 hours after surgery and can be discharged the next day if no complications develop. If an intraoperative CT scan was not performed, one should be obtained before discharge to check the position of the reconstruction plate/titanium mesh.

At discharge, the patient is informed that double vision will be experienced for the first 10 to 14 days and possibly longer. Instructions are given to mobilize the eye as much as possible: monocular orthoptic exercises 3 times per day for at least 4 weeks to prevent adhesions occurring and to stimulate reduction of orbital soft tissue swelling, especially the extraocular muscles.

The patient is followed-up by the involved OMF surgeon, the ophthalmologist, and, as important, by the orthoptist: consecutive BSV and duction measurements at 2 weeks, 6 weeks, 3 months, 6 months, and 12 months after surgery. Successive orthoptic outcome measurements inform the surgeon whether or not additional surgery is required.

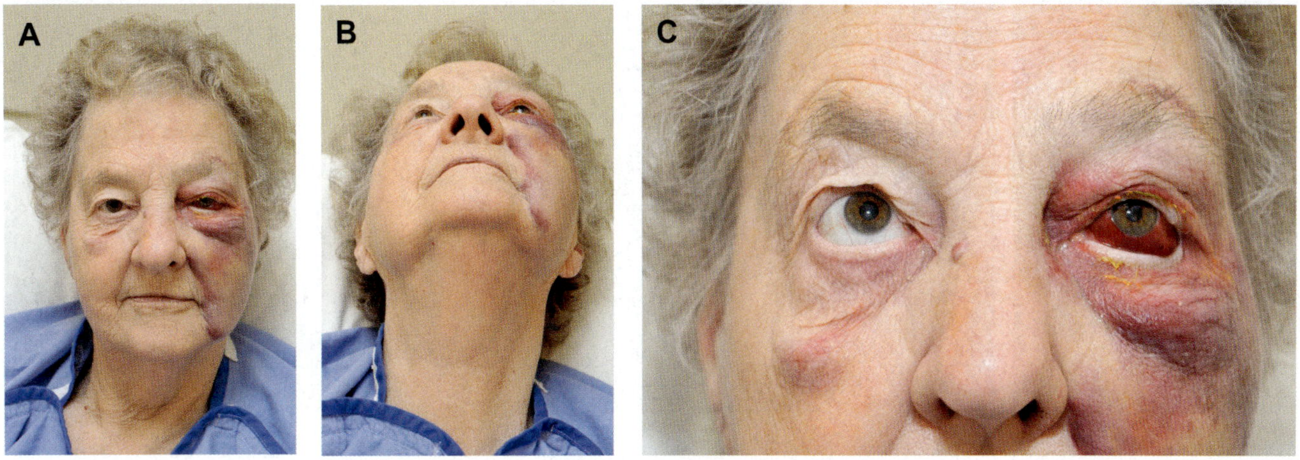

Fig. 5 Case 1: clinical appearance at first presentation: (*A*) en face, (*B*) submental, (*C*) elevation. (*Courtesy of* Leander Dubois, MD, DMD, PhD)

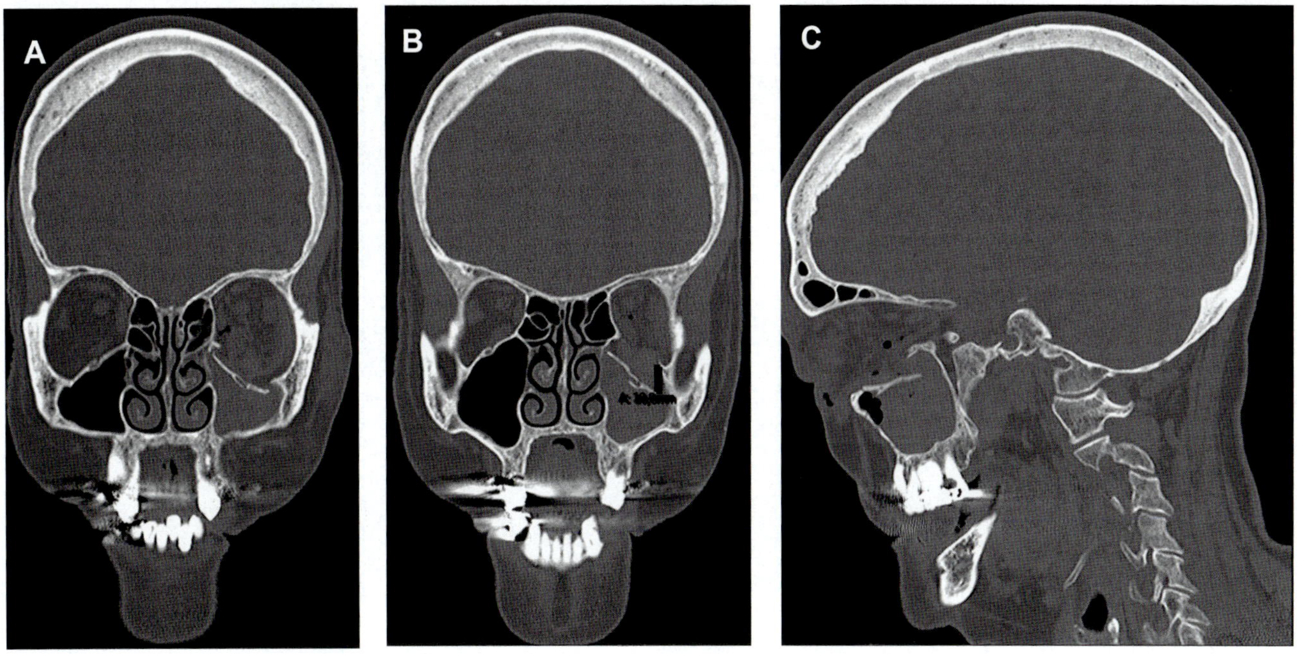

Fig. 6 Case 1: coronal and sagittal views of the CT scan at first presentation (*A–C*). (*Courtesy of* Leander Dubois, MD, DMD, PhD)

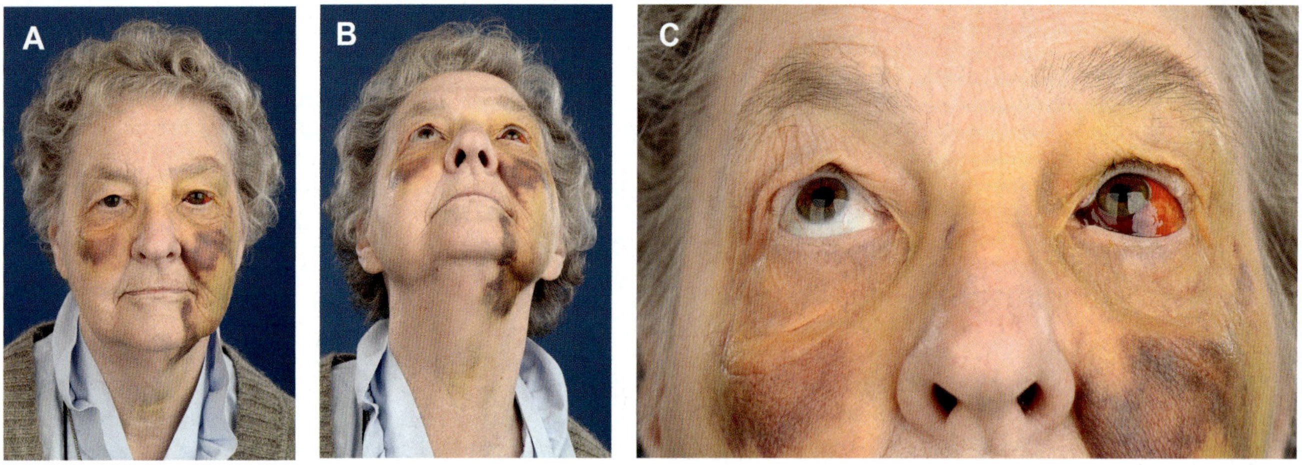

Fig. 7 Case 1: clinical result 2 weeks after trauma, (*A*) en face, (*B*) submental, (*C*) elevation. (*Courtesy of* Leander Dubois, MD, DMD, PhD)

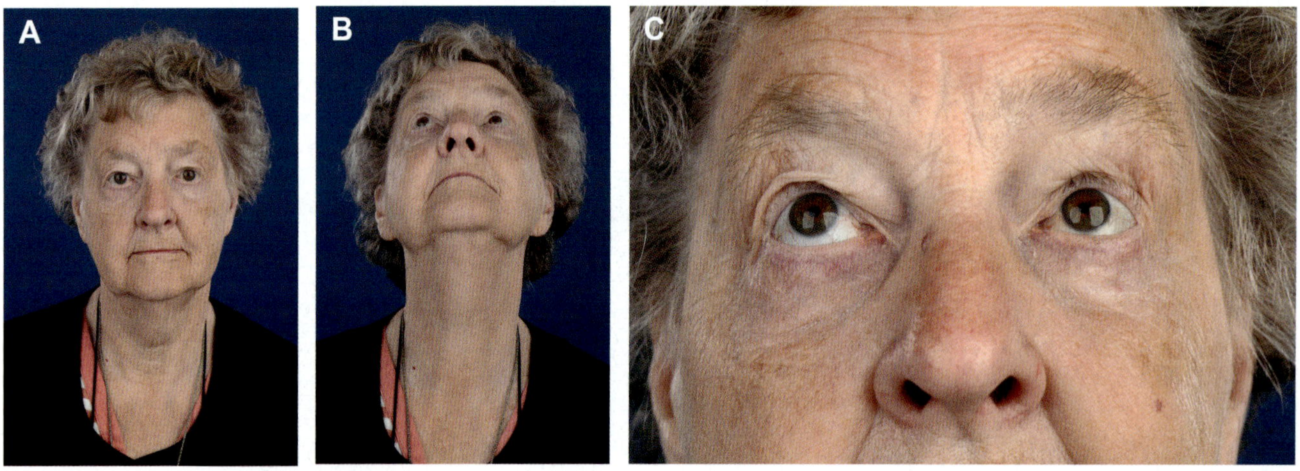

Fig. 8 Case 1: clinical result 1 year after trauma, (*A*) en face, (*B*) submental, (*C*) elevation. (*Courtesy of* Leander Dubois, MD, DMD, PhD)

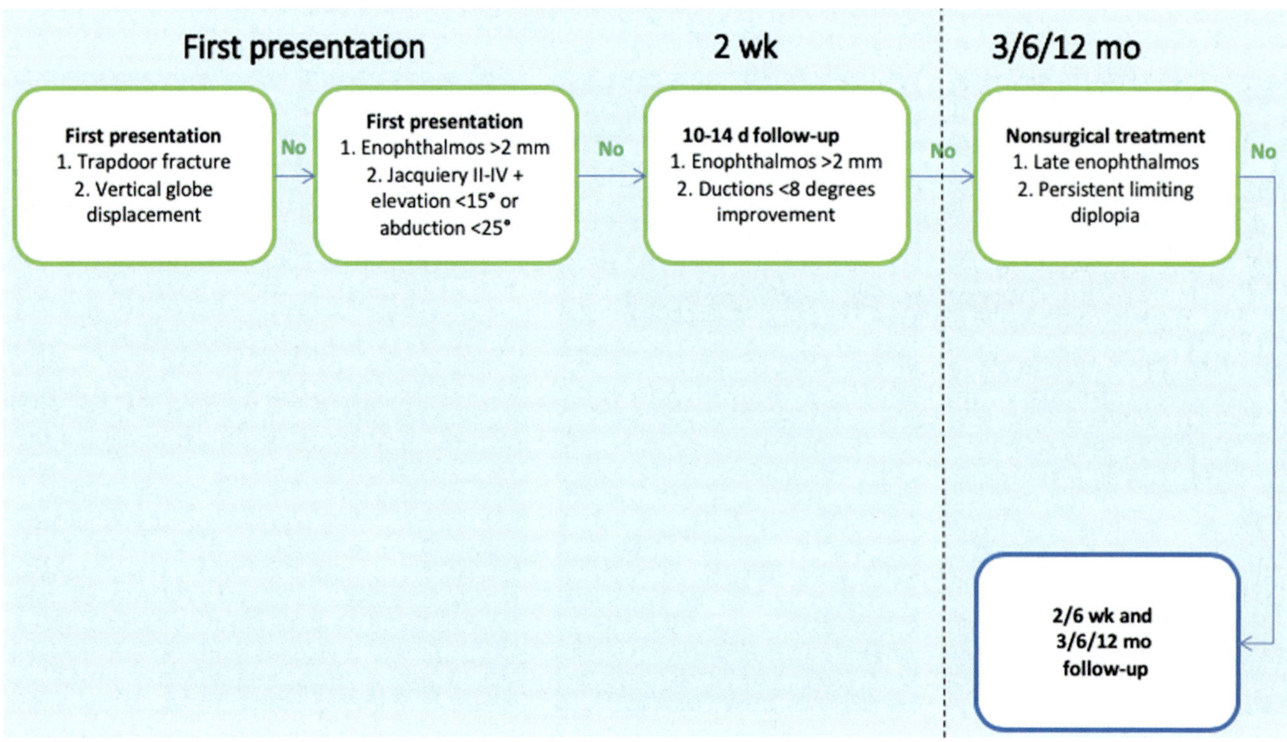

Fig. 9 Case 1: patient-specific flow chart.

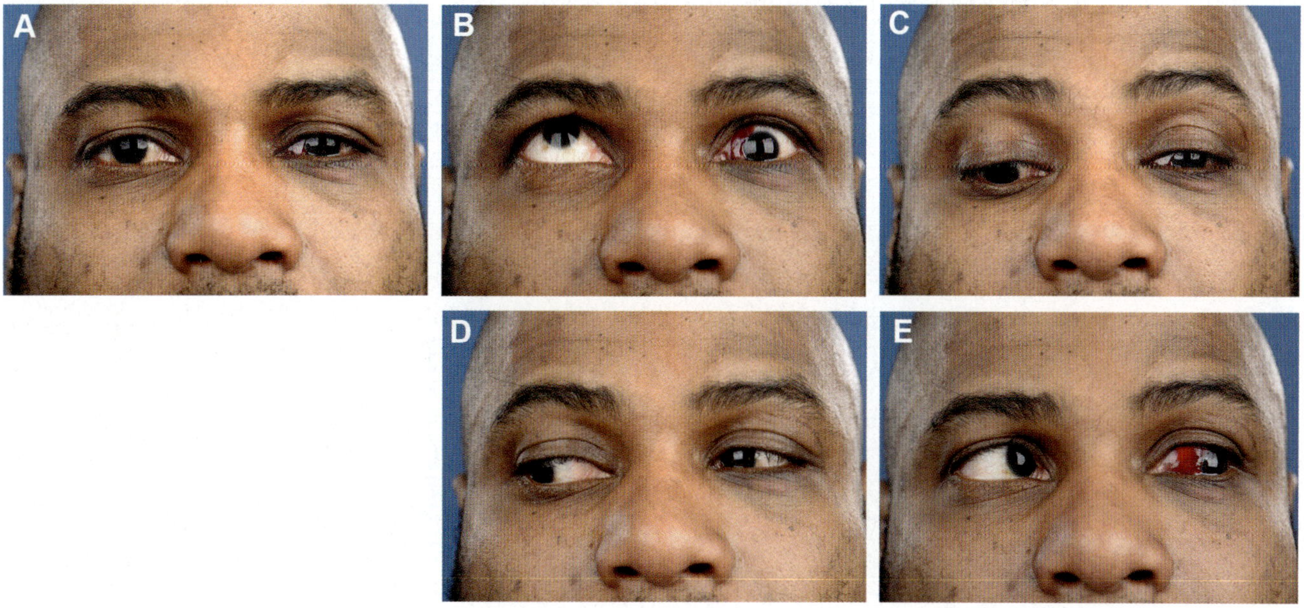

Fig. 10 Case 2: clinical appearance at first presentation, (*A*) en face, (*B*) elevation, (*C*) depression (*D*) adduction, (*E*) abduction. (*Courtesy of* Leander Dubois, MD, DMD, PhD)

Five patient cases are introduced as follows to illustrate the practical implementation of the clinical protocol.

Case 1

An 82-year-old woman with a large orbital floor fracture (>50% of the floor/Jaquiéry class III) on the left side caused by a collapse in the bathroom (Figs. 5A–C and 6A–C). At the orthoptic evaluation, the BSV was 54 and there was limited eye motility in abduction (42° OD/18° OS), elevation (21° OD/15° OS), and depression (56° OD/43° OS). There was no significant enophthalmos (Hertel 18/19). Despite the large fracture, the clinical protocol allows a nonsurgical treatment. Instructions for orthoptic exercises were provided.

After 2 weeks, the ductions and BSV improved significantly (Fig. 7A–C). In the follow-up period of 6 to 12 months the BSV was 100, there was no limited motility, and enophthalmos remained at 1 mm (Fig. 8A–C) The patient completed nonsurgical treatment with a successful clinical result (Fig. 9).

Case 2

A 42-year-old man with an orbital floor trapdoor fracture (class I) on the left side with entrapment of the inferior rectus muscle due to boxing training (Figs. 10A–E and 11A–C). The patient complained of diplopia and blurred vision. At the orthoptic evaluation, there was an absolute elevation restriction (33° OD/1° OS) and a relative depression restriction (51° OD/15° OS). Due to entrapment, the patient required surgery within 48 hours to release the incarcerated tissue; as such, this is an

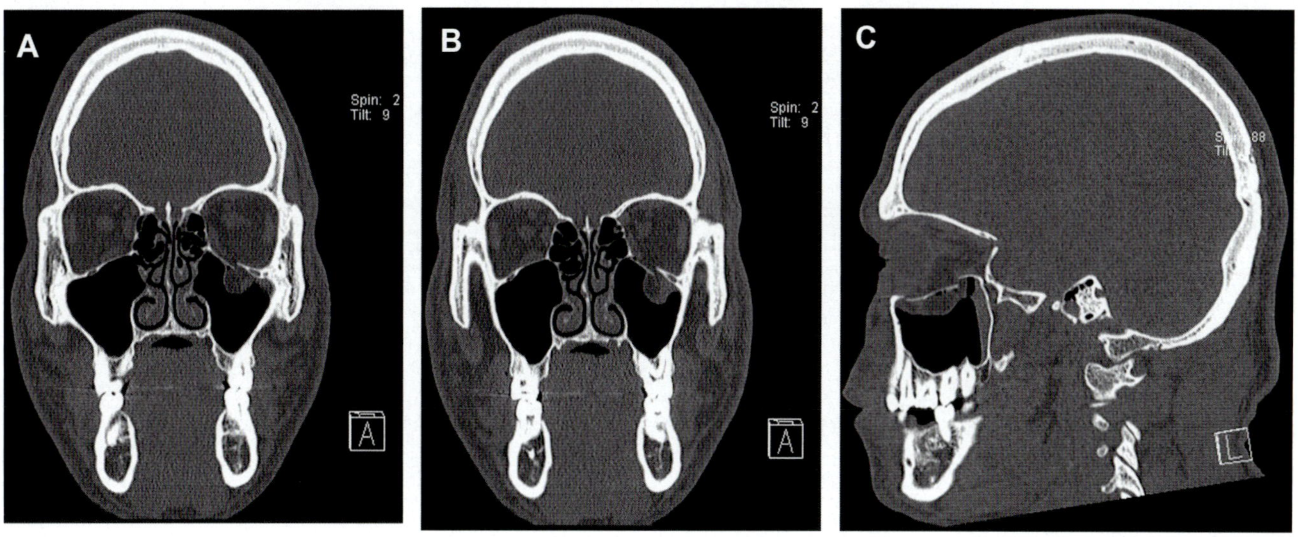

Fig. 11 Case 2: coronal (*A*,*B*) and sagittal (*C*) views of the CT scan at first presentation. (*Courtesy of* Leander Dubois, MD, DMD, PhD)

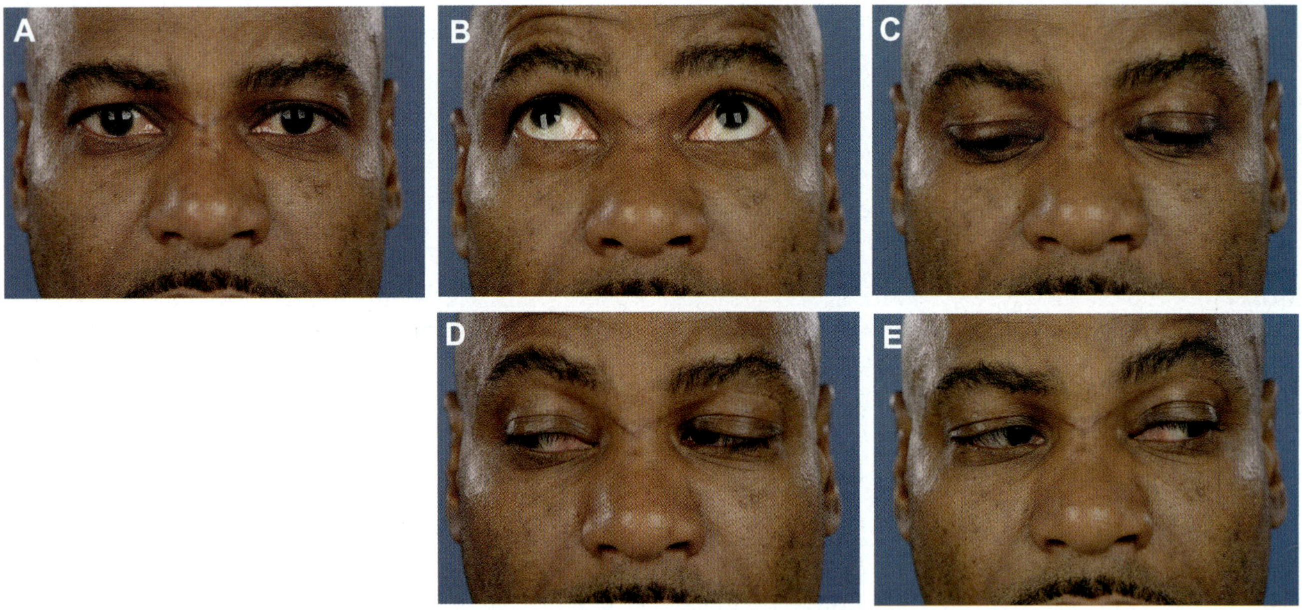

Fig. 12 Case 2: clinical result 1 year after surgery: (*A*) en face, (*B*) elevation, (*C*) depression, (*D*) adduction, (*E*) abduction. (*Courtesy of* Leander Dubois, MD, DMD, PhD)

example of an undisputable indication for early surgical intervention.

The patient received surgery without VSP because of the small fracture. Through a conjunctival approach, the incarcerated muscle and protruding tissue were released, and the orbital floor was reconstructed with a titanium mesh plate. After reconstruction, the forced duction was negative.

Three months after the operation, a mild elevation restriction remained, together with mild diplopia, which was not limiting in daily life. This almost completely diminished after 12 months with elevation 37° OD/33° OS and depression 48° OD/42° OS (Fig. 12A–D). The patient had a successful end result after immediate surgical treatment (Fig. 13).

Case 3

A 21-year-old woman with a dislocated orbital floor and medial wall (class III) combined with a lateral wall fracture on the right side due to interpersonal violence (Figs. 14A–C and

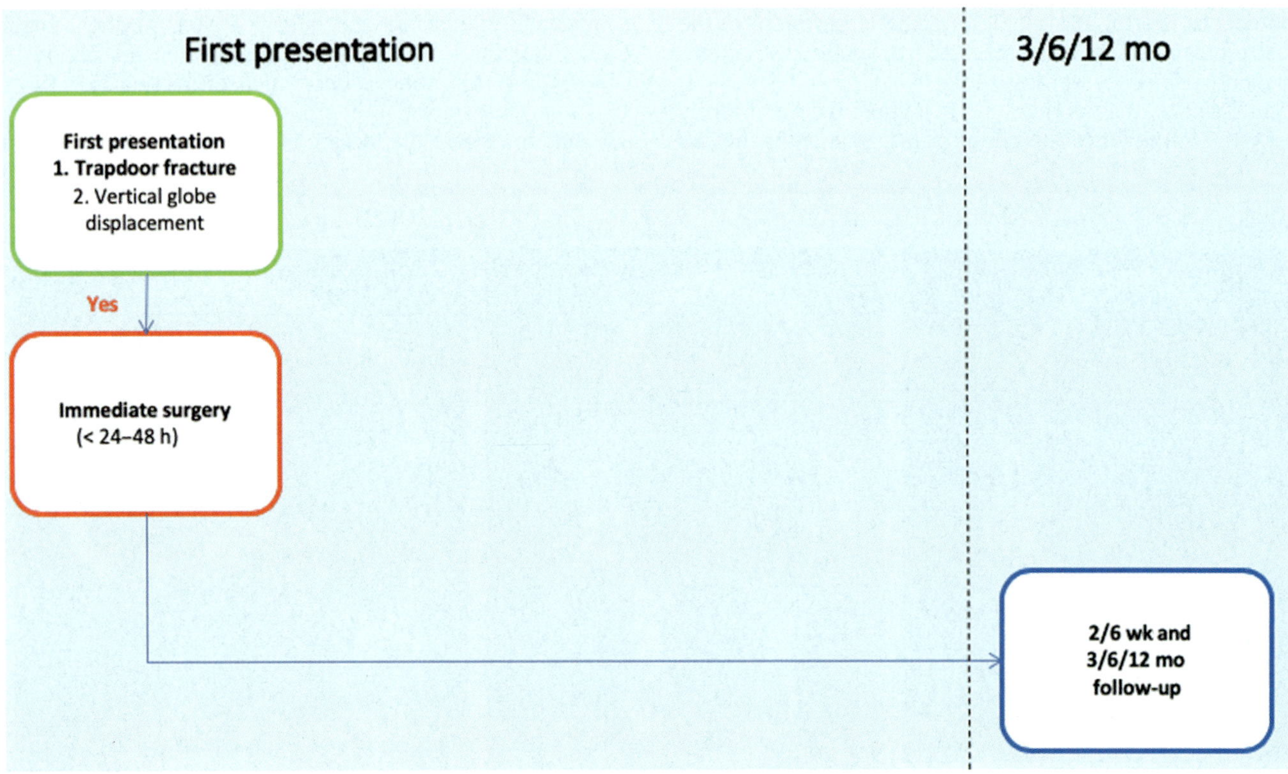

Fig. 13 Case 2: patient-specific flow chart.

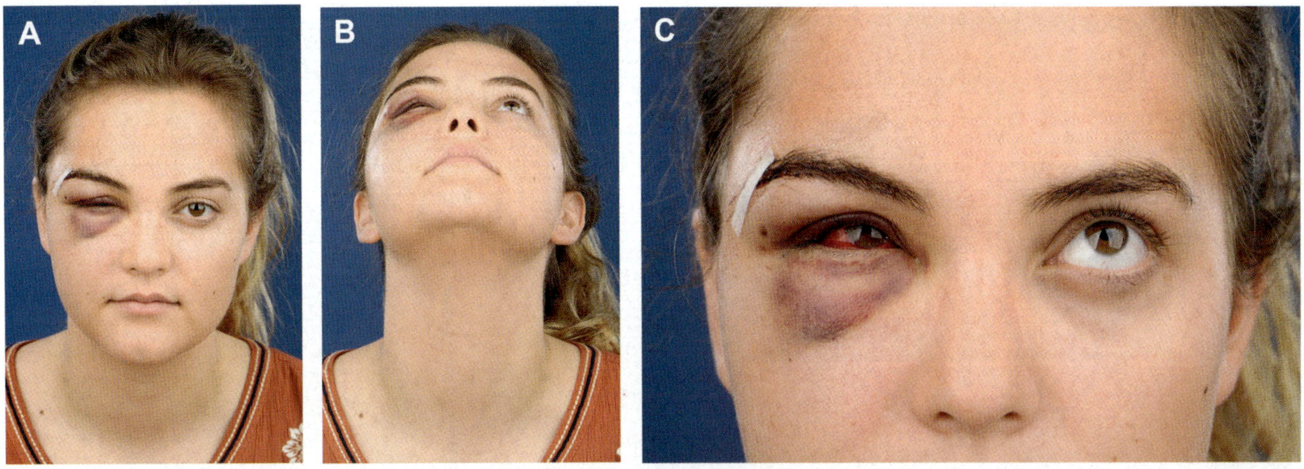

Fig. 14 Case 3: clinical appearance at first presentation: (*A*) en face, (*B*) submental, (*C*) elevation. (*Courtesy of* Leander Dubois, MD, DMD, PhD)

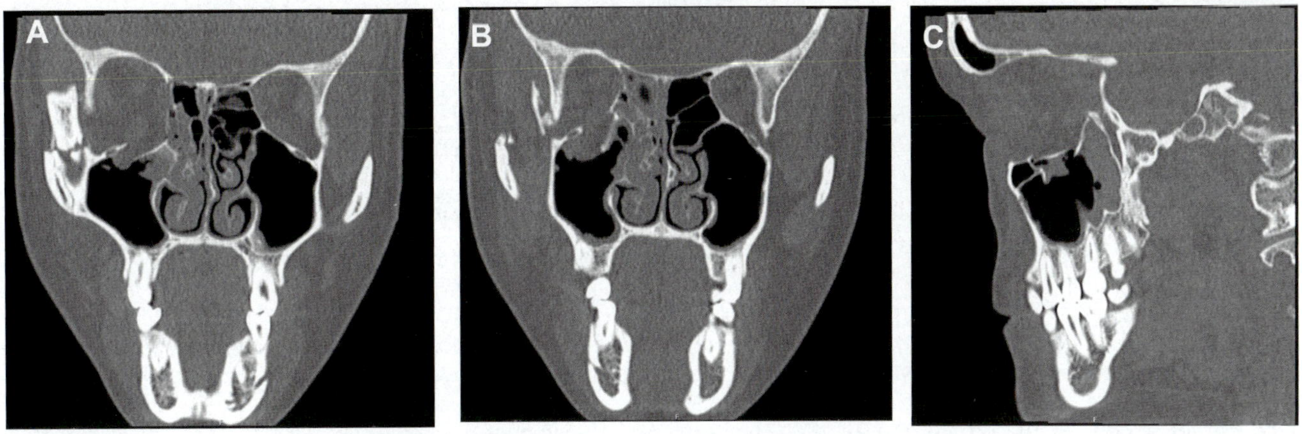

Fig. 15 Case 3: coronal (*A*,*B*) and sagittal (*C*) views of the CT scan at first presentation. (*Courtesy of* Leander Dubois, MD, DMD, PhD)

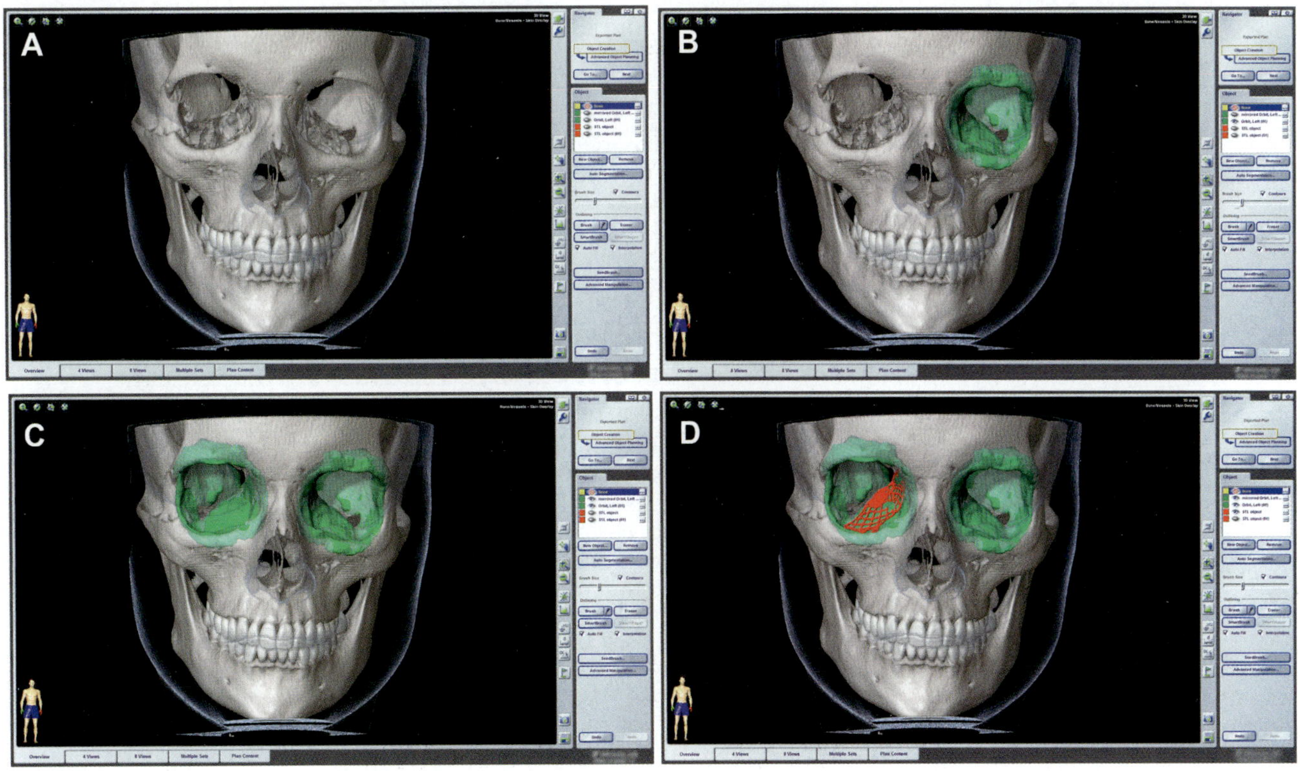

Fig. 16 Case 3: (A) the amount of dislocation of the orbital walls can be easily assessed during the preoperative planning. (B) segmentation of the unaffected side. (C) mirrored to the contralateral side to mimic the pretraumatized anatomy. (D) the STL file of the best-fitting implant imported into the software. (*Courtesy of* Leander Dubois, MD, DMD, PhD)

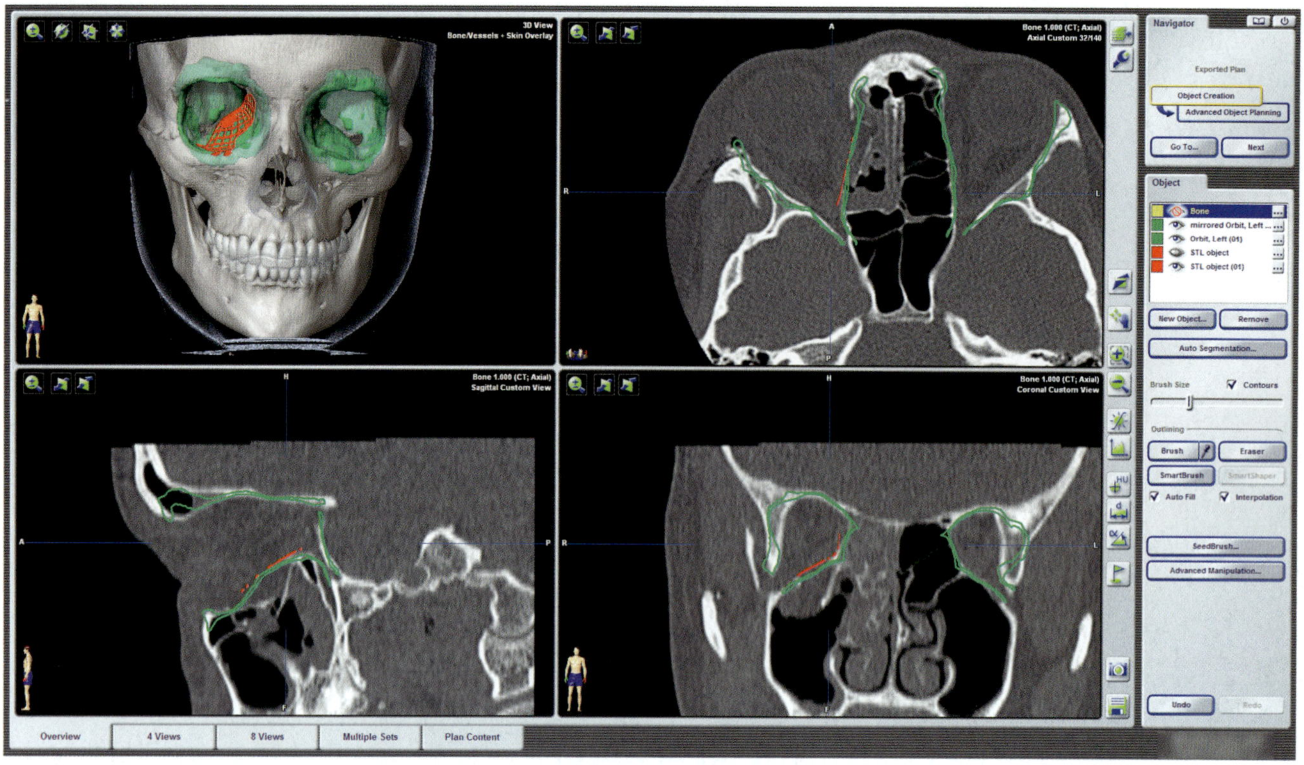

Fig. 17 Case 3: the STL file of the best-fitting implant imported into the software. (*Courtesy of* Leander Dubois, MD, DMD, PhD)

15A–C). The clinical symptoms were diplopia at elevation and depression, limited elevation, and a palpable step at the frontozygomatic suture. There was no significant enophthalmos (Hertel 18/19). At the orthoptic evaluation, limited eye motility was confirmed for elevation (31° OD/40° OS) and depression (40° OD/51° OS) with a BSV score of 38/100 points. Based on the dislocated lateral wall and severe diplopia, it was decided to schedule the patient for early surgical navigation-assisted orbital reconstruction.

The amount of dislocation of the orbital walls can be easily assessed (Fig. 16). The unaffected side is segmented and mirrored to the contralateral side to mimic the pretraumatized

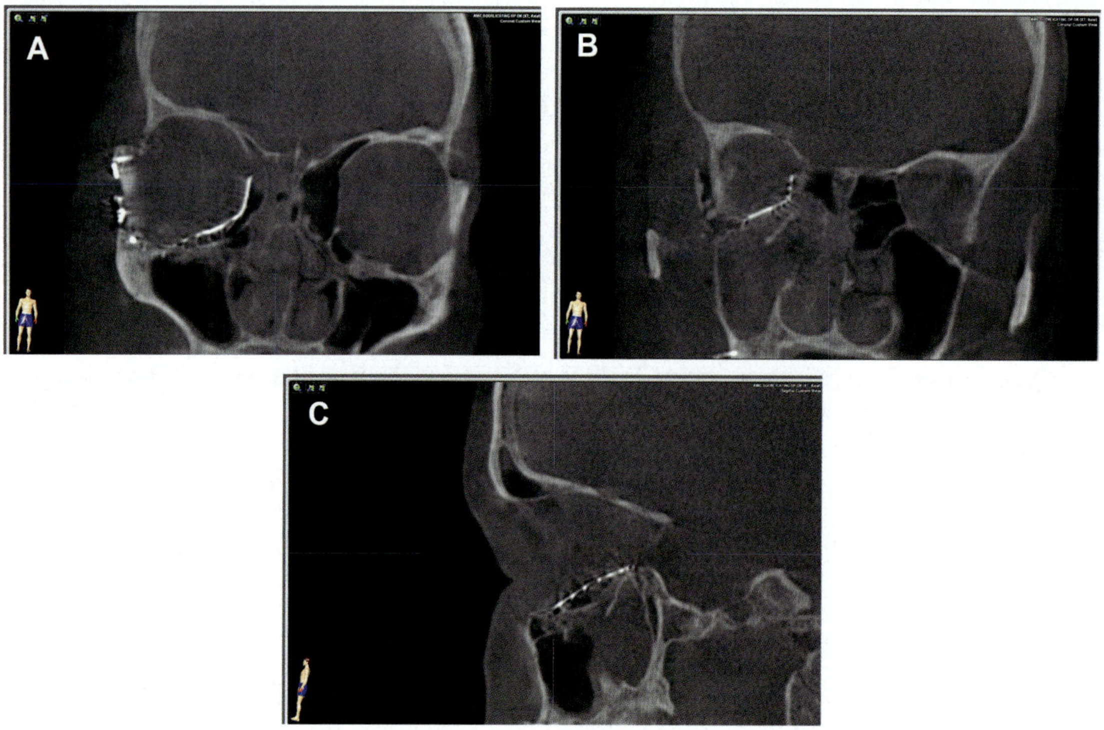

Fig. 18 Case 3: coronal (*A*,*B*) and sagittal (*C*) views of the intraoperative imaging for quality control. (*Courtesy of* Leander Dubois, MD, DMD, PhD)

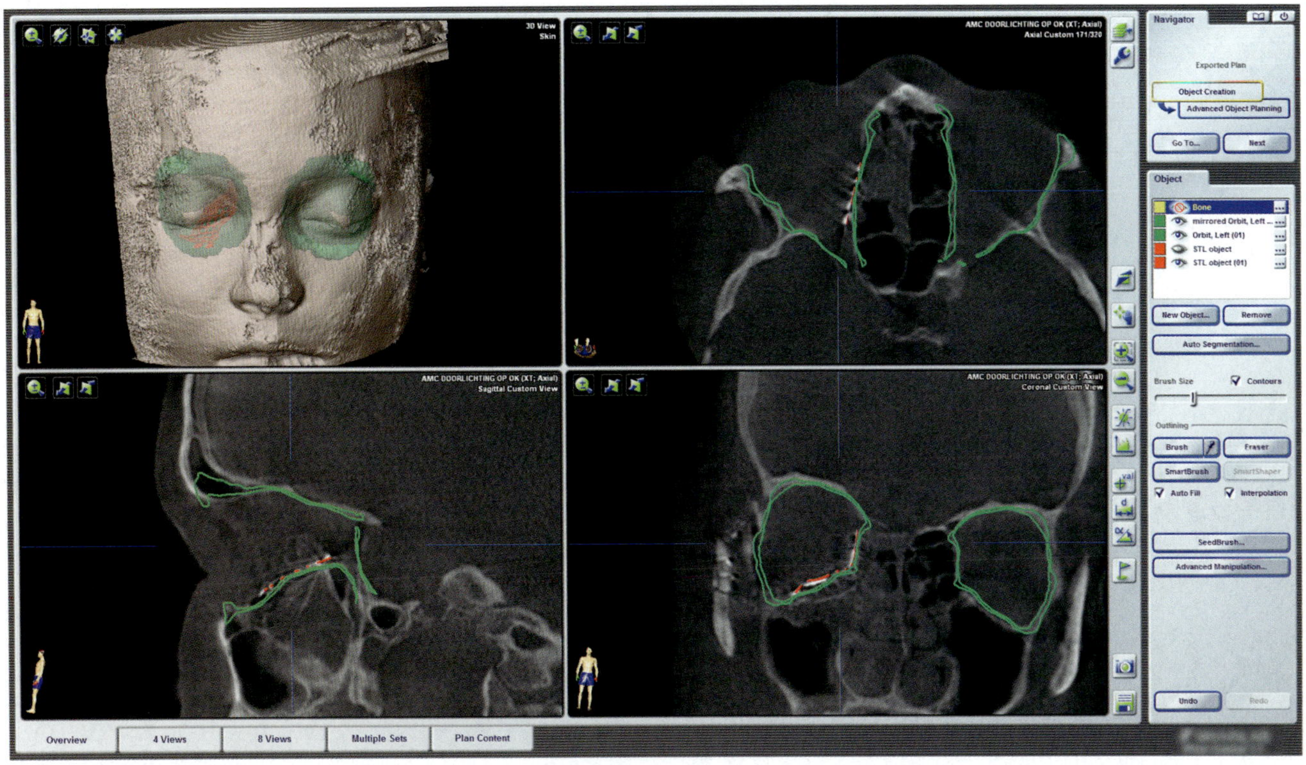

Fig. 19 Case 3: superimposing the planned result with the final result. (*Courtesy of* Leander Dubois, MD, DMD, PhD)

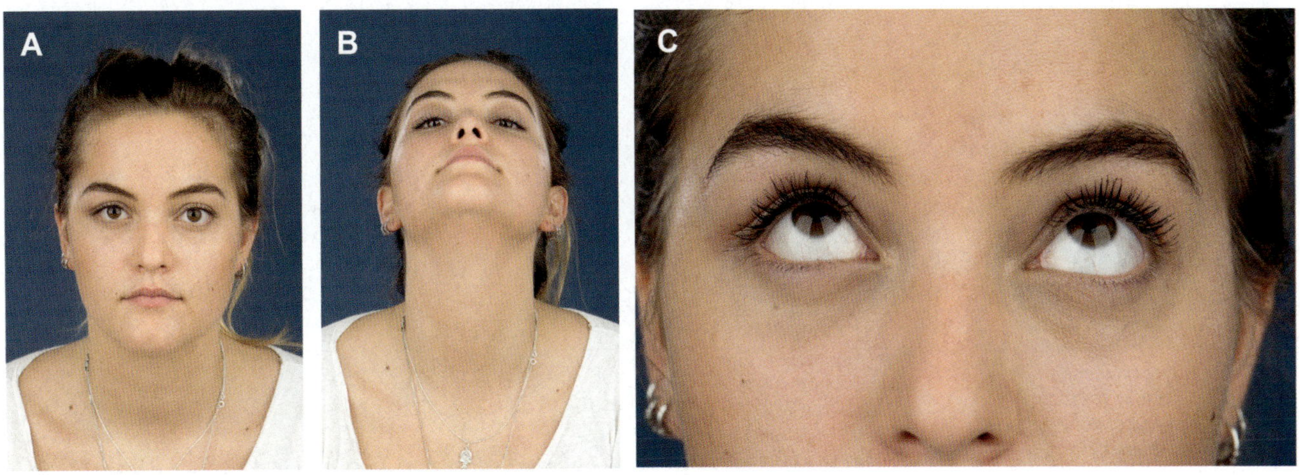

Fig. 20 Case 3: clinical result 1 year after surgery: (*A*) en face, (*B*) submental, (*C*) elevation. (*Courtesy of* Leander Dubois, MD, DMD, PhD)

anatomy . The STL file of the best-fitting implant is chosen and imported into the software (Fig. 17). The additional screw holes or extensions could be cut beforehand to prevent unnecessary intraoperative implant adjustments.

The patient is prepared for navigation. The orbital fracture is reconstructed with a preformed mesh plate. The results are evaluated with an intraoperative scan (Fig. 18A–C). The preoperative planning is superimposed onto the actual result to evaluate the accuracy of the reconstruction (Fig. 19).

The patient was discharged from the hospital the day after surgery. The patient continued her studies 2 weeks after reconstruction. Normal ocular motility was restored directly after surgery. The diplopia dissolved in 3 months. During the follow-up of 12 months, no enophthalmos occurred (Fig. 20A–C). Fig. 21A–D shows the improvement of the BSV over time. The patient benefited from early surgical intervention with an excellent clinical result (Fig. 22). Treatment decision making was based on the involvement and the extent of displacement of the orbital wall fracture(s) in combination with the clearly present limitation of eye motility in the upward and downward gaze.

Case 4

A 23-year-old man with an orbital floor and medial wall fracture (class III) on the left side after a sports accident (Figs.

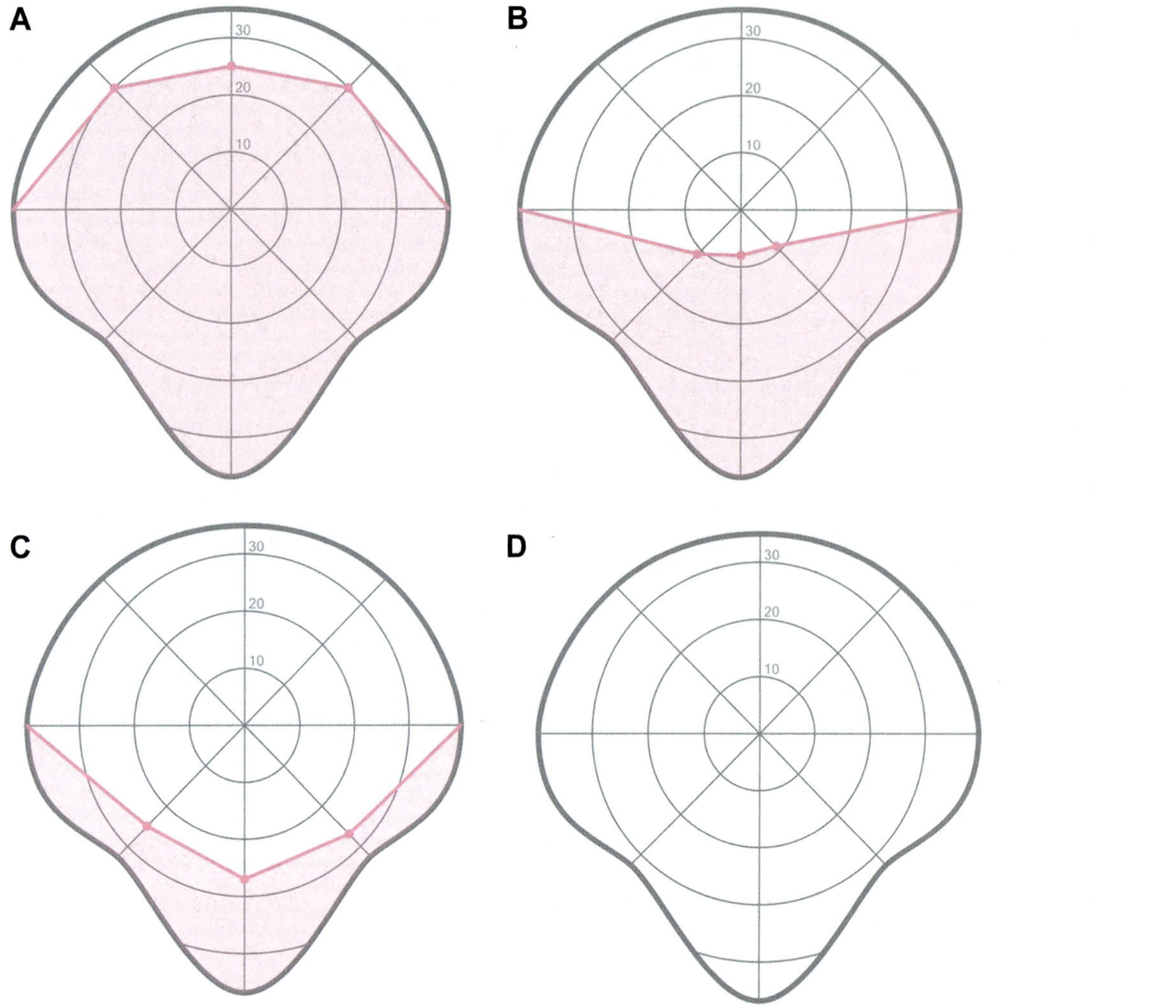

Fig. 21 Case 3: BSV (*A*) preoperative, (*B*) 2 weeks after surgery, (*C*) 6 weeks after surgery, (*D*) 1 year after surgery. The pink area is the field of double vision, the white area is the field of Binocular Single Vision (BSV). (*Courtesy of* Leander Dubois, MD, DMD, PhD)

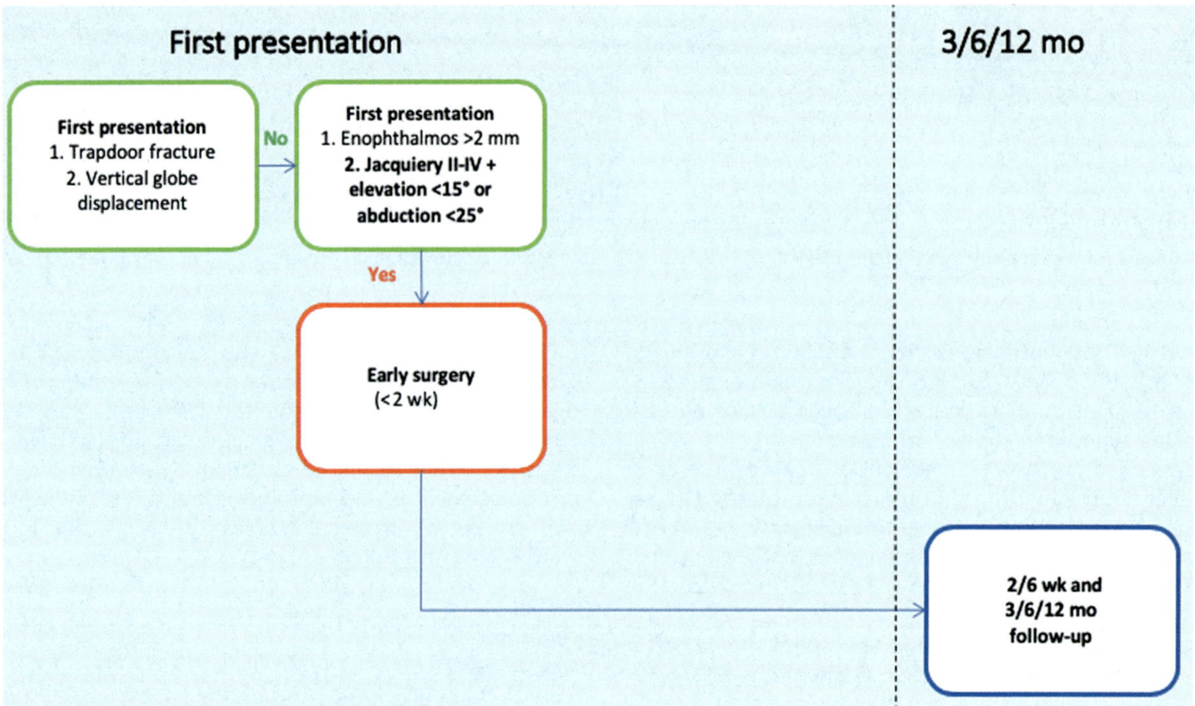

Fig. 22 Case 3: patient-specific flow chart.

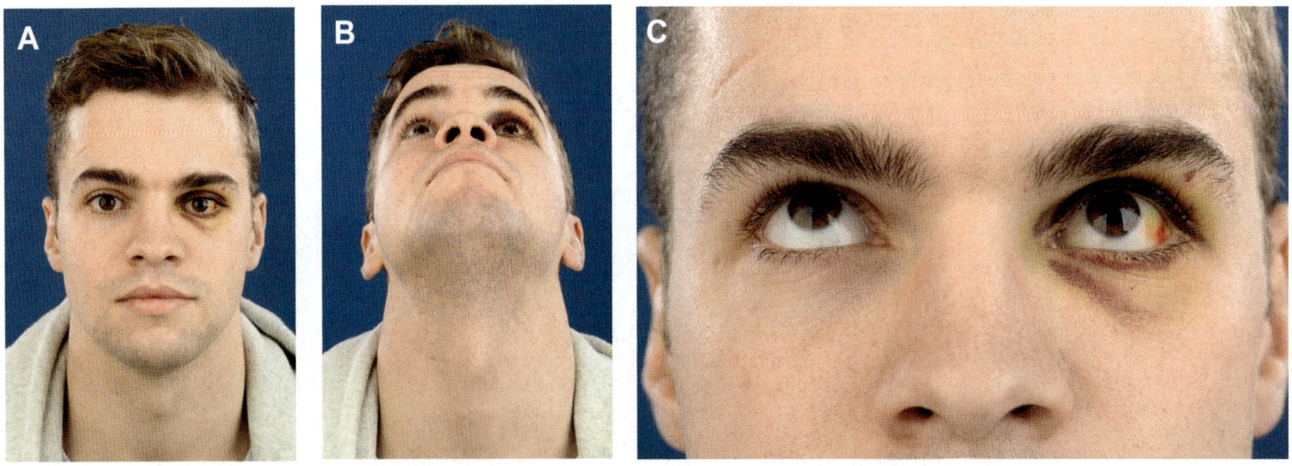

Fig. 23 Case 4: clinical appearance at presentation: (*A*) en face, (*B*) submental, (*C*) elevation. (*Courtesy of* Leander Dubois, MD, DMD, PhD)

23A–C and 24A–C). The patient complained of pain and diplopia only at maximum ductions. At orthoptic evaluation, only the depression was limited (60° OD/48° OS). There was no significant enophthalmos at first presentation (Hertel 16/15). Based on the limited clinical symptoms, the patient initially received nonsurgical treatment. Instructions for orthoptic exercises were provided.

At orthoptic evaluation after 2 weeks, there was improvement in diplopia. However, after the initial swelling had resolved, enophthalmos occurred (Hertel 18/15) (Fig. 25A, B). Based on the enophthalmos, delayed surgery was performed with a titanium mesh plate (Fig. 26A–C). Two weeks after surgery, there was no enophthalmos (Hertel 18/18). The diplopia completely resolved 5 months after surgery. At 12-month follow-up, there was still no enophthalmos with proper ocular motility and no diplopia (Fig. 27A–C). The patient had surgical treatment because of the early enophthalmos according to protocol with a good end result (Fig. 28).

Case 5

A 26-year-old man with an orbital floor fracture on the right side caused by interpersonal violence. At presentation, the patient complained of double vision and mild pain during eye movement (Fig. 29A, B). Radiographic examination showed an orbital floor fracture on the right side with minimal displacement; no evident herniation or incarceration of extraocular muscle tissue (Fig. 30A, B). At the orthoptic evaluation, there was limited elevation (30° OD/38° OS) and a mild depression (49° OD/54° OS), BSV was 73. There was no enophthalmos (Hertel 19/19). Assuming that the diplopia was most likely due to the initial orbital tissue swelling and the finding of only minimal displacement of the orbital floor on the CT scan, it was decided to allow time for recovery of soft tissue damage-contusion with a nonsurgical approach. Instructions for orthoptic exercises were provided.

At clinical and orthoptic evaluation after 2 weeks, there was no improvement of the diplopia and eye motility (elevation 28° OD/37° OS and depression 45° OD/53° OS) despite initial reduction of swelling. The patient underwent an orbital reconstruction several days after this evaluation with a titanium mesh plate (Fig. 31A, B). The clinical appearance 3 months after surgery was satisfactory and stable (Fig. 32A–E). Eye motility recovered and diplopia almost completely dissolved over time and remained stable with a BSV of 95 and the Hertel remained 19/19. Fig. 33A–D shows the

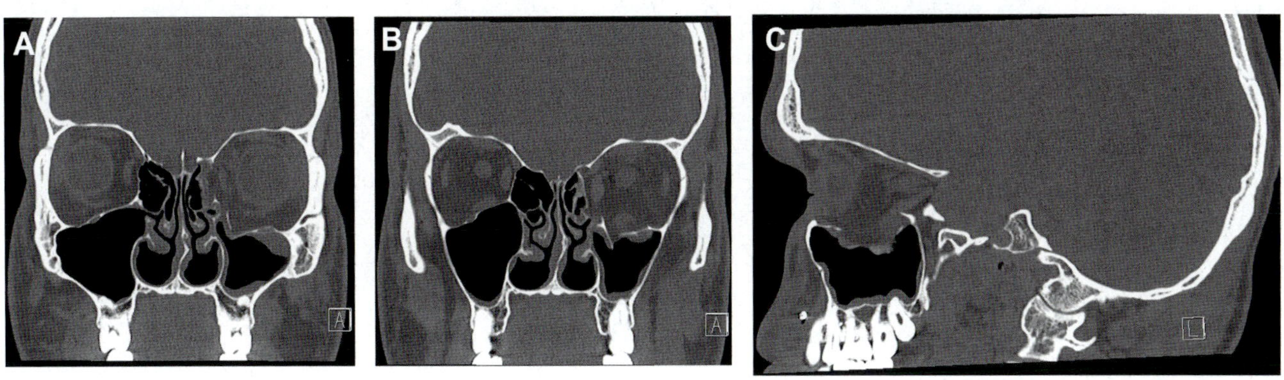

Fig. 24 Case 4: coronal (*A,B*) and sagittal (*C*) views of the CT scan at first presentation. (*Courtesy of* Leander Dubois, MD, DMD, PhD)

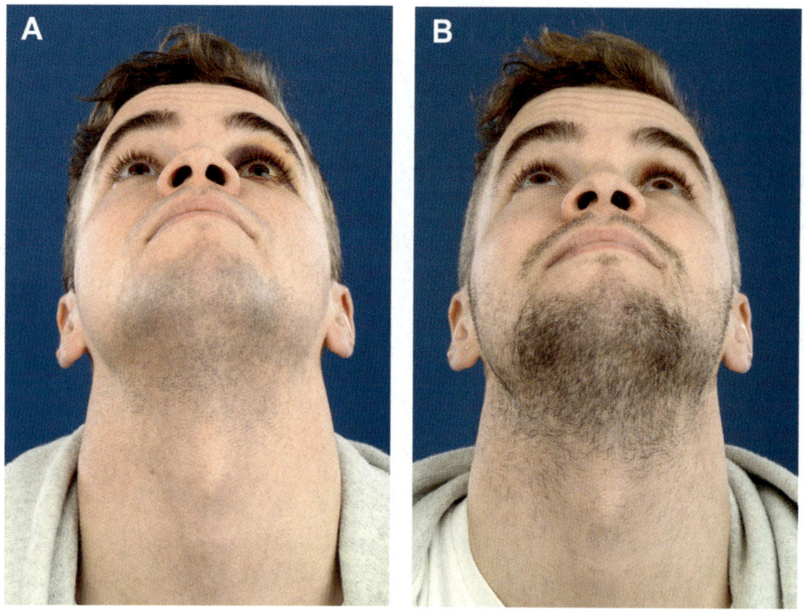

Fig. 25 Case 4: occurrence of enophthalmos over time: (*A*) 5 days after trauma, (*B*) 2 weeks after trauma. (*Courtesy of* Leander Dubois, MD, DMD, PhD)

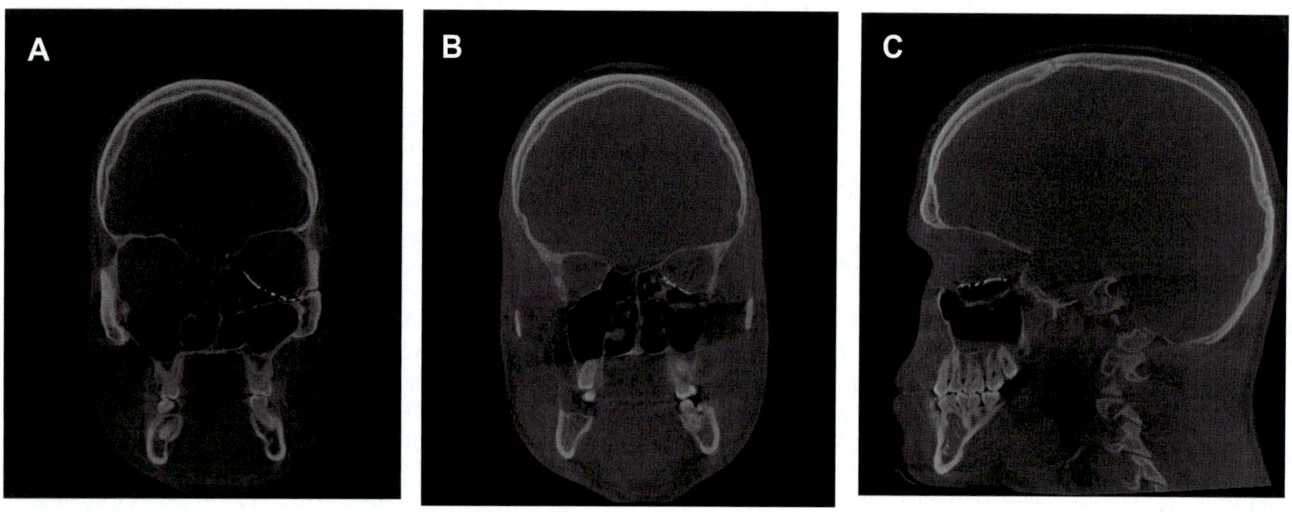

Fig. 26 Case 4: coronal (*A*,*B*) and sagittal (*C*) views of the intraoperative CT scan. (*Courtesy of* Leander Dubois, MD, DMD, PhD)

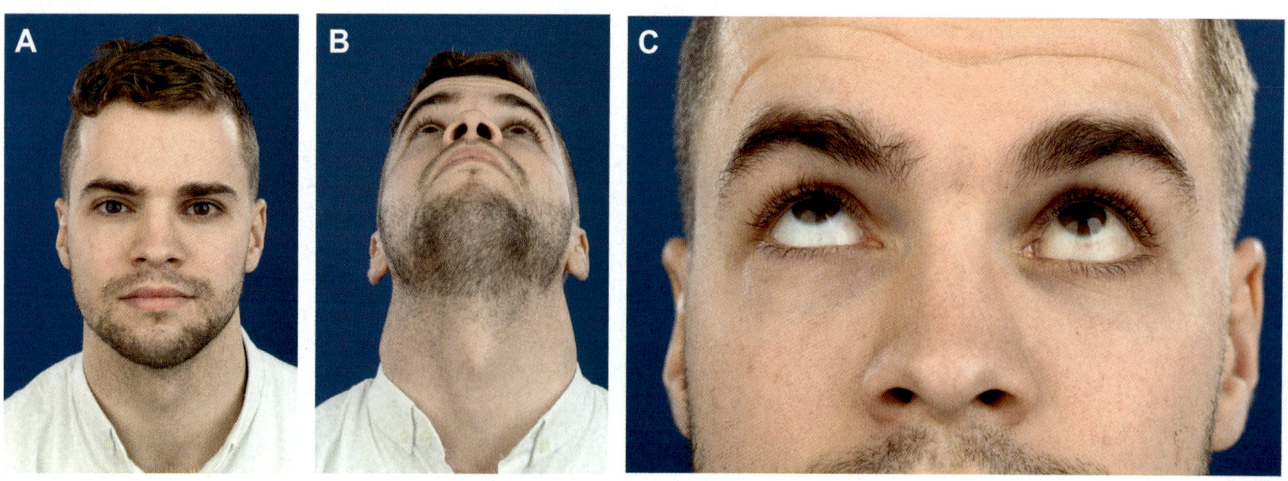

Fig. 27 Case 4: clinical result 1 year after trauma: (*A*) en face, (*B*) submental, (*C*) elevation. (*Courtesy of* Leander Dubois, MD, DMD, PhD)

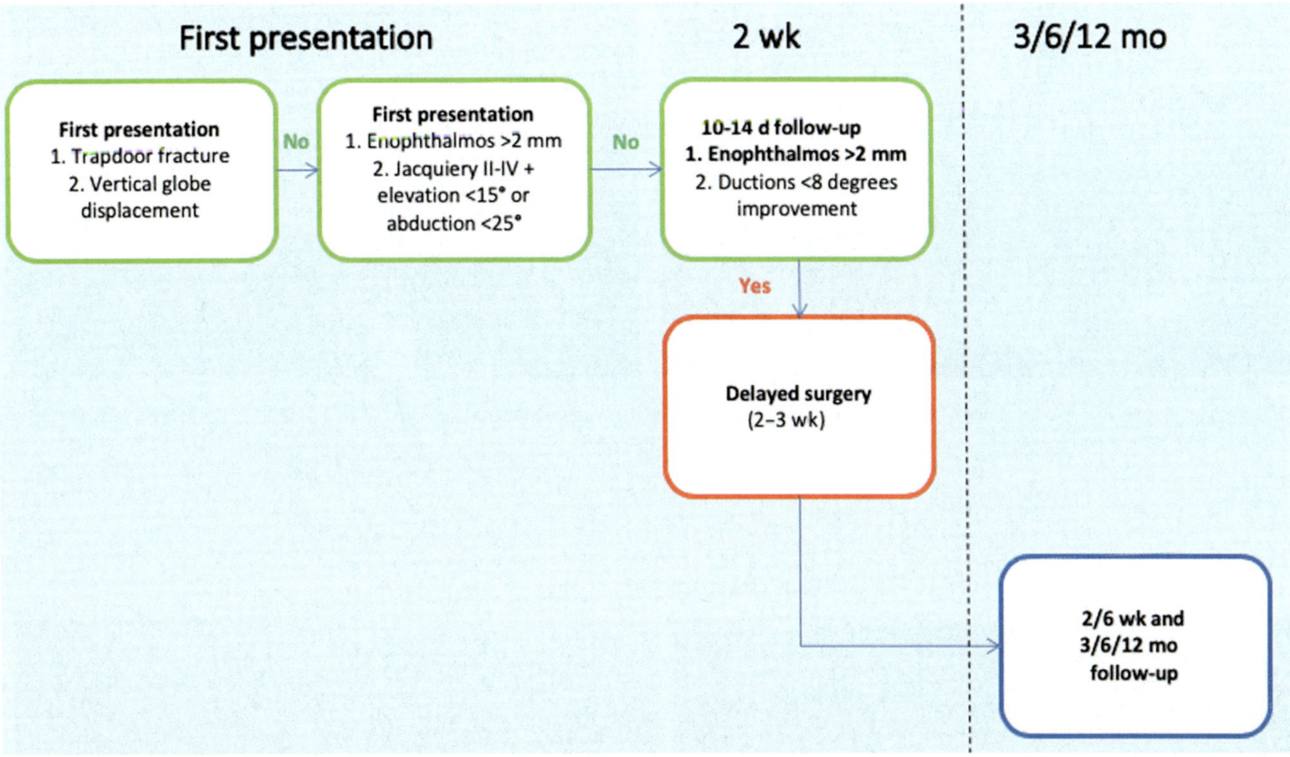

Fig. 28 Case 4: patient-specific flow chart.

improvement of the Hess schemes over time. The patient benefited from a delayed surgical approach (Fig. 34). According to protocol, treatment was carried out on objective and functional parameters, that is, findings.

Pearls and pitfalls

- Pearl: diplopia and limited eye motility have the potential to recover spontaneously after an orbital wall fracture.
- Pearl: the development of clinically significant enophthalmos (>2 mm) after nonsurgical treatment of an extensive orbital wall fracture is rare.
- Pitfall: the CT scan images obtained on first presentation in many cases show extensive bony disruption of the orbital floor. These findings often result in the surgeon scheduling the patient for surgical exploration of the orbit; however, we know that a wait-and-see policy is justified in most of these cases. On the other hand, when postoperative complaints persist, this may not necessarily be caused by the titanium mesh reconstruction material.
- Pearl: a good surgeon will recognize when to postpone surgery.
- Pitfall: severe pain on elevation soon after surgery may be caused by interference of the reconstruction plate with the inferior rectus muscle; to consider a wait-and-see policy in such a case is the wrong decision.
- Pearl: good and satisfactory clinical and functional results are achieved with a predominantly nonsurgical

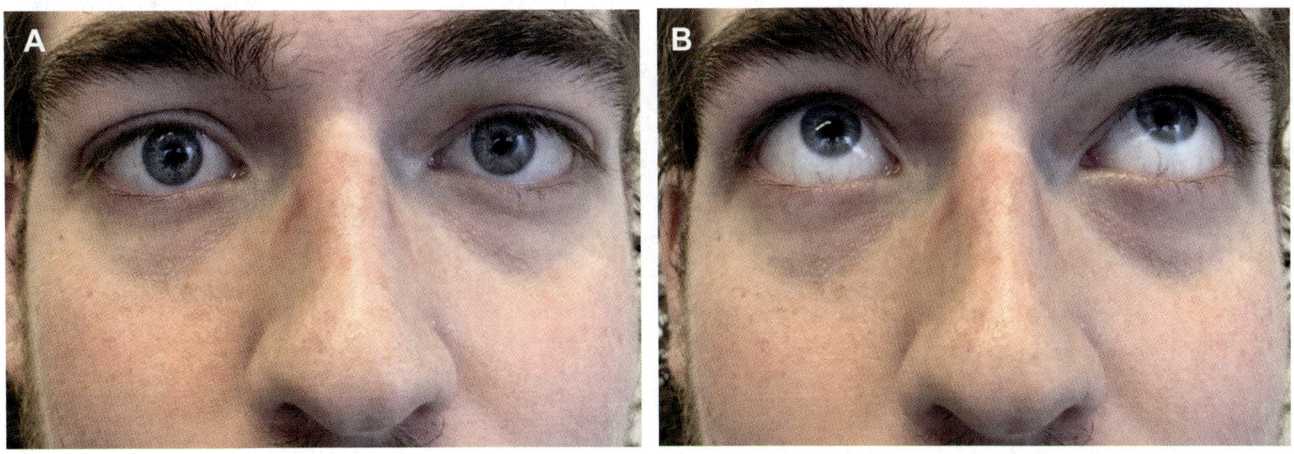

Fig. 29 Case 5: clinical appearance at presentation: (*A*) en face, (*B*) elevation. (*Courtesy of* Peter J.J. Gooris, MD, DMD, PhD, FEBOMFS)

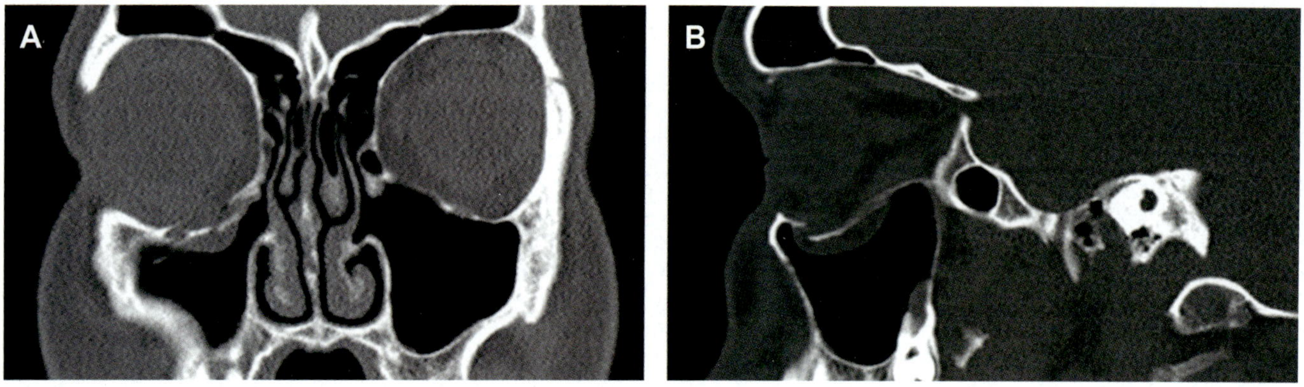

Fig. 30 Case 5: coronal (*A*) and sagittal (*B*) views of the CT scan at first presentation. (*Courtesy of* Peter J.J. Gooris, MD, DMD, PhD, FEBOMFS)

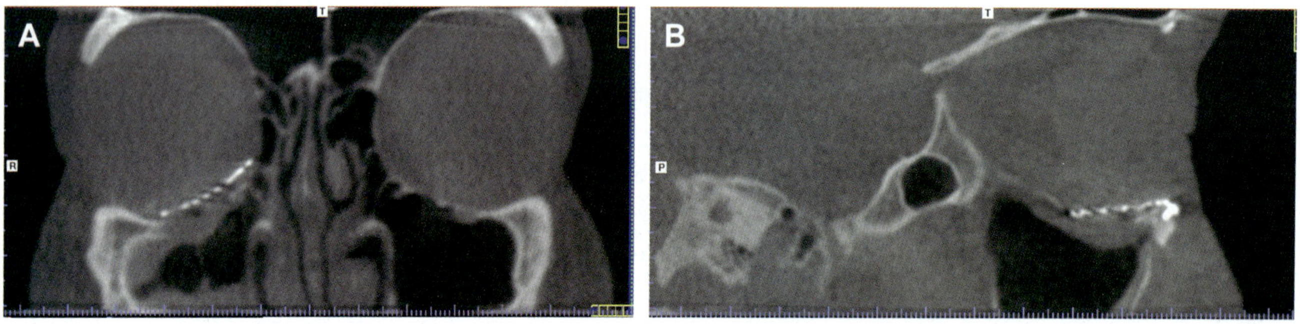

Fig. 31 Case 5: coronal (*A*) and sagittal (*B*) views of the postoperative CT scan. (*Courtesy of* Peter J.J. Gooris, MD, DMD, PhD, FEBOMFS)

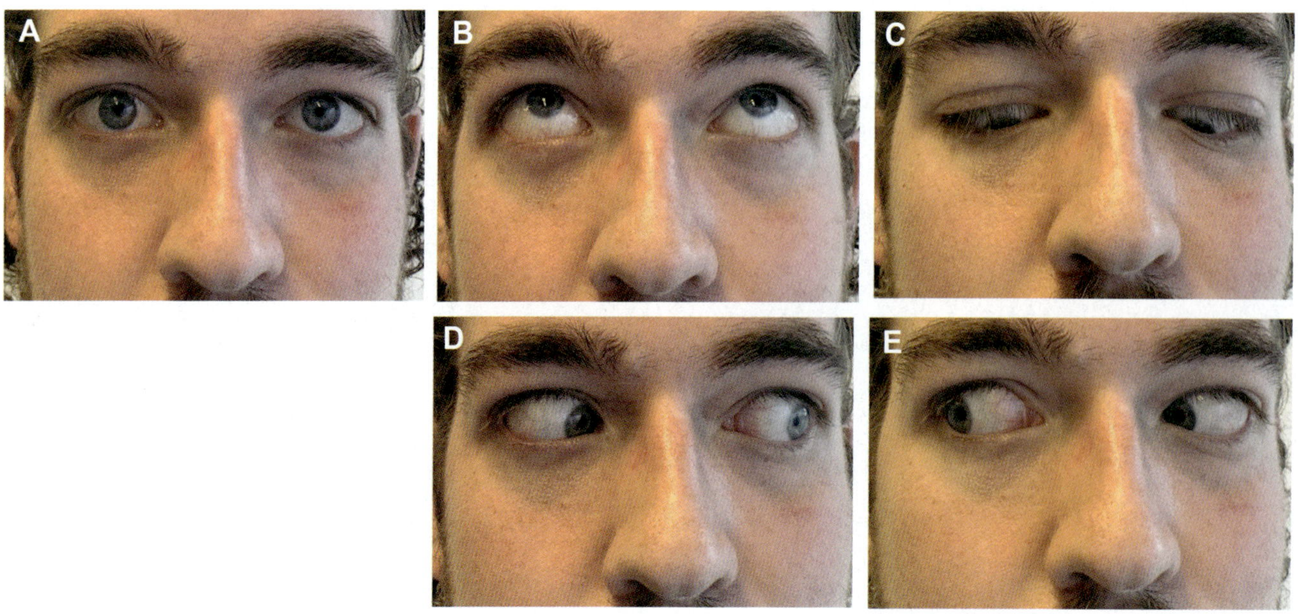

Fig. 32 Case 5: clinical result 3 months after surgery: (*A*) en face, (*B*) elevation, (*C*) depression (*D*) adduction, (*E*) abduction. (*Courtesy of* Peter J.J. Gooris, MD, DMD, PhD, FEBOMFS)

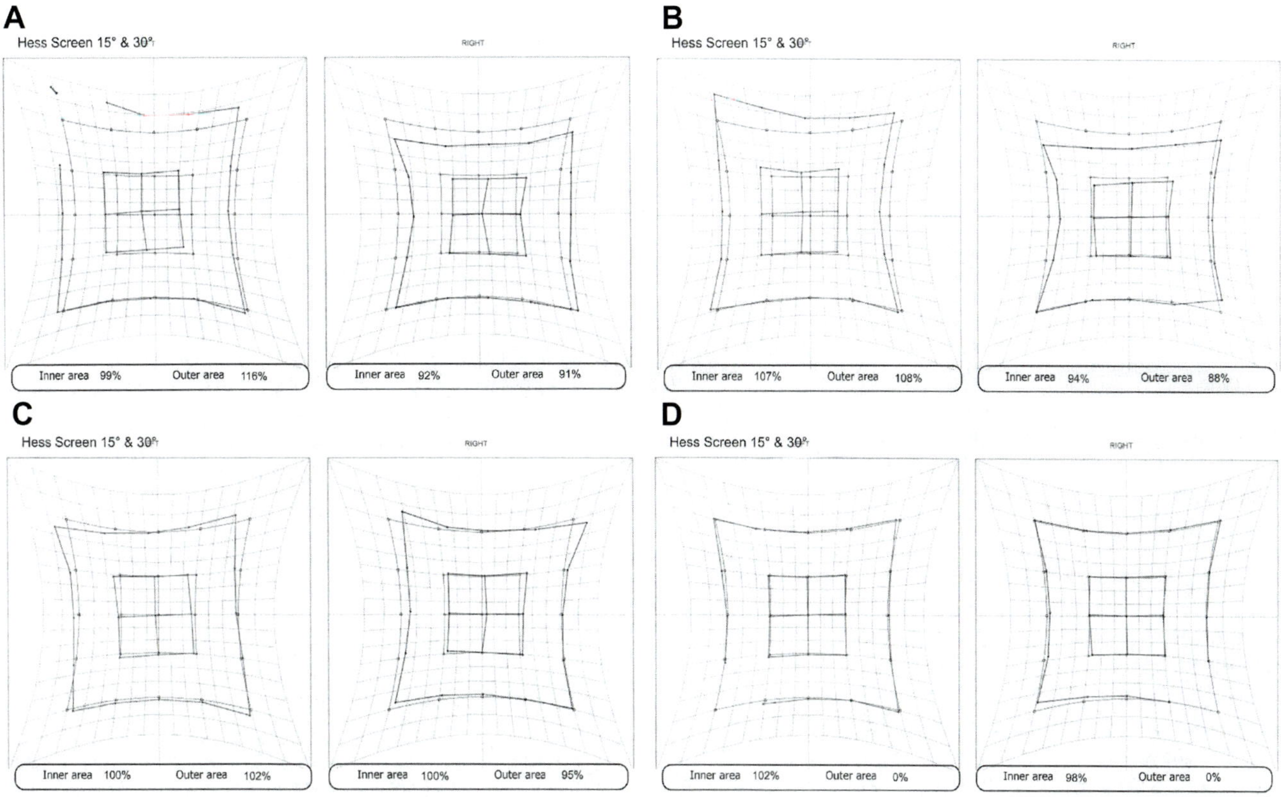

Fig. 33 Case 5: Hess schemes: (*A*) first presentation, (*B*) 2 weeks after trauma, (*C*) 6 weeks after surgery, (*D*) 3 months after surgery. (*Courtesy of* Peter J.J. Gooris, MD, DMD, PhD, FEBOMFS)

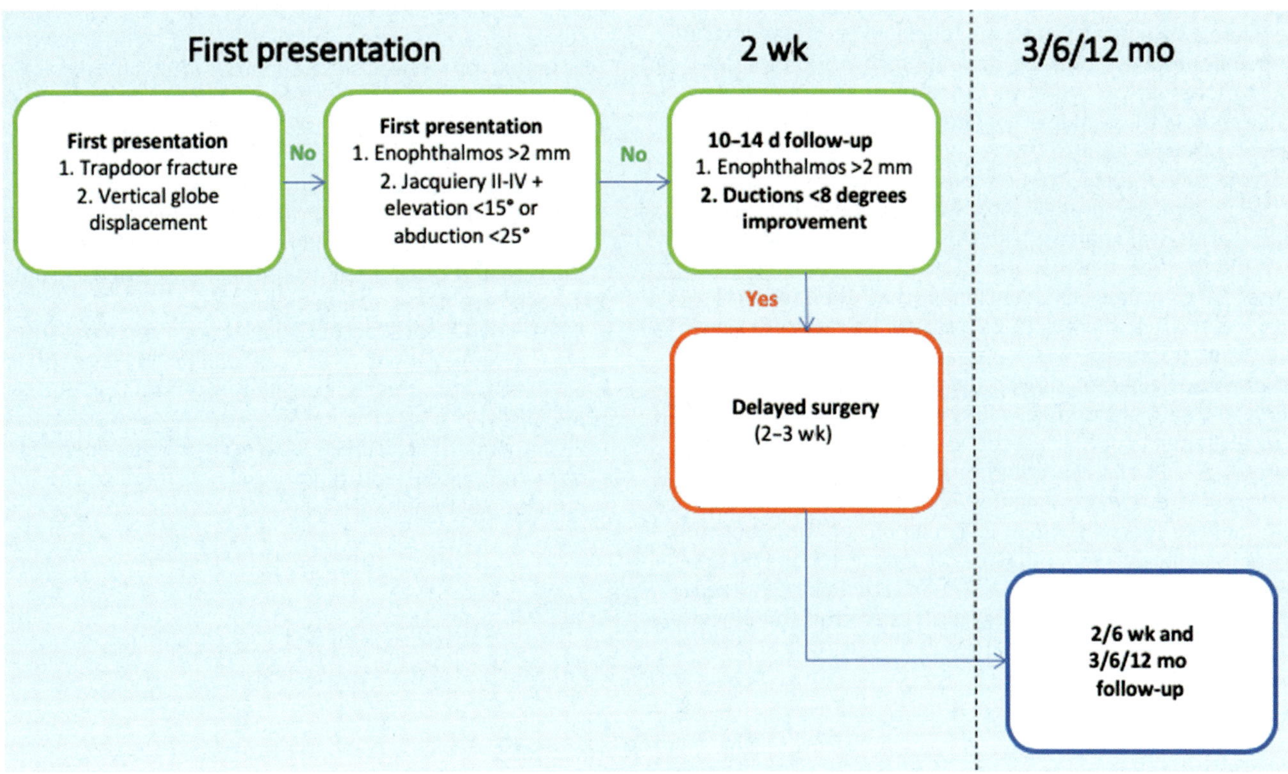

Fig. 34 Case 5: patient-specific flow chart.

approach, which is justified for most orbital wall fractures.

- Pearl: it is recommended to offer the patient with an orbital wall fracture a multidisciplinary approach to determine the most optimal treatment; by extension of this, more knowledge can be amassed about the prevailing issues.

Clinical results in the literature

The main challenge in orbital fracture management is identifying a patient who may benefit from orbital reconstruction above a "wait-and-see policy." The true indications for immediate reconstruction are clear. Extensive research is suggesting that orbital reconstruction is required only when clinical symptoms such as enophthalmos or and diplopia are present and persistent while the criterium for diplopia is predominantly subjective.[6,8,21–25]

We should, if possible, postpone surgery until it is clear that the previously mentioned signs and symptoms develop or are present instead of treating radiographic findings, that is, CT scans. This could potentially prevent more than 60% of surgeries, with the same or better results.[7,8]

Although it is suggested by some investigators that an orbital wall defect exceeding 2 cm^2 or greater than 50% of the surface measured on the CT scan warrants orbital floor reconstruction to prevent enophthalmos, there is no consensus yet on this subject.[26–28]

We now know that as long as the musculo-connective supportive orbital framework of the globe is relatively undamaged, it can be expected that orbital fractures recover spontaneously without significant motility disturbances or enophthalmos.[4,22] Surgical intervention is no guarantee that ocular motility will recover. In fact, surgery implicates additional trauma to the already damaged delicate orbital soft tissue while nonsurgical treatment relies on the regenerative capacity of the body, allowing time for recovery of contused orbital soft tissue.[11,21] Moreover, surgery of the orbital wall does not address the damaged connective tissue or the intrinsic extraocular muscle injury.[6,22]

However, when there is an obvious indication for intervention, the outcome is more favorable when surgery is carried out early.[10,11] This will minimize fibrosis and scarring, which is responsible for late diplopia.

Jansen and colleagues[8] concluded that the nonsurgical approach is a safe and predictable treatment strategy for most orbital wall fractures, which can prevent surgery-related complications. Whether the patient requires surgical or nonsurgical treatment is largely determined by the outcome of the measurements of consecutive orthoptic evaluations. Therefore, a wait-and-see policy is justified; however, when there is insufficient improvement of impairment of extraocular muscle motility, persistent BSV less than 60, or the development of significant exophthalmos, surgical reconstruction should be used.[8] In such cases, VSP, navigation-guided reconstruction, and intraoperative imaging is preferred to achieve the most predictable and optimal result.[12–16]

Summary

The implementation of a clinical protocol for orbital fracture management is presented in this article. We have elaborated on the preoperative workup and the essential role of baseline and consecutive orthoptic evaluations during the posttrauma phase. On the basis of a study model scheme, a decision-making process is explained to determine whether a patient will receive surgical or nonsurgical treatment. Five clinical cases are reported to demonstrate the decision-making process for each treatment.

It appears that there is no strict correlation between the size of the defect on the CT scan and the development of enophthalmos. When there is <2 mm enophthalmos and sufficient improvement in BSV and ductions, as objectivated by repeated orthoptic measurements, the patient can be treated without surgery. For surgical patients, the surgical procedure and postoperative management are briefly mentioned. Allowing time for the contused orbital soft tissue to recover highlights the substantial regenerative capacity; most orbital wall fractures do well without intervention. A multidisciplinary approach is essential to warrant a dependable policy.

clinics care points

- Pearl: allow time for orbital soft tissue to recover; often, diplopia will recover spontaneously while enophthalmus $>$2mm will hardly ever develop and as such will clinically barely noticeable.
- Pitfall: The CT scan images obtained on first presentation in many cases show extensive bony disruption of the orbital floor; these findings are for the surgeon involved often very tempting to schedule the patient for surgical exploration of the orbit while we know that a wait and see policy is justified in most such cases. On the other hand, when postoperative complaints persist, this may not necessarily be caused by the titanium mesh reconstruction material.
- Pearl: a good surgeon will recognize when to postpone surgery Pearl: diplopia and limited eye motility have the potential to recover spontaneously after an orbital wall fracture.
- Pearl: the development of clinically significant enophthalmus ($>$2mm) after a nonsurgical treatment of an extensive orbital wall fracture is rare.
- Pitfall: severe pain on elevation soon postoperative may be caused by interference of the inferior rectus muscle by the reconstruction plate; to consider a wait and see policy in such case is a wrong decision.
- Pearl: good & satisfactory clinical and functional results are achieved with a predominantly nonsurgical approach and this is justified for most orbital wall fractures.
- Pearl: a multidisciplinary approach is recommended to offer the patient with an orbital wall fracture the most optimal treatment.

Disclosure

The authors have nothing to disclose.

References

1. Smith B, Regan WF Jr. Blow out fracture of the orbit: mechanism and correction of internal orbital fracture. Am J Ophthalmol 1957;44:733–9.

2. Converse JM, Smith B, Obear MF, et al. Orbital blow out fractures: a ten-year survey. Plast Reconstr Surg 1967;39:20–36.
3. Putterman AM, Stevens T, Urist MJ. Nonsurgical management of blow-out fractures of the orbital floor. Am J Ophthalmol 1974;77:232–9.
4. Koornneef L. Current concepts on the management of orbital blow-out fractures. Ann Plast Surg 1982;9:185–200.
5. Burnstine MA. Clinical recommendations for repair of isolated orbital floor fractures: an evidence-based analysis. Ophthalmology 2002;109:1207–10.
6. Alhamdani F, Durham J, Greenwood M, et al. Diplopia and ocular motility in orbital blow-out fractures: 10-year retrospective study. J Craniomaxillofac Surg 2015;43:1010–6.
7. Christensen BJ, Zaid W. Inaugural survey on practice patterns of orbital floor fractures for American oral and maxillofacial surgeons. J Oral Maxillofac Surg 2016;74:105–22.
8. Jansen J, Dubois L, Maal TJJ, et al. A nonsurgical approach with repeated orthoptic evaluation is justified for most blow-out fractures. J Craniomaxillofac Surg 2020;48:560–8.
9. Dal Canto AJ, Linberg JV. Comparison of orbital fracture repair performed within 14 days versus 15 to 29 days after trauma. Ophthal Plast Reconstr Surg 2008;24:437–43.
10. Damgaard OE, Larsen CG, Felding UA, et al. Surgical timing of the orbital "blowout" fracture: a systematic review and meta-analysis. Otolaryngol Head Neck Surg 2016;155:387–90.
11. Jazayeri HE, Khavanin N, Yu JW, et al. Does early repair of orbital fractures result in superior patient outcomes? A systematic review and meta-analysis. J Oral Maxillofac Surg 2020;78:568–77.
12. Gellrich N-C, Schramm A, Hammer B, et al. Computer-assisted secondary reconstruction of unilateral posttraumatic orbital deformity. Plast Reconstr Surg 2002;110:1417–29.
13. Novelli G, Tonelli G, Mazzoleni F, et al. Virtual surgery simulation in orbital wall reconstruction: integration of surgical navigation and stereolithographic models. J Craniomaxillofac Surg 2014;42:2025–34.
14. Dubois L, Schreurs R, Jansen J, et al. Predictability in orbital reconstruction: a human cadaver study, part II: navigation-assisted orbital reconstruction. J Craniomaxillofac Surg 2015;43:2042–9.
15. Azarmehr I, Stokbro K, Bell B, et al. Surgical navigation: a systematic review of indications, treatments, and outcomes in oral and maxillofacial surgery. J Oral Maxillofac Surg 2017;75:1987–2005.
16. Schreurs R, Dubois l, Becking AG, et al. Measuring predictability in orbital reconstruction: quantitative assessment of orbital implant position. PLOS One 2016;11:e0150162.
17. Bonawitz S, Crawley W, Shores JT, et al. Modified transconjunctival approach to the lower eyelid: technical details for predictable results. Craniomaxillofac Trauma Reconstr 2016;9:29–34.
18. Gooris PJJ, Muller B, Dubois L, et al. Finding the ledge: sagittal analysis of bony landmarks of the orbit. J Oral Maxillofac Surg 2017;75:2613–27.
19. Gunarajah DR, Samman N. Biomaterials for repair of orbital floor blowout fractures: a systematic review. J Oral Maxillofac Surg 2013;71:550–70.
20. Dubois L, Steenen SA, Gooris PJJ, et al. Controversies in orbital reconstruction – I. Defect-driven orbital reconstruction: a systematic review. Int J Oral Maxillofac Surg 2015a;44:308–15.
21. Aldekhayel S, Aljaaly H, Fouda-Neel O, et al. Evolving trends in the management of orbital floor fractures. J Craniofac Surg 2014;25:258–61.
22. Devoe AG. Fractures of the orbital floor. Trans Am Ophthalmol Soc 1947;45:502–26.
23. Beigi B, Khandwala M, Gupta D. Management of pure orbital floor fractures: a proposed protocol to prevent unnecessary or early surgery. Orbit 2014;33:336–42.
24. Alinasab B, Ryott M, Stjärne P. Still no reliable consensus in management of blow-out fracture. Injury 2014;45:197–202.
25. Bartoli D, Fadda MT, Battisti A, et al. Retrospective analysis of 301 patients with orbital floor fracture. J Craniomaxillofac Surg 2015;43:244–7.
26. Kunz C, Sigron GR, Jaquiéry C. Functional outcome after non-surgical management of orbital fractures: the bias of decision-making according to size of defect: critical review of 48 patients. Br J Oral Maxillofac Surg 2013;51:486–92.
27. Goggin J, Jupiter DC, Czerwinski M. Simple computed tomography-based calculations of orbital floor fracture defect size are not sufficiently accurate for clinical use. J Oral Maxillofac Surg 2015;73:112–6.
28. Jaquiéry C, Aeppli P, Cornelius P, et al. Reconstruction of orbital wall defects: critical review of 72 patients. Int J Oral Maxillofac Surg 2007;36:193–9.

Secondary Corrections of the Orbit

Solitary Fractures

Harald Essig, PD, Dr med, Dr med dent*,
Maximilian Eberhard Hermann Wagner, Dr med univ, Dr med dent,
Michael Blumer, Dr med, Dr med dent

KEYWORDS

• Secondary reconstruction • Orbital reconstruction • Patient-specific implant • Navigation • Intraoperative imaging • Computer-aided design • Virtual reconstruction • Customized implant

KEY POINTS

- Late and secondary orbital reconstructions are more demanding than primary reconstructions due to altered anatomic landmarks and late soft tissue changes—so the ultimate objective should be an adequate primary reconstruction.
- Computer-assisted planning/surgery in combination with intraoperative navigation and/or imaging improve postoperative results.
- Most common indications for secondary orbital reconstructions are globe malposition, binocular diplopia, and impaired eye motility.

Introduction: nature of the problem

Secondary orbital reconstructions mostly affect defects in the area of the orbital floor or the medial wall, because these structures are most susceptible to fractures due to fragility. These defects may cause an increase of the orbital volume and a dislocation of the orbital content; furthermore, an altered globe position may arise (Fig. 1). Clinically, enophthalmos and/or hypoglobus develops (Figs. 2 and 3). As part of primary trauma diagnostics, swelling of the soft tissue in the affected eye socket may compensate this increase in volume for a short time. Even supposedly objective methods such as Hertel or Naugle ophthalmometry are not helpful because the bony structures are not sufficiently taken into account in those cases. In cases where a volume-relevant defect is not treated surgically and swelling has subsided, the bulb can be dislocated permanently and associated complaints may arise. In addition to an aesthetically noticeable asymmetry, functional restrictions are particularly stressful for the patients. These restrictions range from binocular diplopia to motility restrictions and may have a significant impact on everyday quality of life. Such symptoms may be more apparent in insufficiently reconstructed orbits than in fractured orbits with no treatment at all (Fig. 4). This finding is due to more pronounced scarring in previously operated orbits on one hand, on the other hand to foreign material, that has to be removed during secondary orbital reconstruction, and this may complicate the further outcome. The ultimate goal of any reconstruction, primary or secondary, must therefore be to restore the original aesthetic and functional situation as good as possible by means of accurate preoperative diagnostics and planning.

Klinik für Mund-, Kiefer- und Gesichtschirurgie, UniversitätsSpital Zürich, Frauenklinikstrasse 24, Zürich 8091, Switzerland
* Corresponding author.
E-mail address: Harald.Essig@usz.ch

Surgical technique

Preoperative planning

A thorough patient history including the initial trauma and all previous surgeries, as well as physical examination has to be conducted with special focus on visual acuity, pupil function, eye motility, and binocular diplopia. Even though major eye injuries are seldom, an interdisciplinary examination by an ophthalmologist is recommended also for medicolegal reasons. The position of the bulb is assessed using a Naugle or Hertel ophthalmometry and photo documentation. Current indications for secondary orbital corrections are enophthalmos larger than 2 mm and persistent diplopia due to possible tissue entrapment. Optimal timing for the procedure depends on the specific case, but 3 to 6 months after primary reconstruction or trauma is favored by most surgeons. For preoperative planning a three-dimensional (3D) imaging for evaluation of the bony boundary and the orbital soft tissue situation is mandatory. Computed tomography with contrast medium and a layer thickness of less than 1 mm is recommended. Because of the lack of soft tissue resolution, cone-beam computed tomography (CBCT) alone often does not provide sufficient information. The same applies to MRI for the bony boundary. The 3D imaging and the clinical findings facilitate a precise planning of the further procedure.

A recent 3D data set can therefore be used as the basis for further planning. The planning is basically identical to that of a primary orbital reconstruction. Assuming the symmetry of the

Atlas Oral Maxillofacial Surg Clin N Am 29 (2021) 129-137
1061-3315/21/
https://doi.org/10.1016/j.cxom.2020.11.007

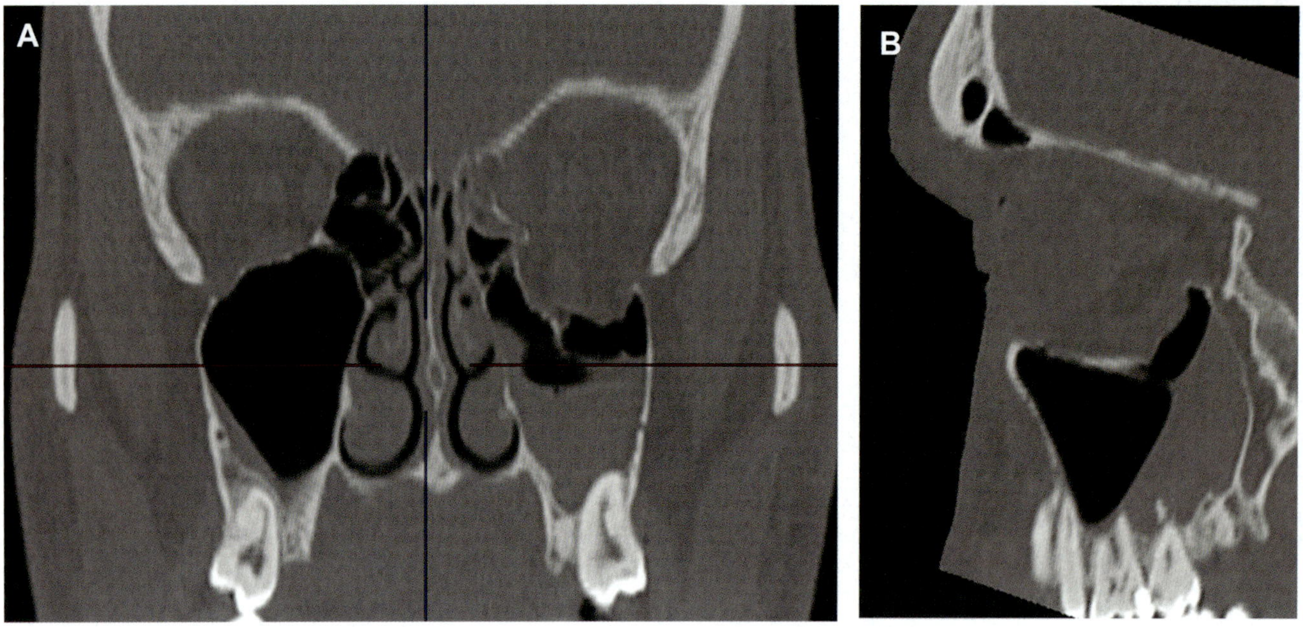

Fig. 1 Coronal (*A*) and sagittal (*B*) view of an orbital 2-wall fracture before primary reconstruction.

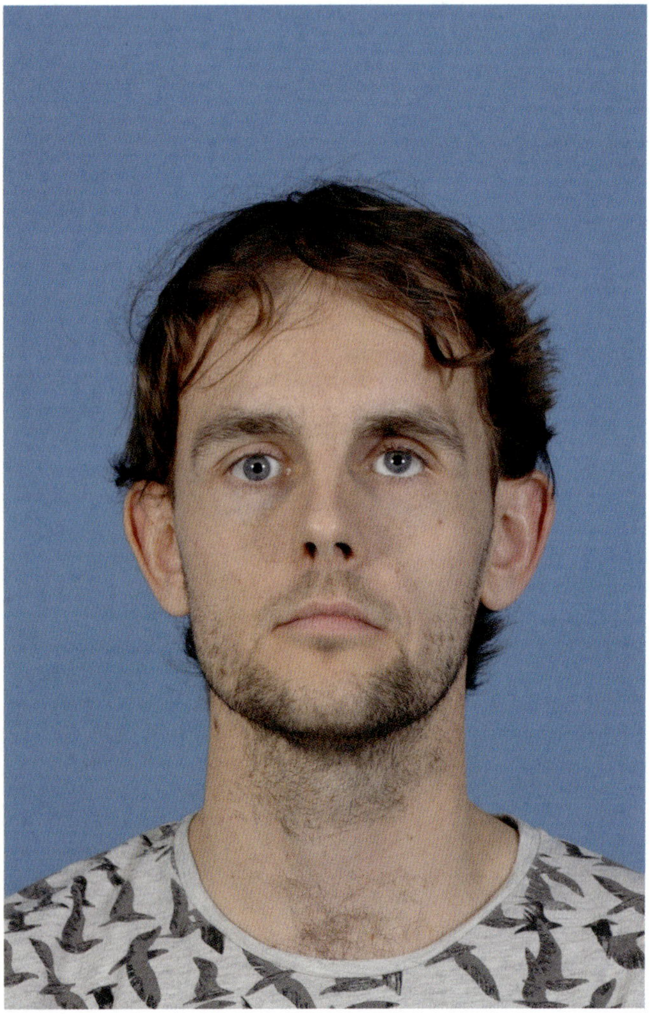

Fig. 2 Frontal view of insufficient reconstructed left orbit. Impaired eye motility, binocular diplopia, and a globe malposition are found. Naugle and Hertel ophthalmometry shows an enophthalmos of 3 mm.

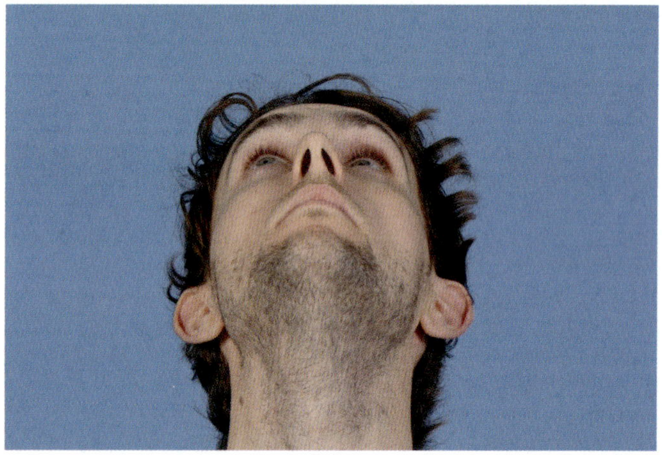

Fig. 3 Bottom view of insufficient reconstructed left orbit. A distinct enophthalmos is found.

midface, the orbital shape of the unaffected side is used. Using a mirroring function of the planning software, this object serves as a template for the virtual reconstruction of the fractured orbit. In primary reconstruction cases, a simple mirroring is usually sufficient. The requirements for patient-specific implants are also similar to those of primary cases: round edges, radiologic visibility, inert material, and reconstruction of significant anatomic areas (ie, posterior ledge, transition zone). The bony frame may be reconstructed in the same shape as before the trauma with the help of determining the orbital volumes based on the bony boundaries, which works well in primary orbital trauma repair. In the case of secondary reconstructions, additional overcorrections of the orbital volume may be necessary due to posttraumatic or postsurgical fat tissue atrophy or increase of the bony orbit (eg, additional roof fracture or loss of lateral wall). The amount of overcorrection has to be estimated individually for each patient and fracture pattern, hence up to now no conclusive literature is available

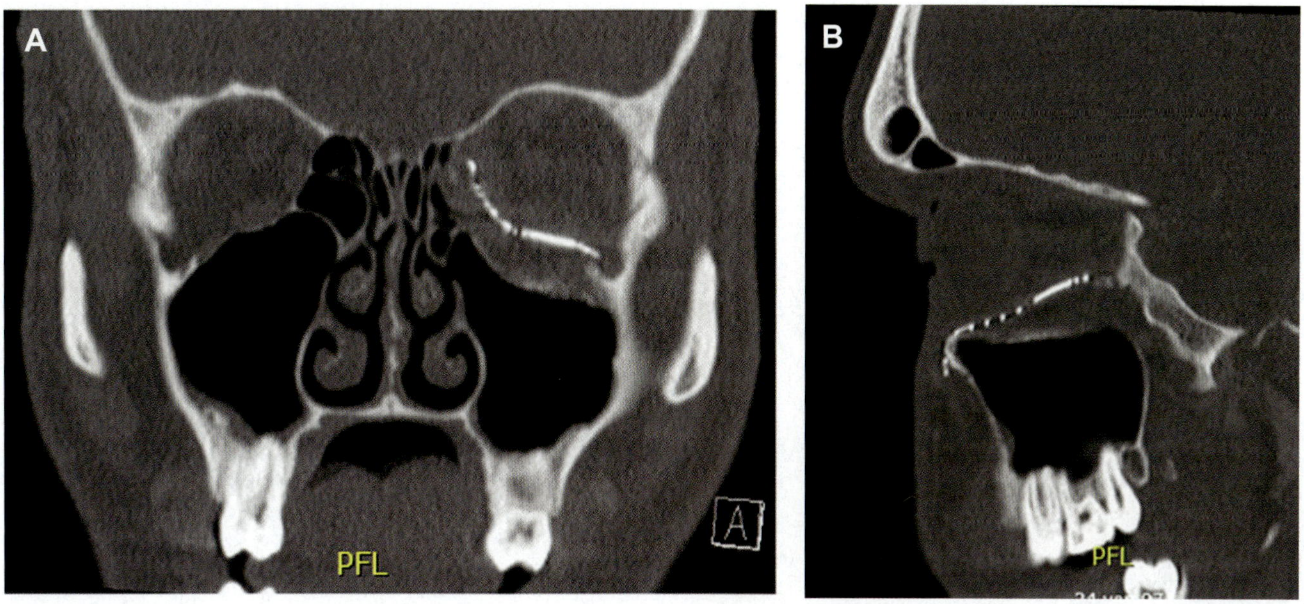

Fig. 4 Coronal (*A*) and sagittal (*B*) view of an orbital 2-wall fracture after insufficient primary reconstruction.

on this matter (Fig. 5). The same applies to imported foreign material. The scope of such an additional virtual volume correction may unfortunately only be determined objectively to a limited extent by volume measurement and still requires a solid experience of the operating surgeon. Ultimately, the goal of preoperative planning is the construction of a virtual model of the orbit, which matches the clinical situation. This virtual model is then the basis for 3D-printing patient-specific bio-models or, ideally, manufacturing patient-specific implants. Many surgeons prefer titanium as standard material due to its

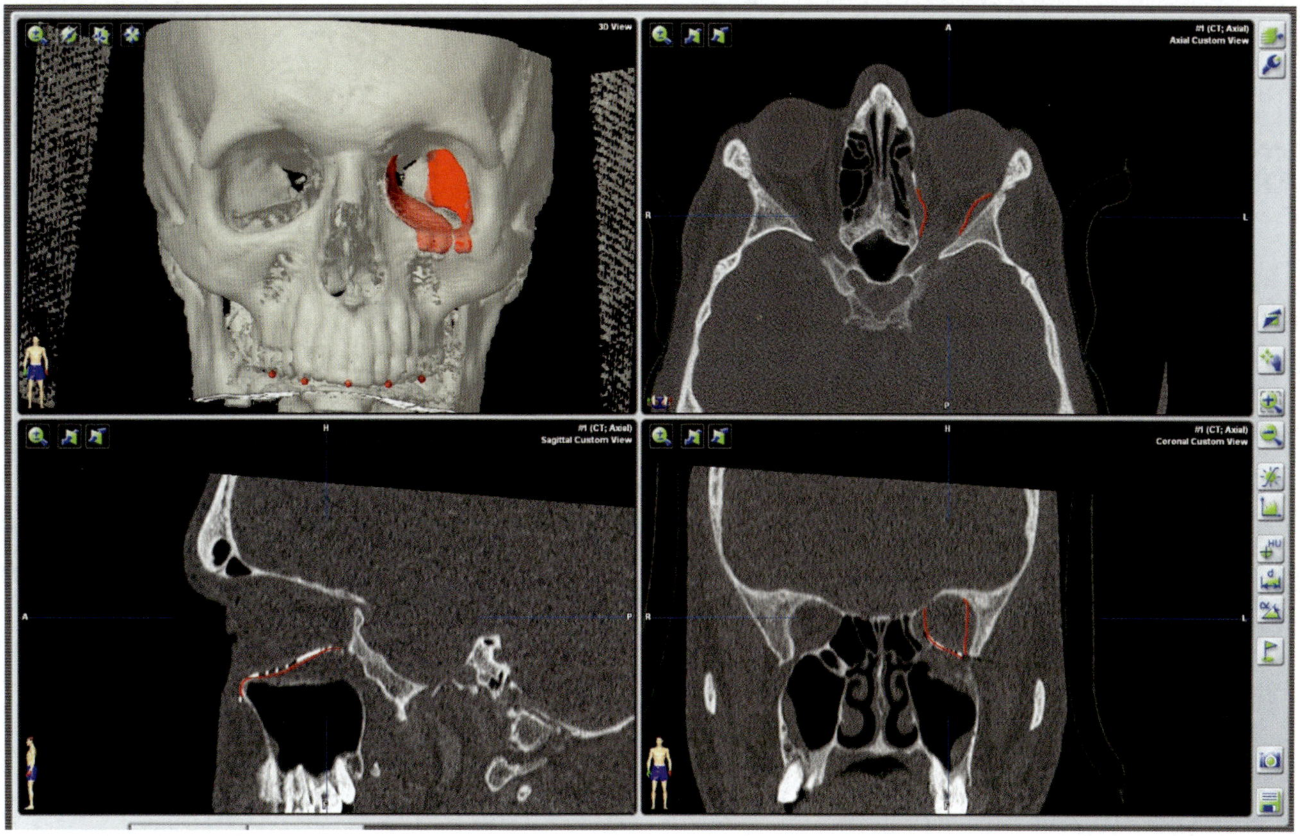

Fig. 5 Preoperative computer-assisted planning shows in red the virtually constructed PSI superimposed on a computed tomography showing the insufficient primary orbital reconstruction. PSI, patient-specific implant.

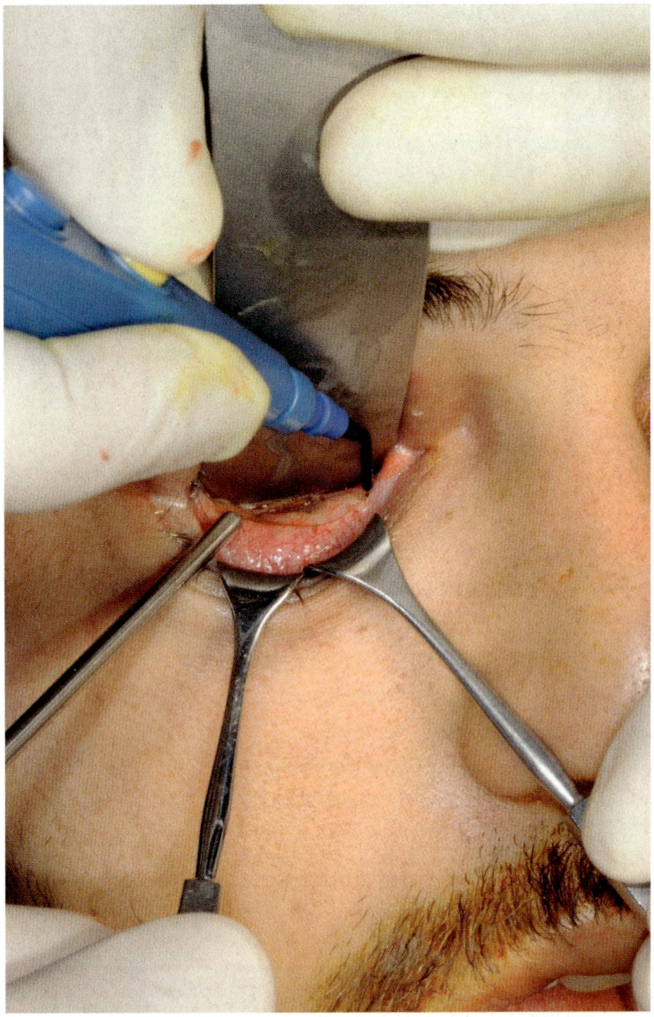

Fig. 6 Arcuate formed incision of the conjunctival tissue using a monopolar needle. The conjunctiva is stretched using lid retractors and a malleable spatula.

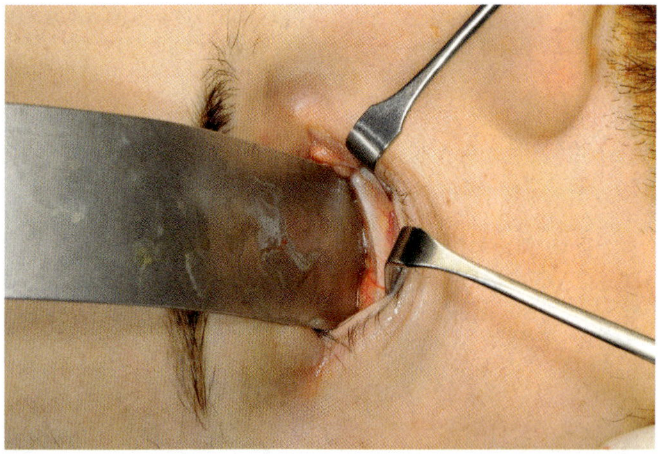

Fig. 8 Identification of the infraorbital margin and incision of the periostium after removal of intraorbital tissue.

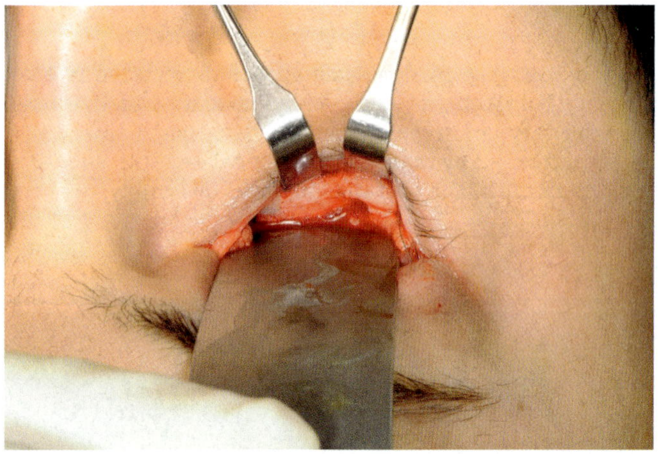

Fig. 9 Dissection and reduction of herniated orbital tissue. The entire bony support area must be identifiable in order to facilitate implant placement without tissue entrapment.

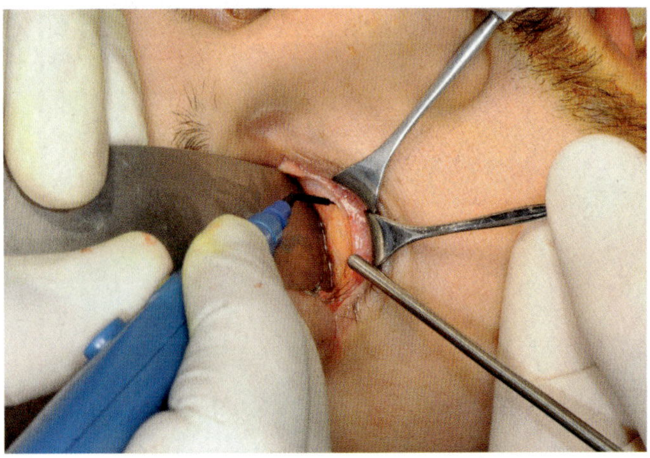

Fig. 7 Subsequent layerwise dissection completing the transconjunctival retroseptal approach.

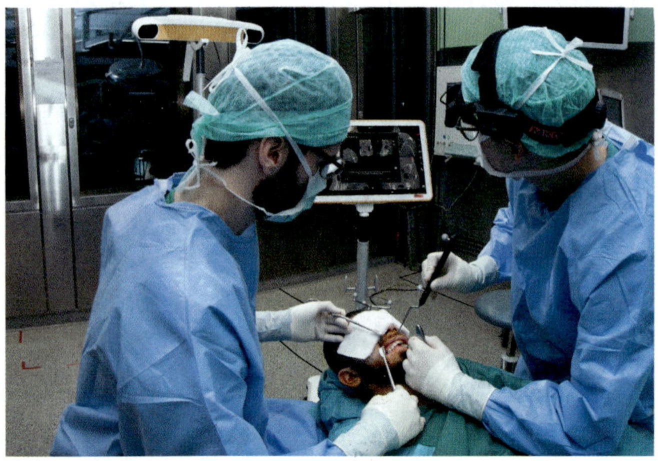

Fig. 10 Intraoperative navigation facilitates secondary orbital reconstruction, offering real-time 3D position control.

biological and technical characteristics (ie, inert, dimensionally stable, radiopacity). The preoperative virtual planning may also be used intraoperatively for real-time navigation or intraoperative 3D imaging with subsequent superimposition as a quality control.

Preparation and patient positioning

When using intraoperative navigation, only hard tissue–based registration is thought to be sufficiently exact for intraorbital navigation. A dental splint with navigational markers (eg, titanium mini screws) may be fabricated preoperatively through a dental technician. With the help of a preoperative 3D data set and the prepared splint, an exact hard tissue registration is possible without further invasive measures. Using this workflow, the most accurate radiation-free position control may be performed. Real-time intraoperative navigation is still an extremely helpful tool, especially for complex reconstructions or less-experienced surgeons.

The patient is placed supine during the procedure and intubated orally in most cases. In cases of intraoperative navigation both the oral cavity and scalp part of the head need to be disinfected in order to place the registration splint and transfixed navigation parts.

The use of a headlamp or an alternative light source tailored to the surgeon is strongly recommended.

Surgical approach

The transconjunctival retroseptal approach seems most suitable, as seldom complications occur. Incision may be done using either a scalpel or a monopolar device. If there are no contraindications, the monopolar offers the advantage of bloodless preparation in layers. In general, the best position for the surgeon is cranially to the patient giving appropriate view for most orbital areas.

Surgical procedure

The lower eyelid is held caudally using lid retractors; the bulb together with the intraorbital soft tissue is gently pulled cranially. Now the conjunctival tissue is incised. It is important to keep a sufficiently large distance from the lid edge, and an arcuate cut should be performed (Fig. 6). Now the subconjunctival layer is also dissected using the monopolar needle (Fig. 7). The intraorbital tissue is carefully pulled up. The eyelid retractors may now be replaced by smaller ones. The periosteum can now be identified easily and incised as well in the area of the infraorbital margin (Fig. 8). Now the orbital floor or the lower parts of the medial wall may be dissected easily (Fig. 9). In cases with large defects in the area of the medial wall, a transcaruncular extension of the transconjunctival approach may be necessary. This way, the entire floor and the medial orbital wall may be reached in a safe and reliable manner. After preparation of the affected region of the orbit and removal of any previously inserted foreign materials, the reconstruction is carried out. A patient-specific titanium implant allows the orbital volume to be reconstructed in a dimensionally stable manner in accordance with the preoperative planning. Intraoperative navigation offers a radiation-free and real-time technique for quality control. For this purpose, a transfixed navigation star is attached to the scalp and the 3D position of the patient in the room is registered by

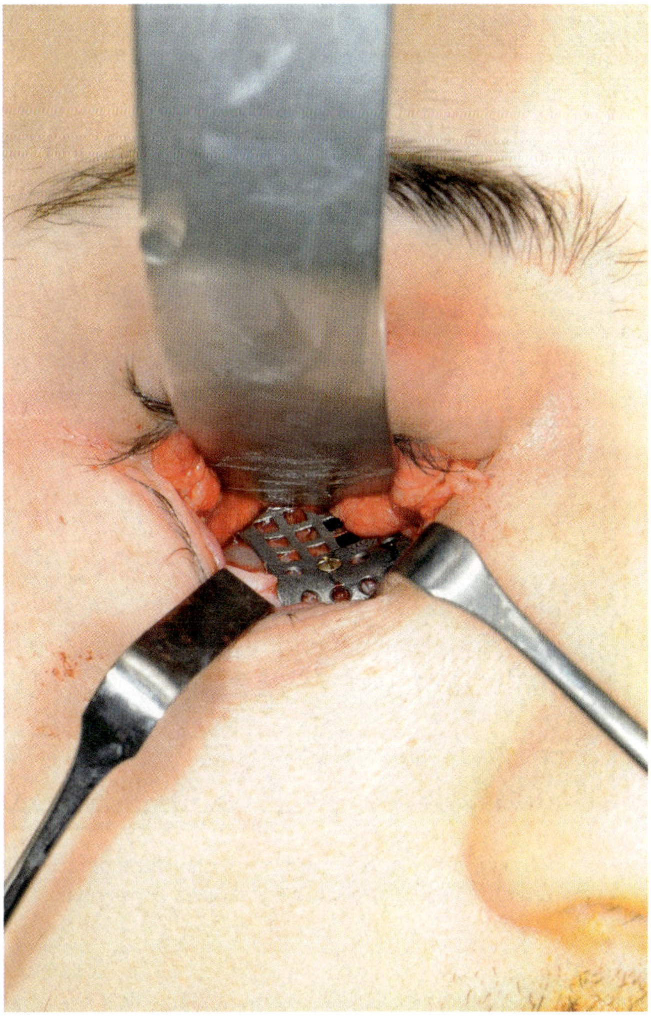

Fig. 11 Implant fixation with mini screws. A forced duction test has to be performed in order to ensure free eye motility. The implant borders have to be visually checked, that there is no tissue entrapment.

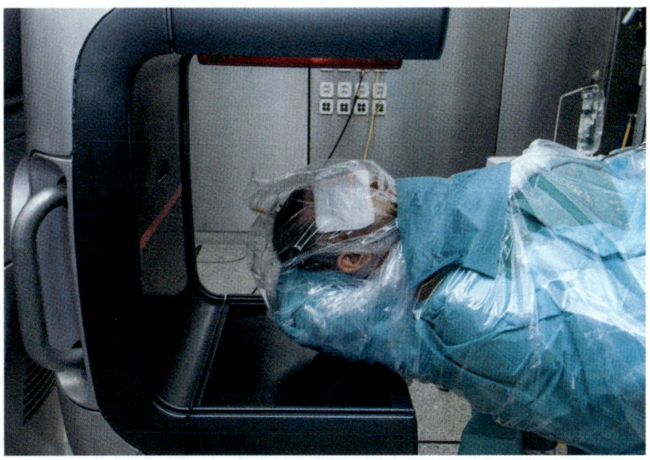

Fig. 12 Intraoperative 3D imaging (ie, CBCT) enables 3D position control of the orbital implant, and furthermore, intraoperative superimposition with the preoperative virtual planning is feasible. Plastic coverage enables instant continuation of the surgery after finishing the imaging process.

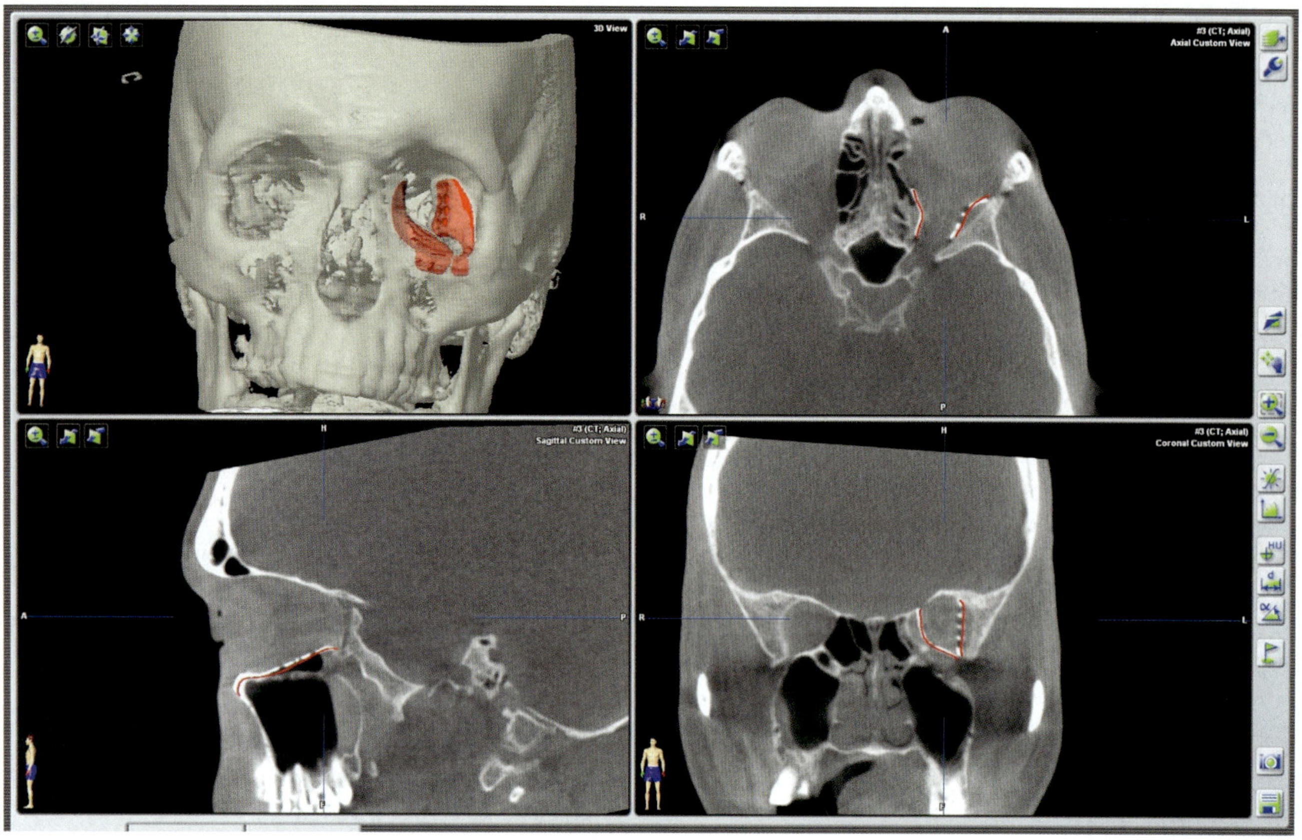

Fig. 13 Intraoperative superimposition of the intraoperative CBCT scan with the preoperative planning shows the accuracy of the secondary orbital reconstruction. In case surgical corrections are needed this may be perfomed instantly.

means of the aforementioned dental splint. This way, a continuous comparison with the virtual planning may already take place during the reconstruction process (Fig. 10). The correct position is first checked clinically. If this seems reasonable, fixation is carried out with at least one osteosynthesis screw in the area of the orbital margin (Fig. 11). The ultimate objective control, however, is the intraoperative 3D imaging (ie, CBCT) (Fig. 12). In addition to direct evaluation of the images, superimposition with the preoperative planning allows for accurate intraoperative quality control (Figs. 13 and 14). With intraoperative imaging corrections may be carried out directly during the same surgery. This way, any secondary

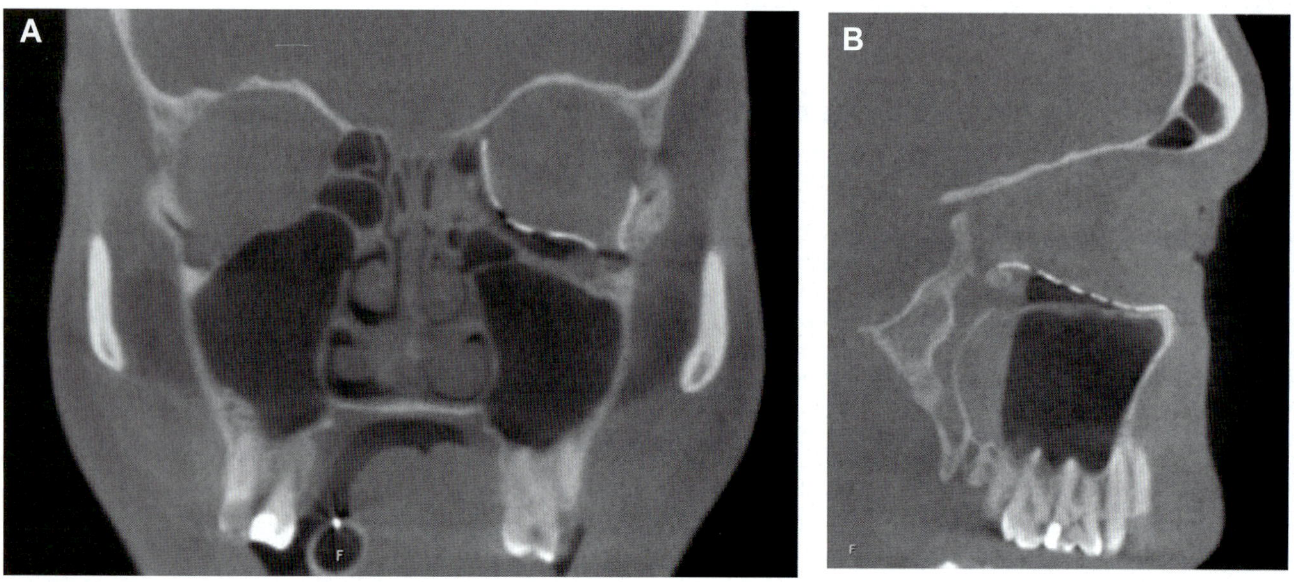

Fig. 14 Coronal (*A*) and sagittal (*B*) view of the intraoperative CBCT scan. Correct position of the implant can be verified.

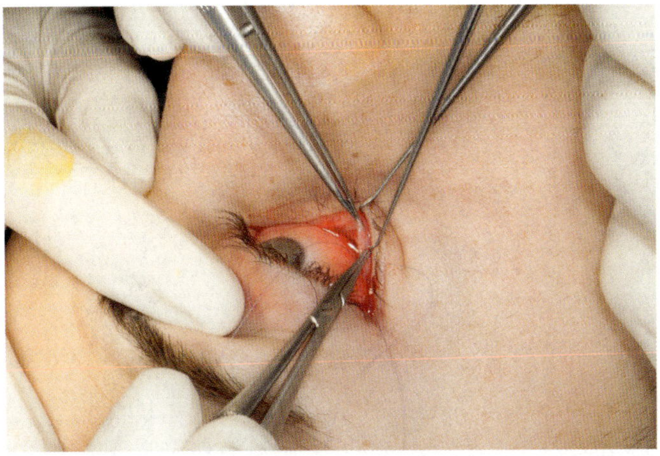

Fig. 15 Wound closure using 7-0 sutures.

intervention is avoided. After satisfactory reconstruction, passive eye motility is checked with the forced duction test. A visual control of the implant borders ensures that no tissue entrapment exists. After rinsing with ringer lactate, the wound is closed using Vicryl 7-0 (Figs. 15–17).

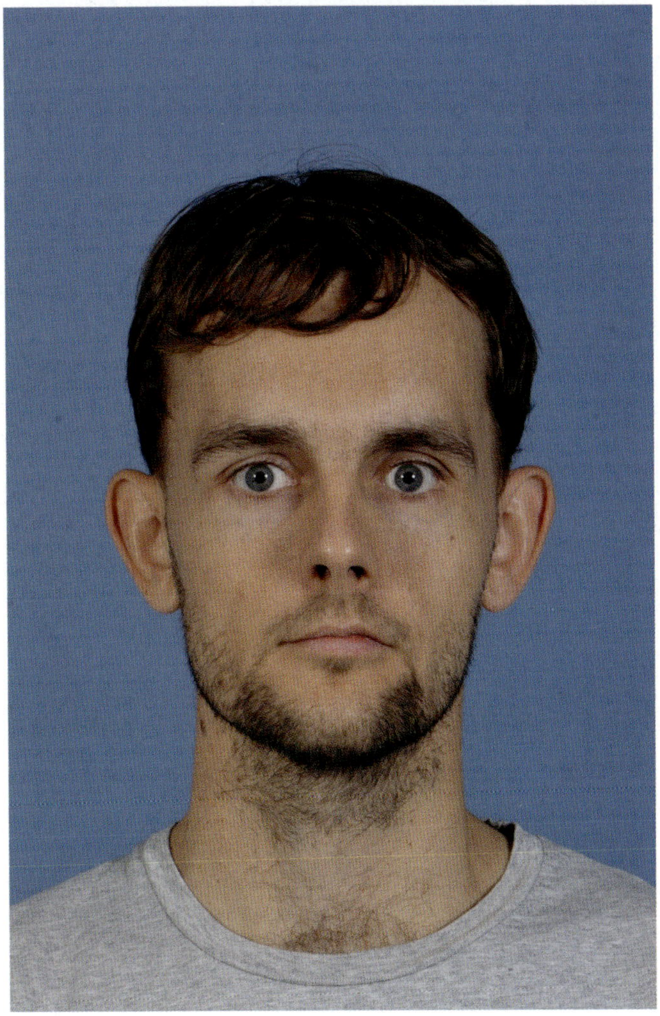

Fig. 16 Frontal view of the secondary reconstructed left orbit with an improved globe position and eye motility. A slight improvement of binocular diplopia was also achieved. Naugle ophthalmometry shows a symmetric result.

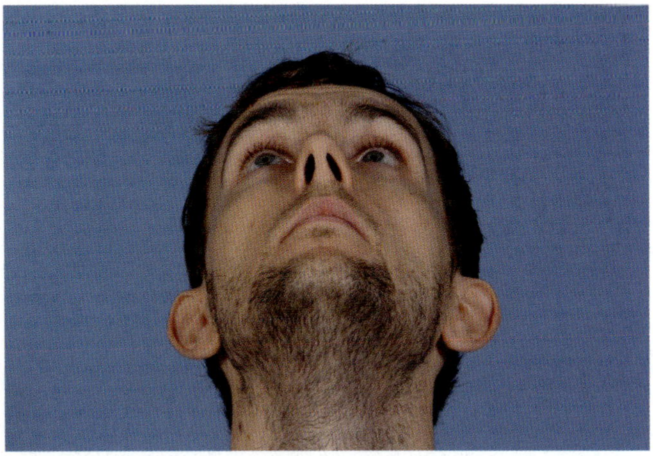

Fig. 17 Bottom view of the secondary reconstructed left orbit with a symmetric globe position.

Potential complications

Scarring in the lower eyelid and consecutive entropion or ectropion may occur, especially in cases with inadequate surgical approach and dissection. Another potential complication is tearing of the lower eyelid, especially in previously operated cases where scarred tissue alters the resilience of the lid. These complications are rare and can be avoided reliably, if dissection is done with sufficient care. Careful dissection is thought to prevent microtrauma to the eye muscles as well as to the orbital tissue. This way extensive fat atrophy hopefully is prevented. Sequelae as binocular diplopia are common in the postoperative inpatient phase due to swelling. Usually diplopia vanishes with decreasing swelling. Blindness of the operated eye is extremely rare and can reliably be avoided with the assistance of modern computer-assisted surgery, patient-specific implants, and sufficient caution by an experienced surgeon.

Pearls and pitfalls

Removal of previously inserted material might be challenging due to scarring. This can differ significantly depending on the used shape and type of material. Scar tissue passes through implant fenestrations and needs to be dissected sharp, which is especially challenging close to structures at risk. The investigators always test free eye motility through a Forced Duction Test *before* implant insertion (as comparative value) and *after* the insertion as ensurement that no orbital tissue is entrapped. Another challenge is the correct estimation of the orbital target volume. Patient-specific implants are thought to ensure a less traumatic orbital reconstruction, a reconstruction that is furthermore in line with preoperative planning. However, intraoperative adaptation is limited. Some studies recommend inserting autogenous bone for correction of orbital volume loss; to the authors' experience, this type of volume contouring is not permanent due to resorption. Titanium blocks in turn may be challenging and difficult to place. In their opinion, thorough preoperative planning of a correct target volume and anatomic shape by an experienced team for planning and surgery constitutes the best solution for achieving optimal results.

Table 1 Clinical results in the literature

	Study Design	Time Posttrauma or Primary Surgery	Cases	Indication	Cause	Reconstruction Material	Surgical Assisting Methods	Complications	Conclusions
Baumann 2015	Retrospective	n.a.	6	Orbital deformity & at least 2-wall defect	5 trauma	4 PEEK	Preoperative CT	1 local infection PEEK	Navigation and CAD/CAM-workflow facilitate late & secondary orbital correction
					1 tumor	2 PSI (titanium)	Preoperative virtual orbit reconstruction CAD/CAM design implants Intraoperative navigation	1 skin perforation in radiated patient	
Park 2016	Retrospective	7 months	16	Enophthalmos	Trauma	Porous polyethylene implants	Preoperative CT	No improvement of eye motility in 2 patients	Reconstruction of posterior margin and floor slope as a key point in prevention of enophthalmos
				Impaired eye motility			Endoscopic assistance		Recommendation of slight exophthalmos at end of surgery
Nkenke 2011	Prospective	6 months	20	Enophthalmos	Trauma	Glass-bioceramic	Preoperative CT	Intraoperative correction of designed implants necessary	Improvement globe position in both groups High costs & fabrication time as drawbacks of designed implants
						Nonpreformed titanium mesh	Preoperative virtual orbit reconstruction 10 CAD/CAM design implants 10 intraoperative formed titanium implants		
Kim 2016	Retrospective	2 d up to 11 y	13	Globe malpositioning Entrapped orbital tissue	Trauma	Majority porous polyethylene-coated titanium mesh	Preoperative CT	Postoperative mydriasis in 1 patient Residual diplopia in 3 patients	Improvement globe position, eye motility & patient satisfaction

Abbreviations: CAD/CAM, computer-aided design/computer-aided manufacturing; n.a., not applicable; PEEK, polyetheretherketone; PSI, patient-specific implant.

Immediate postoperative care

After awaking from general anesthesia, visual acuity, pupil function, eye motility, and binocular diplopia are checked by the surgeon. These functions are subsequently checked every hour within the first 24 hours, in order to avoid optical neuropathy due to an orbital compression. Patients are advised not to blow the nose and be open mouthed when sneezing. In cases of foreign body feeling or pronounced chemosis, eye drops (ie, combination of tobramycin and dexamethasone or carbomer) is administered. In general, an elevated upper body and a cooling device is recommended. As an additional preventive measure kinesiologic taping may be administered, which reduces swelling and tissue sagging. A perioperative antibiotic therapy, oral or intravenous for 5 days, is pursued.

Rehabilitation and recovery

Swelling subsides mostly in the first few days to the first 2 weeks at the latest. During this period diplopia may arise or increase in intensity and patients should be well educated. Conclusive clinical assessments of postoperative results, especially when extensive secondary reconstruction was performed, are feasible often after several weeks or even months. During a complex postoperative course, interdisciplinary support (ie, ophthalmology) may accelerate the healing process.

Clinical results in the literature

Latest literature on secondary orbital repair is sparse (Table 1). Many studies use digital planning and intraoperative quality control; differences exist mainly in selection of reconstruction material. Frequent indications for secondary orbital reconstruction are globe malposition, diplopia, and impaired eye motility. Surgical outcomes regarding enophthalmos reduction are in general good, certainly with the help of navigation and patient-specific implants.

Summary

Indications for secondary orbital corrections are enophthalmos larger than 2 mm, impaired eye motility, and binocular diplopia due to incorrect implant placement or possible tissue entrapment. Late and secondary orbital reconstructions are more demanding than primary reconstruction cases due to altered anatomic landmarks and late soft tissue changes. In addition to the primary reconstruction workflow with mirroring and virtual reconstruction of the fractured orbit, volume corrections may be necessary in order to prevent globe malposition.

Disclosure

The authors have nothing to disclose.

Suggested reading list

Gellrich NC, Schramm A, Hammer B, et al. Computer-assisted secondary reconstruction of unilateral posttraumatic orbital deformity. Plast Reconstr Surg 2002;110(6):1417–29.

Blumer M, Rostetter C, Johner J-P, et al. Associated Ophthalmic Injuries in Patients With Fractures of the Midface. Craniomaxillofacial Trauma & Reconstruction 2020;13:168.

Wagner ME, Gellrich NC, Friese KI, et al. Model-based segmentation in orbital volume measurement with cone beam computed tomography and evaluation against current concepts. Int J Comput Assist Radiol Surg 2016;11(1):1–9.

Lauer G, Pradel W, Schneider M, et al. Efficacy of computer-assited surgery in secondary orbital reconstruction. J Craniomaxillofac Surg 2006;34(5):299–305.

Essig H, Dressel L, Rana M, et al. Precision of posttraumatic primary orbital reconstruction using individually bent titanium mesh with and without navigation: a retrospective study. Head Face Med 2013; 9:18.

Gander T, Essig H, Metzler P, et al. Patient specific implants (PSI) in reconstruction of orbital floor and wall fractures. J Craniomaxillofac Surg 2015;43(1):126–30.

Baumann A, Sinko K, Dorner G. Late reconstruction of the orbit with patient-specific implants using computer-aided planning and navigation. J Oral Maxill Surg 2015;73(12 Suppl):S101–6.

Gander T, Blumer M, Rostetter C, et al. Intraoperative 3-dimensional cone beam computed tomographic imaging during reconstruction of the zygoma and orbit. Oral Surg Oral Med Oral Pathol Oral Radiol 2018;126(2):192–7.

Kim JS, Lee BW, Scawn RL, et al. Secondary orbital reconstruction in patients with prior orbital fracture repair. Ophthalmic Plast Reconstr Surg 2016;32(6):447–51.

Nkenke E, Vairaktaris E, Spitzer M, et al. Secondary reconstruction of posttraumatic enophthalmos: prefabricated implants vs titanium mesh. Arch Facial Plast Surg 2011;13(4):271–7.

Park J, Kim J, Lee J, et al. Secondary reconstruction of residual enophthalmos using an endoscope and considering the orbital floor and medial wall slope. J Craniofac Surg 2016;27(4):992–5.

Gander T, Rostetter C, Blumer M, et al. Use of a monopolar microneedle device in a transconjunctival, retroseptal approach. J Craniomaxillofac Surg 2017;45(12):1934–7.

Blumer M, Gander T, Kruse Gujer A, et al. Influence of mirrored computed tomograms on decision-making for revising surgically treated orbital floor fractures. J Oral Maxillofac Surg 2015;73(10): 1982 e1–9.

Secondary Correction of Midface Fractures

Jonathan Chodroff, DDS, MD, MEd [a,*], Nadir Elias, DMD, MSc [b,1], Michael Whitcomb, DMD, MD [a], Cong Vo, DDS, MD [a], Richard Bryan Bell, MD, DDS, FRCS (Ed) [c,d]

KEYWORDS

• Secondary midface deformity • NOE fractures • Telecanthus • Enophthalmos • Navigation • Medial canthal deformity • Virtual surgical planning • Malocclusion

KEY POINTS

- The goal of secondary reconstruction of the midface is to restore harmony with a primary focus of restoration of form and function.
- An organized assessment of the facial structures is crucial to a successful outcome. These include the orbit, the nasal-ethmoid complex and the zygoma.
- Within the orbit, secondary correction most often relates to malposition of the globe within the bony orbit.
- When the naso-orbito-ethmoid complex is involved, proper positioning of the medial canthus is critical to avoid persistent telecanthus.
- Virtual surgical planning, intraoperative navigation, and custom implants can be helpful for complex secondary reconstructions of the midface, especially in panfacial injuries.

Introduction

Secondary deformities of the midface pose a significant challenge for even the most experienced of surgeons. Although the first operation provides the best opportunity for an ideal outcome, this not always is possible. There often is significant distortion in anatomy, inadequate bony foundation, and macerated soft tissue, especially in patients with avulsion injuries. Avulsion injuries result in a failure to achieve complete reduction and stabilization of fractures during the initial reconstruction.

The goal of secondary reconstruction is to restore harmony, with a primary focus of restoration of form and function. This is achieved in a manner similar to the approach taken during the primary reconstructive phase. In the assessment and treatment of secondary reconstruction patients, the main focus is to restore orbital volume and bizygomatic width and projection and to achieve proper occlusion. An organized assessment of the facial structures is crucial to a successful outcome. These include the orbit, the nasal-ethmoid complex, and the zygoma. Each of these anatomic subunits should be evaluated for functional deficits. Within the orbit, the deficits most often encountered are secondary to malposition of the globe within the bony orbit. These deficits include hypoglobus, dystopias, entropion or ectropion, and diplopia. Malpositioning of the zygomaticomaxillary complex (ZMC) also may lead to these deficits. Additionally, patients with secondary deformities of midface may present with malocclusion and limitations in opening and closing. When the naso-orbito-ethmoid (NOE) complex is involved, improper positioning of the medial canthus may lead to a persistent telecanthus. Furthermore, improper reduction of the nasal complex and lacrimal system results in impaired nasofrontal and lacrimal drainage and poor nasal projection. All these factors are compounded in panfacial fractures. The aim of this article is to review the approaches to the assessment and management of patients who present for the correction of secondary defects to the midface.

Secondary correction of enophthalmos

When present, postoperative enophthalmos may be observed at follow-up appointments after repair of many midface fractures, including the NOE, ZMC, and orbital complex. As the edema from the original injury and subsequent surgery subside, the globe settles into a depressed position relative to the contralateral side due to increased orbital cavity volume. This usually is due to inadequate reduction and loss/atrophy of intraorbital adipose tissue.

If not obtained in the immediate postoperative period, computed tomography (CT) imaging should be acquired in order to determine those areas of the orbital complex that are the most significant contributors to orbital

[a] Department of Oral and Maxillofacial Surgery, Oregon Health & Science University, 3181 Southwest Sam Jackson Park Road, Floor 7D, Portland, OR 97239, USA

[b] Legacy Emanuel Medical Center, Head and Neck Institute, Portland, OR, USA

[c] Earle A. Chiles Research Institute at Robert W. Franz Cancer Center, Providence Cancer Institute, 4805 Northeast Glisan Street, Suite 2N35, Portland, OR 97213, USA

[d] Providence Head and Neck Cancer Program and Clinic, Providence Cancer Institute, Portland, OR, USA

* Corresponding author.

E-mail address: Chodroff@ohsu.edu

Twitter: @rbryanbell (R.B. Bell)

[1] Present address: 3809 North Vancouver Avenue, Portland, OR 97227.

Atlas Oral Maxillofacial Surg Clin N Am 29 (2021) 139–150
1061-3315/21/
https://doi.org/10.1016/j.cxom.2020.11.008

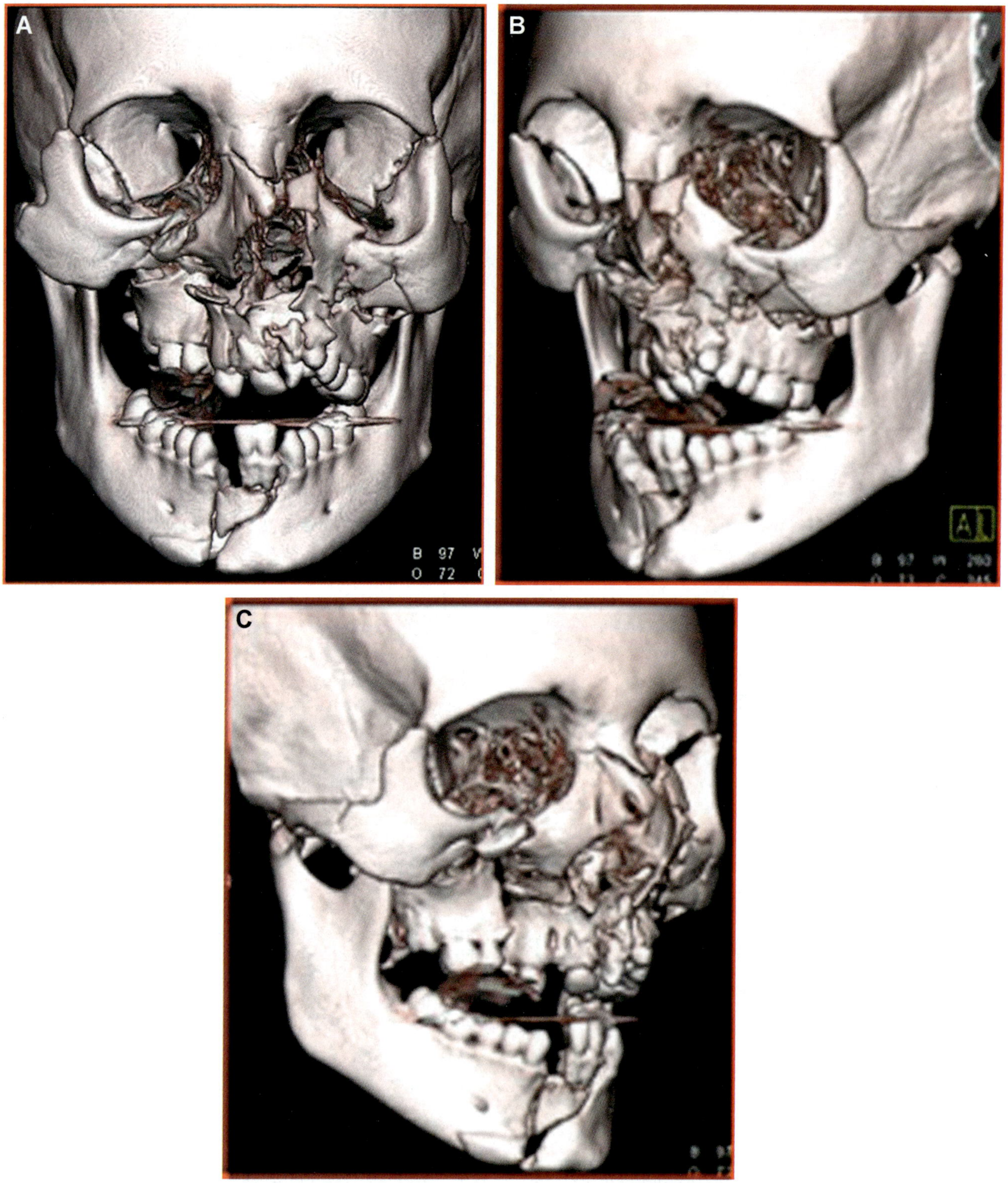

Fig. 1 A 16-year-old girl was involved in a high-speed motor vehicle collision resulting in panfacial fractures. She initially was treated at an outside institution with open reduction and internal fixation of her facial fractures before being referred to the Oral and Maxillofacial Surgery Service at Legacy Emanuel Medical Center for secondary reconstruction. (*A–C*) A 3-D reconstruction of her CT scans demonstrates significantly displaced panfacial fractures, including Le Fort III, NOE complex, and mandible. Note typical findings associated with displaced panfacial injuries, including shortening, widening, and flattening of the facial skeleton.

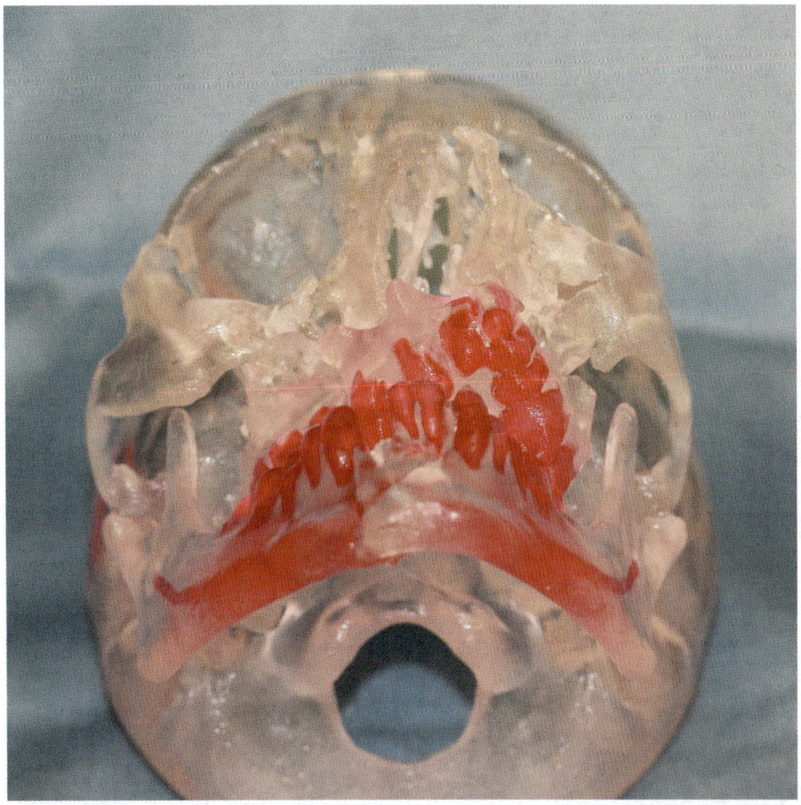

Fig. 2 Stereolithographic model of initial injury. Note widening, flattening, and shortening of the face with bilateral orbital disruption and increased orbital volume.

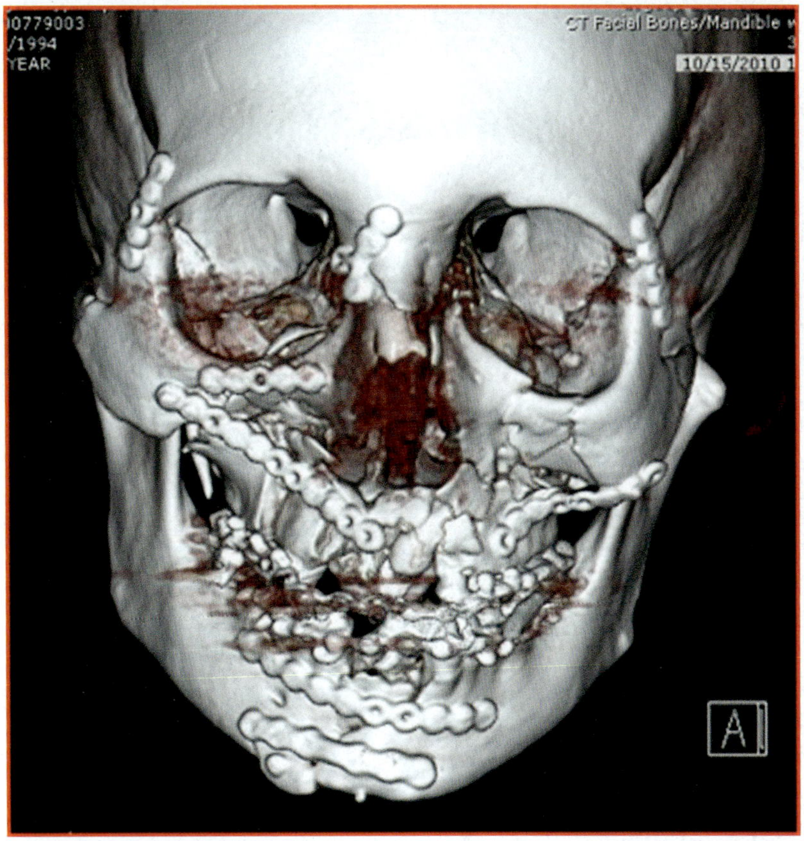

Fig. 3 Postoperative CT reconstruction of initial repair at outside hospital. Note lack of reduction with persistent widening, flattening, and shortening of the facial skeleton; increased orbital volume; and displaced mandibular condyles located lateral of the mandibular fossa bilaterally.

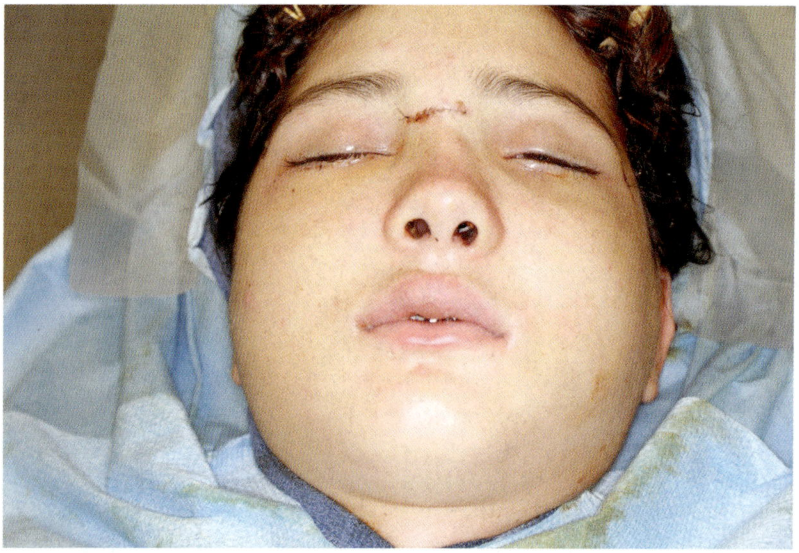

Fig. 4 Appearance of patient upon transfer to Legacy Emanuel Medical Center. Note telecanthus, decreased facial projection, and bizygomatic widening.

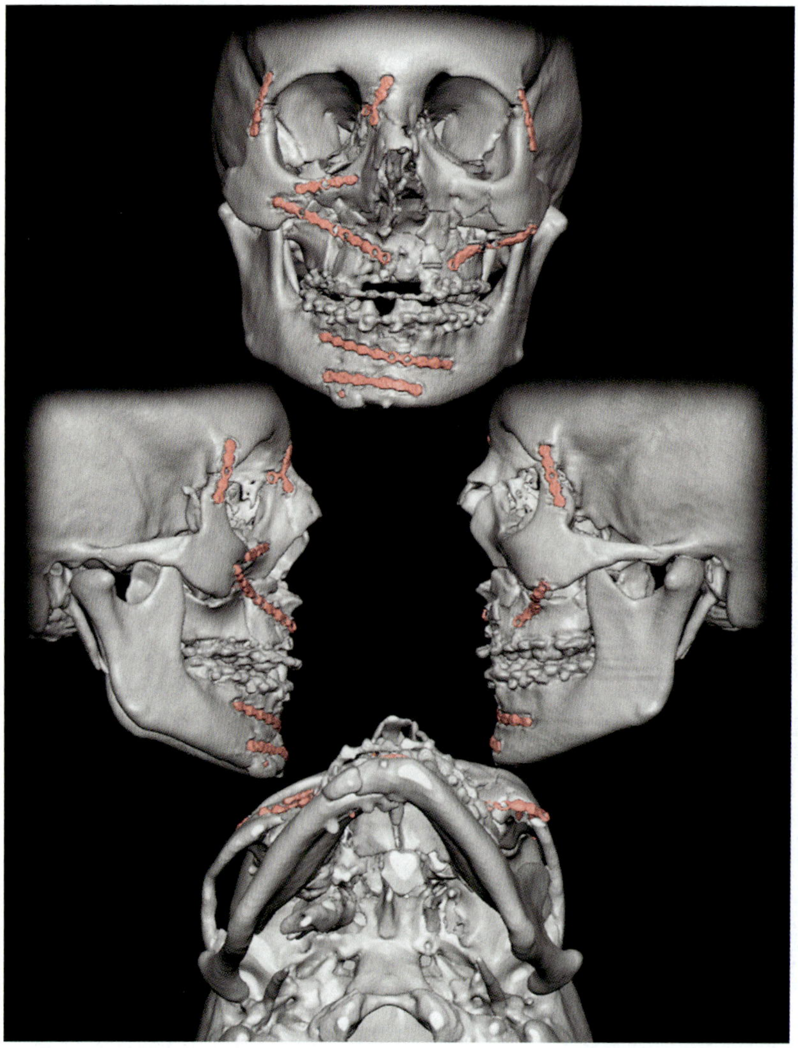

Fig. 5 CT reconstruction prior to secondary reconstruction.

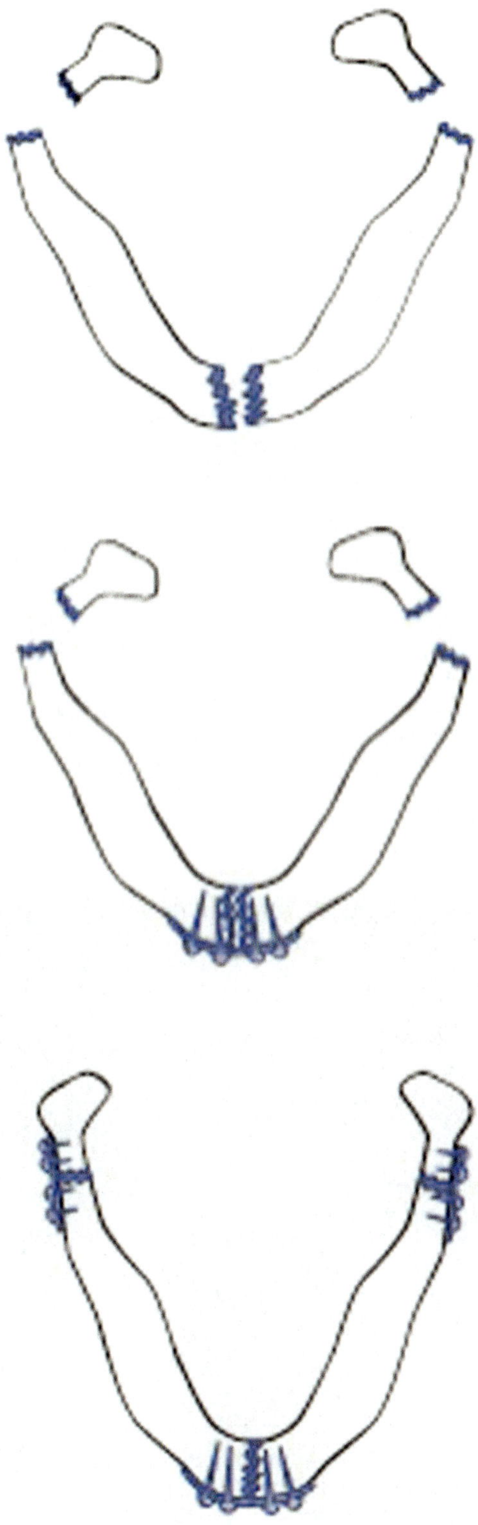

Fig. 6 Diagram illustrating the importance of lower face reconstruction in re-establishing proper facial width. Condyles should be placed place into the glenoid fossa and the midface then is reconstructed on the repositioned mandible.

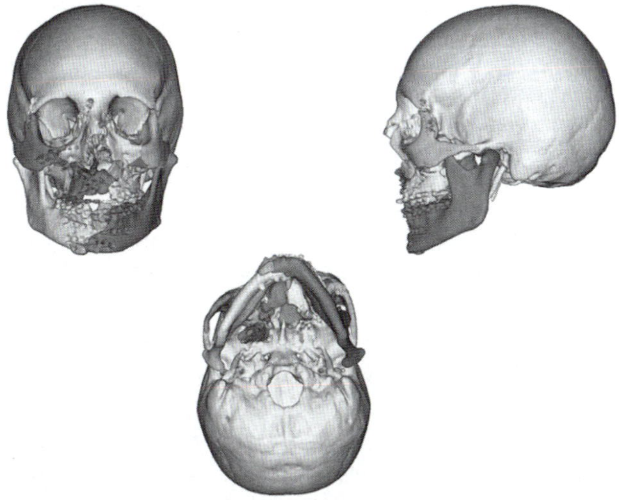

Fig. 7 VSP images demonstrating segmentalized major anatomic components to be repositioned.

volume expansion. Enophthalmos alone can be a subtle finding that is observed by the trained eye. The average layperson, however, notes an abnormal appearance with an enophthalmos of 3 mm to 4 mm.[1] Binocular diplopia is the strongest indicator that secondary repair is required. Although a variety of approaches can be utilized, the favored approach is the transconjunctival approach because this technique is less prone to cause additional cosmetic defects, such as ectropion. Secondary repair of such a defect can be difficult after initial healing, because scar tissue often complicates the approach and limits the forward mobility of the globe. For this reason, thorough subperiosteal dissection along the orbital floor, medial wall, and lateral wall beyond the site of injury frequently is required. Historically, orbital volume was restored using autogenous bone grafts. More

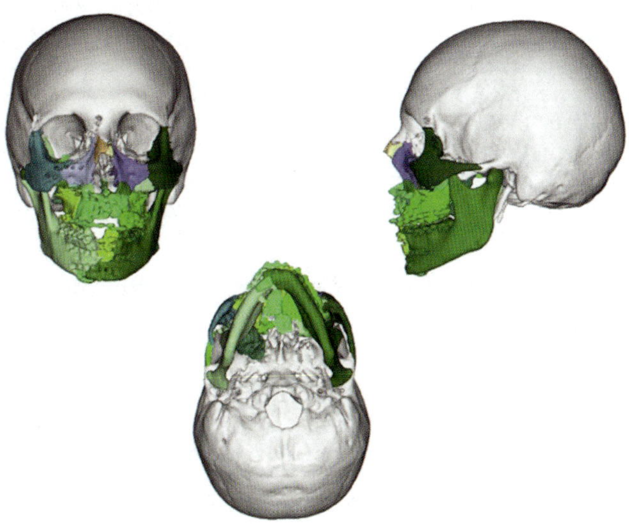

Fig. 8 VSP images demonstrating repositioned bony segments to re-establish facial projection and height and symmetry at the zygomas, orbits, maxilla, and mandible.

recently, orbital volume most often is reduced via placement of alloplastic implants composed of materials, such as titanium, porous polyethylene, or a combination of the 2. There also now is the option of using virtual surgical planning (VSP) to manufacture custom implants that can achieve a passive fit in situations where there is significant distortion of normal anatomy that is not amenable to reconstruction with stock materials.[2] Although secondary repair can aid in globe position, if persistent diplopia is noted, then strabismus surgery or prism glasses may be required in order to restore the patient to their premorbid functional status.[3]

Secondary correction of the zygomaticomaxillary complex

Secondary correction of ZMC injuries is indicated when inadequate reduction during the primary surgery produces a deficiency in malar projection. This usually is a result of inadequate restoration of proper contour of the zygomatic arch. Anatomically, the zygomatic arch is fairly straight. Failure to restore this arch form often leads to increased facial width and decreased projection.

Often the degree of ZMC displacement and/or lack of anatomic reduction dictates the amount of malar projection and contributes to the apparent flattening/widening of the face on the ipsilateral side. The characteristics of a patient's skin and body habitus, however, also can affect this finding. Observing a patient from a cephalad position allows one to assess the patient's malar projection bilaterally and palpation further assess the relative contributions from hard and soft tissues. Historically, such malar deficiencies were treated with local rearrangement of adipose tissue. This often has produced the undesirable result of lower eyelid shortening and hollowing and no longer is utilized. Once the deficiency has been identified, correction can be pursued with reosteotomy at the sites of improper reduction or more commonly with placement a malar implant via a vestibular approach.[4,5] The implant should be inserted in a subperiosteal plane and evaluated from frontal, profile, and cephalad views in order to best approximate symmetry with the contralateral side, trimming, and contouring the implant, as necessary, and eventually fixating the implant as needed. Although rarer, the possibility of a proper bony reduction in the setting of a purely soft tissue deficiency also should be considered, most often a result of malar fat pad atrophy and/or improper suspension of the soft tissue. Secondary correction of such soft tissue deficiencies can be compensated for by using adipose tissue grafting, dermal fillers, and/or rhytidectomy techniques.[6]

Secondary correction of naso-orbito-ethmoid fractures

The NOE complex is a delicate 3-dimensional (3-D) anatomic structure.[7] Damage to this region may result in severe facial dysfunction and malformation. NOE fractures involve the central upper midface. This consists of the confluence between the paired nasal bones that form the nasal sidewalls and medial orbital rims.

When secondary repair of NOE fractures is necessary, the repair should be planned methodically focusing on restoring facial function and form. Specific attention should be applied on the medial canthus and intercanthal relationship. The pivotal structure that is present in this region is the medial canthal tendon. This tendon supports the canthus and enables proper union between the eyelid and the globe. The canthal tendon serves to suspend the upper and lower tarsal plates across the eye and is critical in maintaining a sharp medial canthal angle.[8] Therefore, in order to achieve a proper aesthetic result after NOE fracture repair, the medial canthal tendon must be fixated securely to the small bone fragments to which it has remained attached in Markowitz types I and II fractures or reattached to stable bone in Markowitz type III fractures.[9]

Traumatic telecanthus and hypertelorism are the most frequent late complications from inadequate management of medial canthal tendons. The unaesthetic aspect of telecanthus is created not only by the increased intercanthal distance but also by the rounded palpebral fissure and the flattened nose. Therefore, in order to achieve proper and definitive correction, the entire nasal skeleton requires reshaping. This is accomplished by reosteotomy and medial repositioning of the bone fragment that anchors the displaced medial canthal attachment.[10] This osteotomy should include the lacrimal crest and its associated attachment of the inner canthal ligament. If the ligamentous insertion is not violated, it should be preserved because the normal anatomic configuration is extremely difficult to reproduce operatively. Fixation of the mobilized nasal segments is performed using the same techniques as in

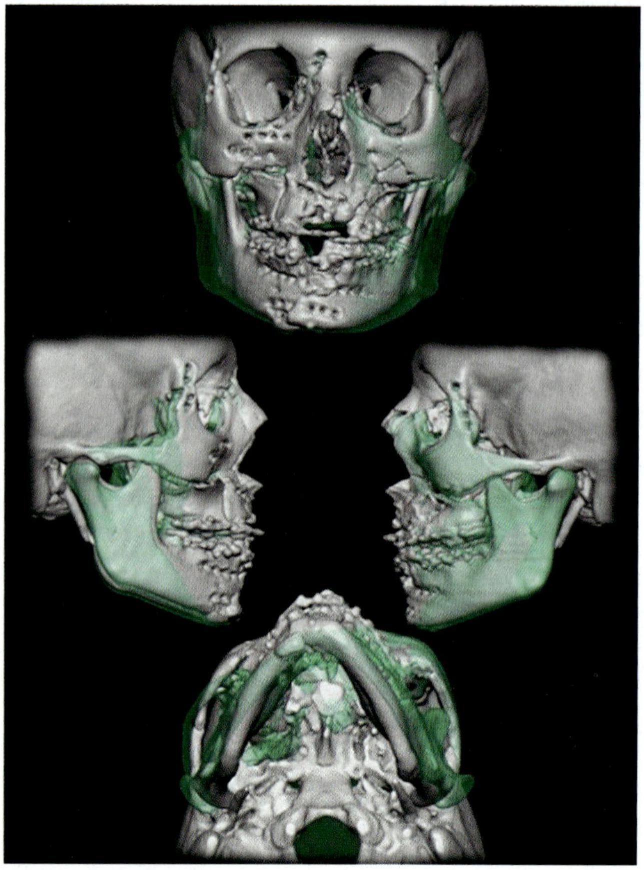

Fig. 9 VSP was utilized for secondary surgical reconstruction. Preoperative position of the maxilla and mandible (*green*) versus planned positioning (*gray*).

primary repair. A transnasal wire secures the nasal bone fragment against outward rotation, even if a canthopexy is performed. In addition, if 1 canthus is superior to the other, the inferior canthus should be elevated to achieve symmetry.[11] If the medial canthal tendon is detached completely during secondary surgery, the medial canthal tendon itself must be reduced with a separate transnasal canthopexy. The ligament is grasped with a 28-gauge wire at its origin, proximal to where the 3 limbs have not yet separated. This wire is passed transnasally and the point of insertion must be above and behind the nasolacrimal duel.[12] If the bone in this area does not permit creation of an insertion point, a midface miniplate can be used as an alternative.[13] Tightening of the transnasal canthopexy always should be the last step in secondary corrections because placement of bone grafts is facilitated by free canthal ligaments.[14]

Unfortunately, there often is significant scar contracture and soft tissue thickening after NOE repairs, which can give the appearance of pseudotelecanthus.[10] An oblique transnasal wiring technique with V-Y epicanthoplasty incision can minimize scar formation and contracture.[15] In addition, maximal skeletal narrowing should be achieved in order to create a nearly normal intercanthal distance. Even with maximal narrowing, however, repair of telecanthus usually falls short of premorbid appearance. Irreparable telecanthus can be slightly masked by increasing the nasal profile with a dorsal nasal bone graft.[16] Less invasively, favorable soft tissue adaptation has been described using a thermoplastic stent contoured and overextended in the naso-orbital region.[17]

Considerations in panfacial fractures

Panfacial injuries provide a set of challenges for secondary reconstruction due to the extensive nature of these fractures. Initial repair also is complicated by can by significant facial injury and edema, thereby making access and intraoperative evaluation of facial projection difficult.[18] Generally, this fracture pattern results in flattening and widening of the face due to depression of the midface and increased bigonial width secondary to mandible fractures involving the symphysis or parasymphysis. Primary reconstruction is aimed toward restoring facial projection by rebuilding the vertical and horizontal buttresses of the face.[19,20] Secondary reconstruction is

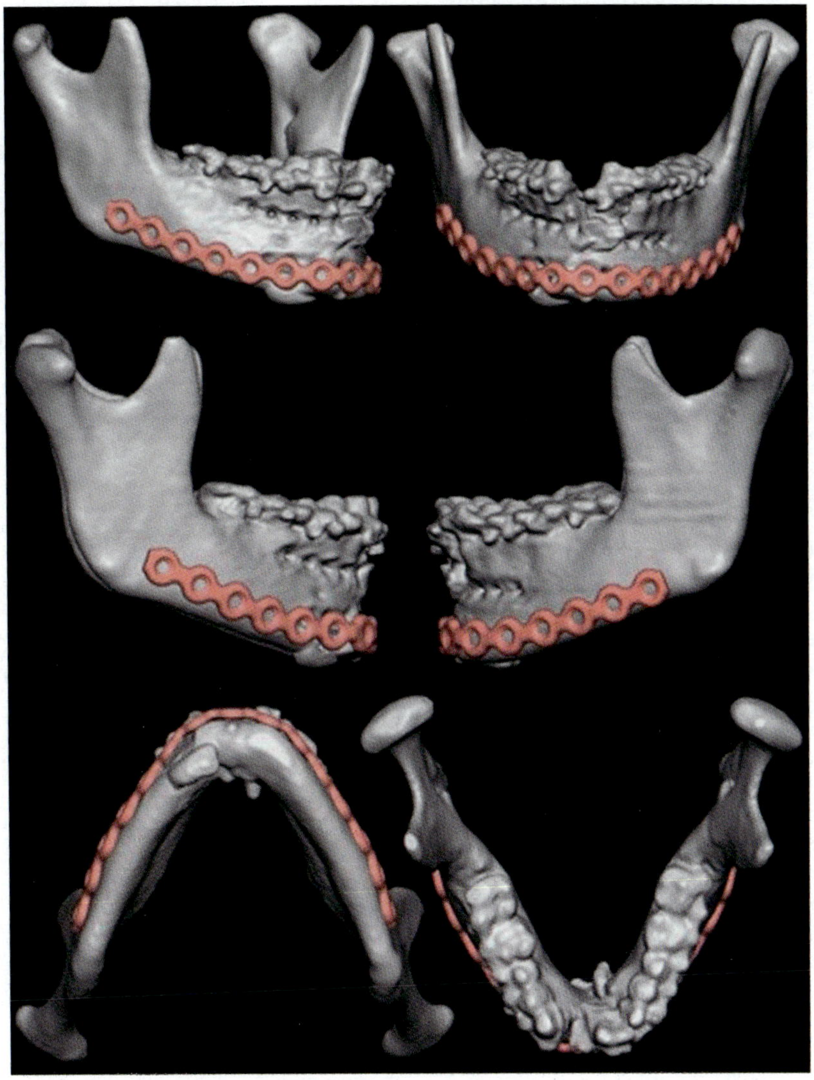

Fig. 10 Virtual reconstruction plate to optimize mandibular width.

necessitated weeks to months after the initial repair due to inadequate functional or cosmetic results. Sometimes, the facial injuries can go untreated due to the inexperience of surgery specialists at the primary care center. Additionally, incomplete or inadequate repair can be secondary to lack of resources at such institutions. These include VSP intraoperative CT and intraoperative navigation.

Regardless, panfacial fractures requiring secondary reconstruction usually feature common complications that can be addressed with a variety of surgical strategies, discussed previously. Malocclusion is the most commonly encountered complication. Cuddy and colleagues reviewed 33 patients with panfacial fractures that went untreated for 4 or more weeks, and malocclusion was present in 100% of the patients.[21] Depending on the degree of severity, malocclusion can be treated by guiding elastics, orthodontics, or orthognathic surgery. In Cuddy and colleagues' review, all patients had Le Fort I osteotomies done as the last step of reconstruction. Alternatively, other investigators have suggested establishing occlusion via Le Fort I osteotomy first, then reconstructing the remainder of the midface subunits with the techniques, discussed previously and reviewed later.[22] This strategy can simplify an otherwise complex reconstruction.

Sequelae involving the midface include malar flattening, enopthalmos or hypoglobus, and telecanthus. Malar flattening typically is due to a depressed or posteriorly rotated ZMC fracture. Concomitant orbital floor fractures also may cause enophthalmos and hypoglobus secondary to the increase in orbital volume.

Minor malar deformities can be corrected using onlay grafting and recontouring or using custom implants. If a significant deficiency exists, projection can be restored by performing a ZMC osteotomy and then positioning/fixating the zygoma in a more ideal location. A bicoronal flap and maxillary vestibular and lower lid incisions typically are necessary for access. Complete subperiosteal dissection is important to fully mobilize the zygoma. Osteotomies are done using a combination of a sagittal saw and osteotomes. A saw cut typically is made first at the zygomaticofrontal suture, followed by osteotomy of the orbital floor with an osteotome. The saw then is used for osteotomies at the infraorbital rim, anterior maxilla, zygomaticomaxillary junction, and zygomatic arch. It is important to remember that mobilization and repositioning of the zygoma may create an orbital floor defect, which needs reconstruction with an orbital floor plate or calvarial bone graft to avoid subsequent enophthalmos. Similarly, gaps that are created at the osteotomy sites should be filled with bone graft after fixation is completed.

The NOE region can prove the most difficult to reconstruct due to lack of a sagittal buttress in the area. Common complications are telecanthus and dorsal nasal defects. Persistent telecanthus is due to the lateral displacement of the medial orbital bones where the medial canthal tendon attaches or inadequate canthopexy. Autogenous strut grafts can be used to restore projection of the nasal dorsum and at the same time can camouflage telecanthus.

The complexity of panfacial fractures makes using adjunctive tools essential. VSP from CT scans with fine cuts (<1 mm) allows for fabrication of custom plates, implants, or cutting guides.[22] Intraoperative navigation also can be used to verify the positioning of bony segments prior to fixation. If the tooth-bearing skeleton is involved, dental impression and mounted casts can be invaluable in restoring proper occlusion. Typically, establishment of occlusion alone can restore the appropriate facial projection.

In cases of significant bone loss, either autogenous block graft or free flap reconstruction should be considered, particularly when implant-retained dental prostheses are desired. Residual soft tissue deficits can remain after bony reconstruction, and soft tissue augmentation can be achieved by a combination of soft tissue suspension and autogenous grafting.

Although it is ideal to avoid secondary reconstruction of panfacial fractures, the aforementioned circumstances necessitate at least some type of revision procedure. The advantage of secondary reconstruction is that it allows time for meticulous surgical planning and input from the patient that typically is not afforded during the primary repair.

Virtual surgical planning and custom implants in secondary reconstruction

VSP, intraoperative navigation, and custom implants can be helpful in secondary reconstructions of the midface. These technological advances have been shown to improve efficiency and precision for complex craniomaxillofacial surgical operations.[21–29]

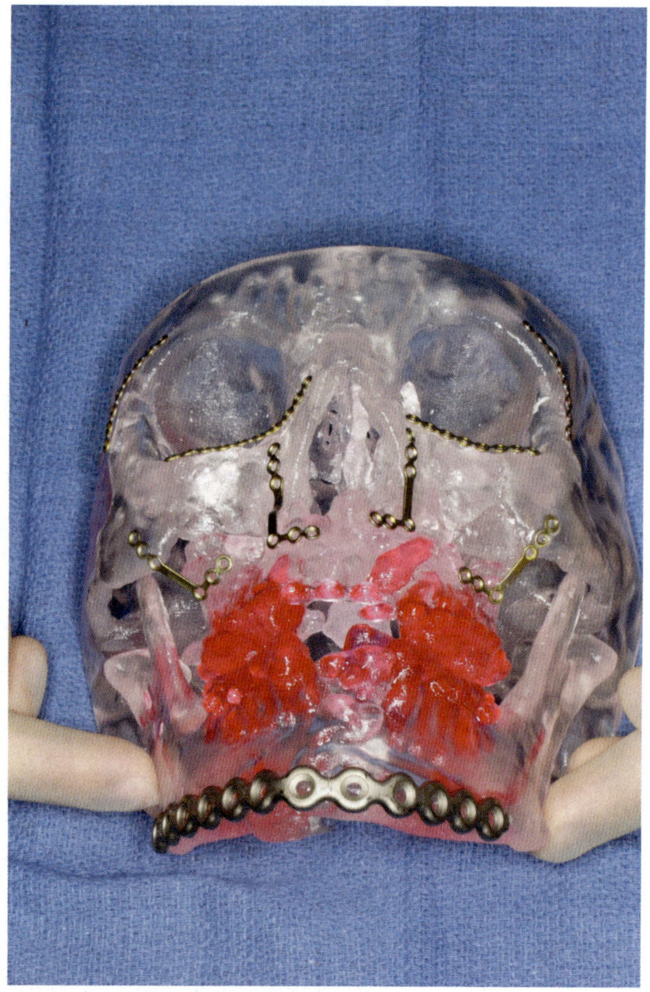

Fig. 11 Stereolithographic model of virtually reconstructed maxilla and mandible with prebent titanium plates to facilitate accurate transfer of the virtual plan to the patient.

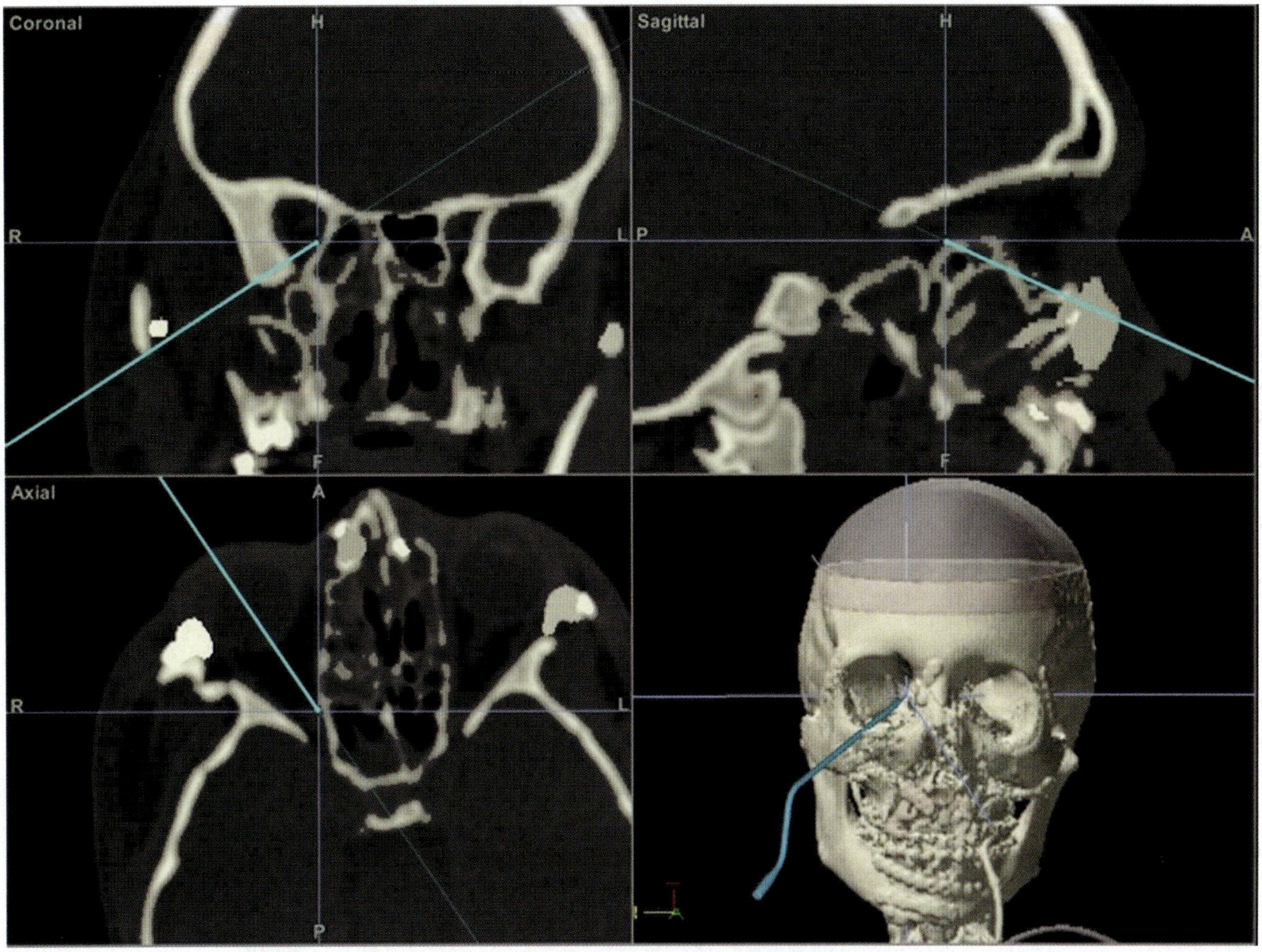

Fig. 12 Intraoperative navigation image to assess adequate position of orbital plate to reconstruct the critical posterior medial ethmoidal and superior antral bulges for restoration premorbid orbital volume.

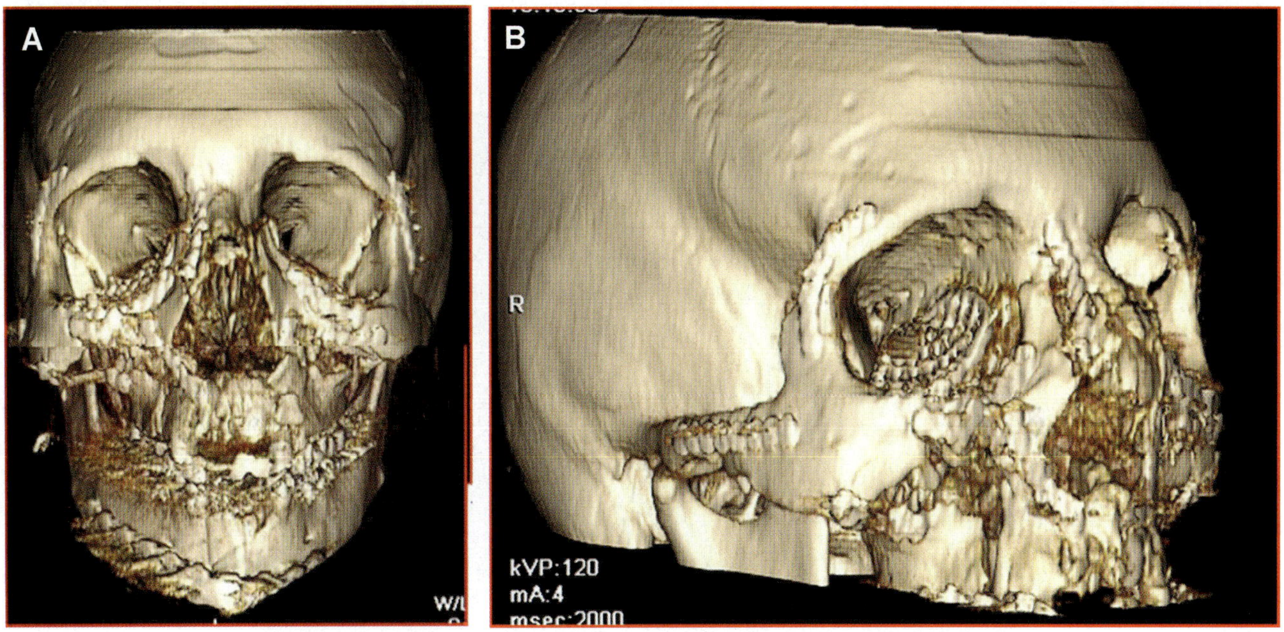

Fig. 13 A 3-D reconstruction of intraoperative CT scan demonstrating favorable restoration of facial width, height, and projection—(*A*) frontal view and (*B*) oblique view.

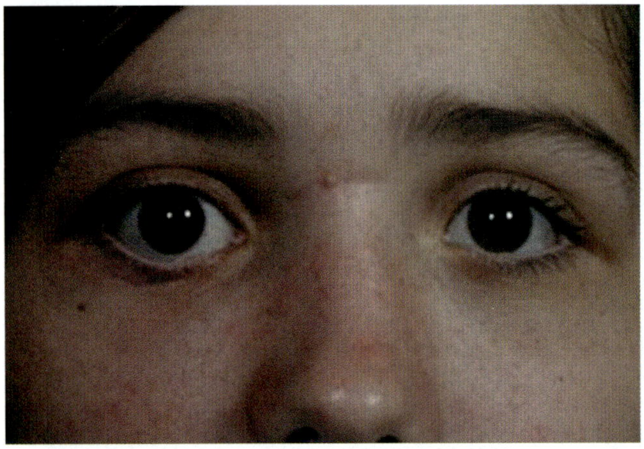

Fig. 14 Postoperative clinical appearance after secondary reconstruction reveals lower lid retraction and entropion associated with loss of bone at the infraorbital rim.

Combining multiplanar CT scans with 3-D reconstruction software permits the surgeon to visualize the complex anatomy of the midfacial region and can overcome the unintentional imprecisions associated with traditional intraoperative spatial repositioning.[23] Prior to VSP, anatomic reduction relied on a surgeon's capacity to mentally translate the 3-D movements. Unfortunately, bony repositioning in the midface is difficult to verify in real time to the naked eye. VSP allows the surgeon the ability to plan an accurate spatial bone correction, taking into account the many degrees and angles of movement. The advent of custom fixation plates has allowed for accurate fixation of the bony segments in their desired position.

Accuracy can be expanded on by using intraoperative simultaneous visualization of both the surgical field and the 3-D virtual planning superimposed on the CT images by means of tracked instruments. Interoperative navigation permits the ability the surgeon to verify in real time the precision of the

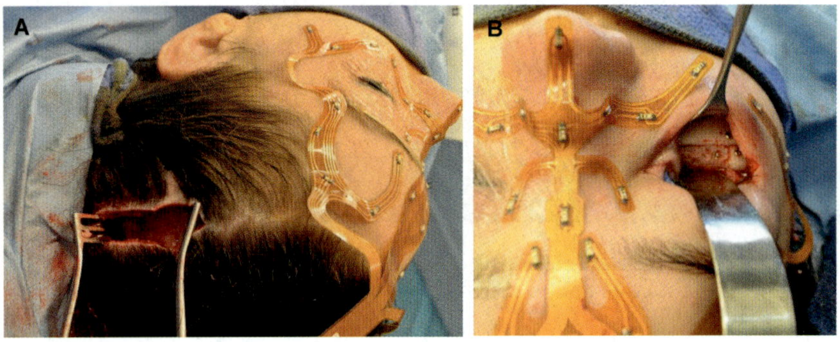

Fig. 15 (*A*) Calvarial bone grafting in combination with inferior lid resuspension was performed in order to normalize globe position, improve lid projection, and decrease scleral show, calvarial bone graft harvest; (*B*) inset of bone graft via lower eyelid approach.

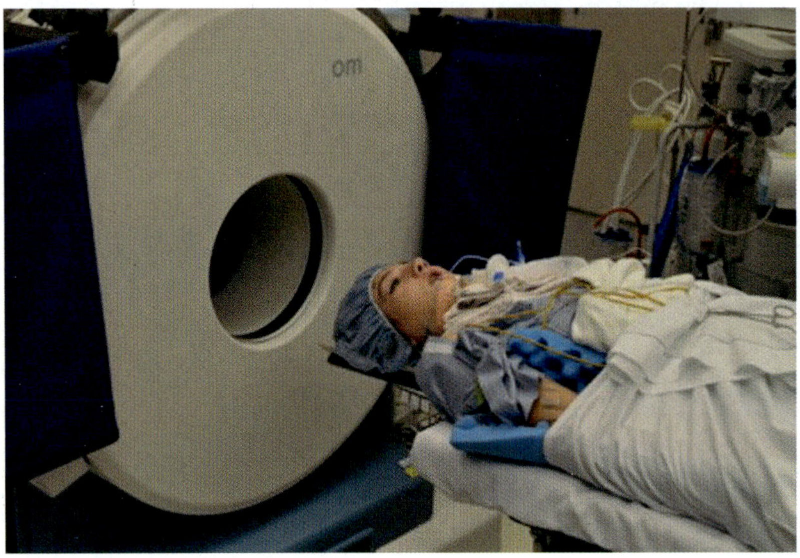

Fig. 16 .Patient undergoing intraoperative CT to confirm accurate orbital reconstruction.

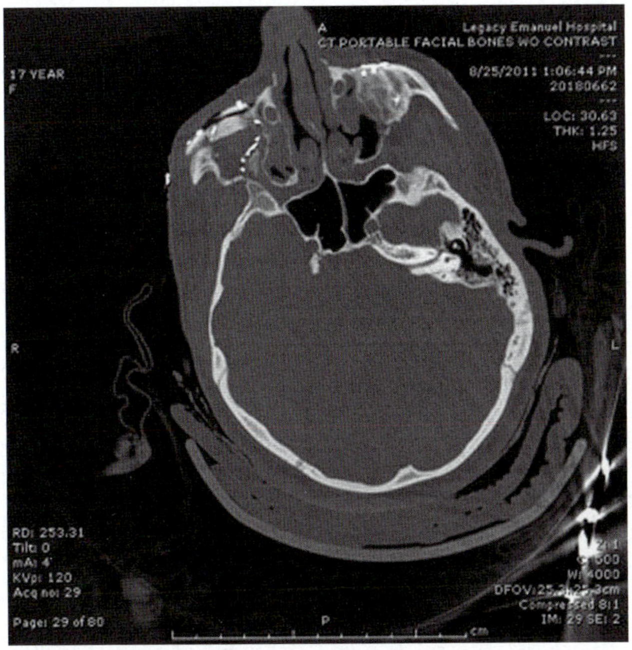

Fig. 17 .Intraoperative CT image demonstrating accurate position of orbital bone graft and normalized orbital volume.

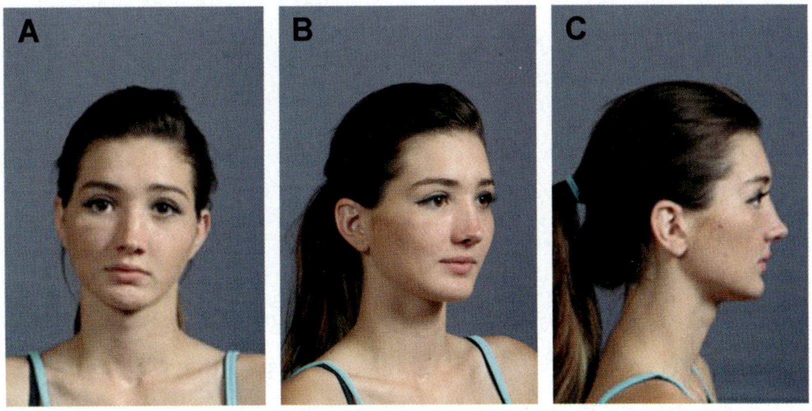

Fig. 18 Final postoperative appearance of patient after secondary reconstruction: (*A*) frontal, (*B*) oblique, and (*C*) lateral views.

repair. This is helpful particularly in the poorly visualized posterior-medial orbital wall reconstruction. Accurate reconstruction of this anatomy is critical in supporting and projecting the ocular globe and, thus, limiting chances of postoperative enophthalmos.[21]

The advent of computer-aided design/computer-aided manufacturing technology has allowed surgeons to directly translate and integrate 3-D VSP without the need for navigation assistance.[24] This process is achieved through patient-specific surgical cutting guides and patient-specific implants. Custom cutting guides are useful for midface deformities that require multispatial repositioning, as orbital hypertelorism or secondary correction of telecanthus.[25] Patient-specific implants, most commonly made with poly-ether-ether-ketone implants or titanium, can be custom designed to a patient's anatomy. This technology eliminates the often laborious and, at times, inaccurate method of hand manipulating stock implants intraoperatively. Furthermore, in unilateral defects, surgeons can use mirroring software to reproduce the unaffected facial side and reestablish facial symmetry.[26]

VSP is a valuable instrument that may be used to help surgeons in the planning and intraoperative stages. VSP has been shown to increase the precision and accuracy of implant and hardware positioning. Moreover, the advent of patient-specific implants has transformed how surgeons manage complex 3-D defects and secondary reconstructions of the midface.

Case study

A 16-year-old girl was involved in a high-speed motor vehicle collision resulting in panfacial fractures. She initially was treated at an outside institution with open reduction and internal fixation of her facial fractures before being referred to the Oral and Maxillofacial Surgery Service at Legacy Emanuel Medical Center (Portland, Oregon) for secondary reconstruction (Figs. 1–18).

Clinics care points

- If not obtained in the immediate post-operative period, CT imaging should be acquired in order to determine those areas of the orbital complex that are the most significant contributors to orbital volume expansion.
- The average layperson will note an abnormal appearance with an enophthalmos of 3-4mm.
- Soft tissue deficiency, most often a result of malar fat pad atrophy and/or improper suspension of the soft tissue during ZMC repair can be compensated for by using adipose tissue grafting, dermal fillers, and/or rhytidectomy techniques.
- The unaesthetic aspect of telecanthus is created not only by the increased intercanthal distance, but also by the rounded palpebral fissure and the flattened nose.
- Irreparable telecanthus can be slightly masked by increasing one's nasal profile with a dorsal nasal bone graft.
- The naso-orbital-ethmoid region can prove to be the most difficult to reconstruction due to lack of a sagittal buttress in the area.
- In unilateral defects midface defects, surgeons can use mirroring software to reproduce the unaffected facial side and reestablish facial symmetry.

Disclosure

The authors have nothing to disclose.

References

1. Koo L, Hatton MP, Rubin PA. When is enophthalmos "significant"? Ophthal Plast Reconstr Surg 2006;22(4):274–7.
2. Baumann A, Sinko K, Dorner G. Late reconstruction of the orbit with patient-specific implants using computer-aided planning and navigation. J Oral Maxillofac Surg 2015;73(12 Suppl):S101–6.
3. McRae M, Augustine HFM, Budning A, et al. Functional outcomes of late posttraumatic enophthalmos correction. Plast Reconstr Surg 2018;142(2):169e–78e.
4. Layoun W, Guyot L, Richard O, et al. Augmentation of cheek bone contour using malar osteotomy. Aesthetic Plast Surg 2003;27(4):269–74.
5. Yaremchuk MJ, Doumit G, Thomas MA. Alloplastic augmentation of the facial skeleton: an occasional adjunct or alternative to orthognathic surgery [published correction appears in Plast Reconstr Surg. 2011 Jul;128(1):340. Doumit, Gabe [corrected to Doumit, Gaby]]. Plast Reconstr Surg 2011;127(5):2021–30.
6. Hilinski JM, Cohen SR. Soft tissue augmentation with ArteFill. Facial Plast Surg 2009;25(2):114–9.
7. Nguyen M, Koshy JC, Hollier LH. Pearls of nasoorbitoethmoid trauma management. Semin Plast Surg 2010;24(4):383–8.
8. Rosenberger E, Kriet JD, Humphrey C. Management of nasoethmoid fractures. Curr Opin Otolaryngol Head Neck Surg 2013;21:410e416.
9. Markowitz BL, Manson PN, Sargent L, et al. Management of the medial can- thal tendon in nasoeithmoid orbital fractures: the importance of the central fragment in classification and treatment. Plast Reconstr Surg 1991;87:843e853.
10. Frodel JL Jr. Management of posttraumatic pseudotelecanthus. Facial Plast Surg 2015;31(03):280–8.
11. Herford AS. Secondary treatment of naso-orbital ethmoid injuries. Facial Plast Surg 2017;33(06):591–7.
12. Sargent L. Nosoethmoid orbital fractures: diagnosis and treatment. Plast Reconstr Surg 2007;120(2):16S–31S.
13. Shibuya TY, Chen VY, Oh YS. Naso-orbito-ethmoid fracture management. Oper Tech Otolaryngol 2008;19:140e144.
14. Young P, Rice D. Management of a type II nasoeth-moid orbital fracture and near-penetration of theintracranial cavity with transnasal canthopexy. Ear Nose Throat J 2007;86(6):344–60.
15. Kim TG, Chung KJ, Kim YH, et al. Medial canthopexy using Y-V epicanthoplasty incision in the correction of telecanthus. Ann Plast Surg 2014;72:164–8.
16. Gunter JP, Rohrich RJ. Augmentation rhinoplasty: dorsal onlay grafting using shaped autogenous septal cartilage. Plast Reconstr Surg 1990;86(01):39–45.
17. Han, Peter S, et al. Complications and Treatment of Delayed or Inadequately Treated Nasoorbitoethmoid Fractures. Seminars in plastic surgery. Vol. 33. No. 02. Thieme Medical Publishers, 2019.
18. Zachariades N, Mezitis M, Michelis A. Posttraumatic osteotomies of the jaws. Int J Oral Maxillofac Surg 1993;22:328–31.
19. Manson PN, Hoopes JE, Su CT. Structural pillars of the facial skeleton: an approach to the management of Le Fort fractures. Plast Reconstr Surg 1980;66:54–62.
20. Gruss JS, Mackinnon SE. Complex maxillary fractures: role of buttress reconstruction and immediate bone grafts. Plast Reconstr Surg 1986;78:9–22.
21. Cuddy K, Khatib B, Bell RB, et al. Use of intraoperative computed tomography in craniomaxillofacial trauma surgery. J Oral Maxillofac Surg 2018;76(05):1016–25.
22. Cuddy K, Dierks EJ, Cheng A, et al. Management of zygomatico-maxillary complex fractures utilizing intraoperative 3-dimensional imaging: the ZYGOMAS protocol. J Oral Maxillofac Surg 2020;S0278-2391(20):31094–6.
23. Azarmehr I, Stokbro K, Bell RB, et al. Contemporary Techniques in orbital reconstruction: a review of the literature and report of a case combining surgical navigation, computer-aided surgical simulation, and a patient-specific implant. J Oral Maxillofac Surg 2020;78(4):594–609.
24. Khatib B, Cuddy K, Cheng A, et al. Functional anatomic computer engineered surgery protocol for the management of self-inflicted gunshot wounds to the maxillofacial skeleton. J Oral Maxillofac Surg 2018;76(3):580–94.
25. Azarmehr I, Stokbro K, Bell RB, et al. Surgical navigation: a systematic review of indications, treatments, and outcomes in oral and maxillofacial surgery. J Oral Maxillofac Surg 2017;75(9):1987–2005.
26. Markiewicz MR, Bell RB. The use of 3D imaging tools in facial plastic surgery. Facial Plast Surg Clin North Am 2011;19(4): 655–682, ix.
27. Bui TG, Bell RB, Dierks EJ. Technological advances in the treatment of facial trauma. Atlas Oral Maxillofacial Surg Clin N Am 2012; 20(1):81–94.
28. Markiewicz MR, Dierks EJ, Bell RB. Does intraoperative navigation restore orbital dimensions in traumatic and post-ablative defects? J Craniomaxillofac Surg 2012;40(2):142–8.
29. Bell RB. Computer planning and intraoperative navigation in cranio-maxillofacial surgery. Oral Maxillofacial Surg Clin N Am 2010; 22(1):135–56.

Advanced Concepts of Orbital Reconstruction

A Unique Attempt to Scientifically Evaluate Individual Techniques in Reconstruction of Large Orbital Defects

Ruud Schreurs, MSc [a,*], Alfred G. Becking, DDS, MD, DMD, PhD, FEBOMS [b], Jesper Jansen, MD, DMD, PhD [b], Leander Dubois, DDS, MD, DMD, PhD [b]

KEYWORDS

- Computer-assisted surgery • Orbit • Orbital reconstruction • Endoscopy • Virtual surgical planning • Intraoperative imaging • Intraoperative navigation • Cadaver study

KEY POINTS

- The use of a cadaver model allows assessment of the effect of individual steps of computer-assisted surgery on orbital implant positioning.
- The accuracy and consistency of implant positioning without computer-assisted surgery are low, which enphasizes the need for intraoperative control.
- 3D virtual surgical planning leads to a better implant position through enhanced insight in anatomy and fracture details, and detailed knowledge on the ideal implant position.
- Deviations from the ideal implant position can be identified with intraoperative imaging and the implant's position can be improved accordingly.
- Real-time navigation proves to be the safest, fastest and most accurate method of intraoperative navigation for orbital reconstruction.

Introduction

In most, if not all, clinical research papers and presentations on novel techniques in orbital reconstruction, combinations of different techniques have been used to highlight technological progress and increased quality of surgical outcomes in terms of predictability and reliability.[1–6] In the Amsterdam University Medical Centers, The Netherlands, a comprehensive research started in 2014 with the development of a human cadaver model for assessment of orbital reconstruction. This model was used in sequence to evaluate every single technological step in the process of orbital reconstruction. This article is a resume of this series of investigations and publications in which the additive value of individual steps used in computer-assisted surgery, including various intraoperative navigation techniques, in orbital reconstruction has been assessed.

[a] Orbital Research Group (ACOR), 3D Laboratory, Department of Oral and Maxillofacial Surgery, University Medical Center Amsterdam, University of Amsterdam, Academic Center of Dentistry Amsterdam, Meibergdreef 9, 1105 AZ, Amsterdam, the Netherlands
[b] Orbital Research Group (ACOR), Department of Oral and Maxillofacial Surgery, University Medical Center Amsterdam, University of Amsterdam, Academic Center of Dentistry Amsterdam, Meibergdreef 9, 1105 AZ, Amsterdam, the Netherlands
* Corresponding author.
E-mail address: r.schreurs@amsterdamumc.nl

The interventions evaluated were as follows:

1. Conventional transconjunctival reconstruction (baseline)[7]
2. Reconstruction with transsinusoidal endoscopy[7]
3. Reconstruction with virtual surgical planning[8]
4. Reconstruction with intraoperative imaging[9]
5. Reconstruction with intraoperative image-guided navigation[10]
6. Reconstruction with intraoperative marker-based navigation[11]
7. Reconstruction with intraoperative real-time navigation[12]

Materials and methods

Materials and methods of assessment were almost identical in all studies. Fixed human cadaver heads were obtained from the Department of Medical Biology, Section of Clinical Anatomy and Embryology of the Amsterdam University Medical Centers. Computed tomography (CT) scans of the cadaver heads were performed at baseline (with intact orbits, T0) (SOMATOM Sensation 64; Siemens Healthineers, Erlangen, Germany). Scan parameters included collimation of 20 × 0.6 mm, 120 kV, 350 mAs, pitch 0.85, field of view 30 cm, matrix 512 × 512, reconstruction slice thickness of 0.75 mm with overlapping increments of 0.4 mm, bone kernel H70s, and bone window W1600 L400. The orbital floor and medial wall were fully exposed through a standard transconjunctival incision and retroseptal preparation. Following the

Atlas Oral Maxillofacial Surg Clin N Am 29 (2021) 151–162
1061-3315/21/
https://doi.org/10.1016/j.cxom.2020.10.003

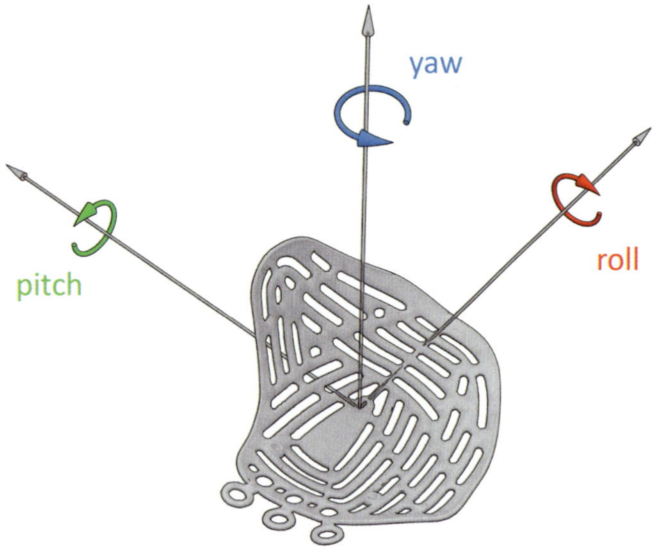

Fig. 1 Orbital implant positioning frame. The roll (*red*), pitch (*green*), and yaw (*blue*) rotation around the reference axes are visualized. (Courtesy of Ruud Schreurs, MSc, Alfred G. Becking, MD, DMD, PhD, FEBOMS, Jesper Jansen, MD, DMD, PhD and Leander Dubois, MD, DMD, PhD.)

Jaquiéry classification, complex orbital defects (class III–IV) were created with piezoelectric surgery (Mectron SpA, Carasco, Italy).[13]

After creation of the orbital defects (T1), and postoperatively after implant placement (T2), consecutive CT scans were acquired using the aforementioned scanning protocol. After T2 imaging was acquired, the orbital reconstruction plates were removed, and the screw holes were covered with dental filling material (DuraLay; Reliance Dental Mfg Co, Worth, IL, USA) to make them invisible. In all studies, preformed orbital titanium mesh implants (KLS Martin, Tuttlingen, Germany) were used; the stereolithographic models (STL files) of these implants were imported in the iPlan Cranial software environment (version 3.0.5; Brainlab AG, Munich, Germany). The optimal position of the implant was virtually planned and served as the target position during reconstruction. The faces of the human cadaver heads were covered to prevent recognition in consecutive studies, and the various studies were carried out with time intervals of several months to years.

Validation studies were performed to investigate the accuracy and precision of different methods for orbital reconstruction. The acquired implant position was compared with the target implant position of the planning. For this purpose, a reference frame for the preformed orbital implant was created (Fig. 1).[14] This reference frame made quantification of the difference between acquired and planned implant position possible: the individual rotational (roll, pitch, and yaw, in degrees) and translational (in millimeters) deviations served as the outcome parameters for all studies. In studies 1 to 5, 19 orbits were reconstructed by 2 surgeons; 10 orbits were reconstructed by 1 surgeon in study 6, and 20 orbits (of another cadaver group) were reconstructed by 2 surgeons in study 7. The results of studies 2 to 5 were compared with the baseline results (study 1). Studies 6 and 7 were compared with the results of study 5, because image-guided navigation could be considered the reference method for evaluating these enhanced navigation methods.

Conventional transconjunctival reconstruction (study 1)

In the first surgical session, all orbits were reconstructed without further technological additions, with a transconjunctival approach. Preformed orbital implants were positioned according to the best judgment of the surgeon and fixed with osteosynthesis screws. It is important to know that the surgeon had no access to information on the preoperative virtual planning, but only to a multiplanar visualization and 3-dimensional (3D) reconstruction of the CT scan acquired after creation of the orbital defects (T1). The information available to the surgeon and hardware used are visualized in Fig. 2. This study acted as a baseline study for comparison of implementation of the technologies evaluated.

Reconstruction with transsinusoidal endoscopy (study 2)

The orbital reconstructions in this surgical session were performed with the additional use of a transsinusoidal endoscope. The standard transconjunctival approach was again used to position the implant. To facilitate inspection with an endoscope, a gingivobuccal incision and a 5-mm antrostomy were created in the canine fossa concavity using a Piezotome (Mectron SpA). The sinus mucosa was removed, so the defect and position of the implant could be visualized from the maxillary sinus with a 30° endoscope (KARL STORZ SE & Co KG, Tuttlingen, Germany). In Fig. 3, the available information during surgery and the hardware used are visualized. The results of this session were compared with the baseline study (study 1).

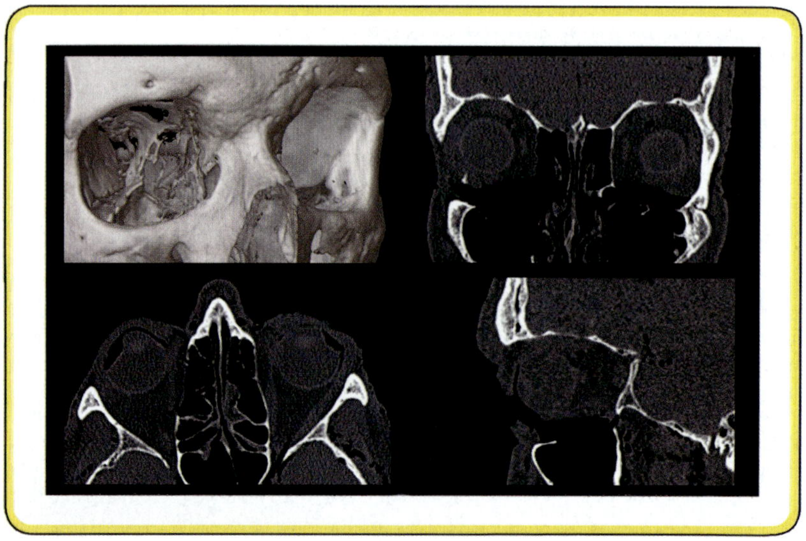

Fig. 2 Information available to the surgeon during conventional transconjunctival reconstruction. The multiplanar reconstruction and 3D reconstruction of the T1 CT were accessible; no additional hardware was used. (Courtesy of Ruud Schreurs, MSc, Alfred G. Becking, MD, DMD, PhD, FEBOMS, Jesper Jansen, MD, DMD, PhD, and Leander Dubois, MD, DMD, PhD.)

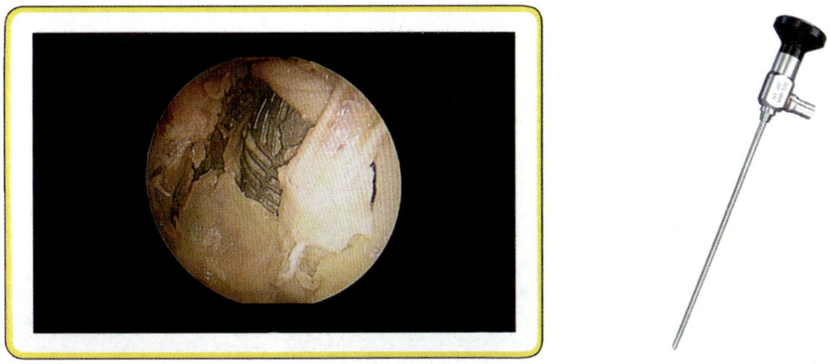

Fig. 3 Additional information at hand in reconstruction with transsinusoidal endoscopy (*left*), and hardware used (*right*). The multiplanar reconstruction and 3D reconstruction from study 1 (see Fig. 2) were accessible as well. (Courtesy of Ruud Schreurs, MSc, Alfred G. Becking, MD, DMD, PhD, FEBOMS, Jesper Jansen, MD, DMD, PhD, and Leander Dubois, MD, DMD, PhD.)

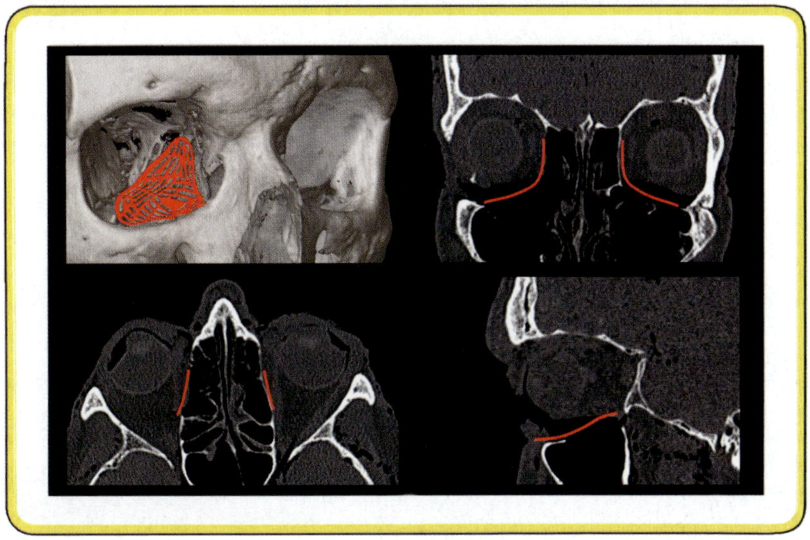

Fig. 4 The virtual surgical planning for reconstruction that was visible to the surgeon during reconstruction in study 3. No hardware tools were used in the workflow. (Courtesy of Ruud Schreurs, MSc, Alfred G. Becking, MD, DMD, PhD, FEBOMS, Jesper Jansen, MD, DMD, PhD, and Leander Dubois, MD, DMD, PhD.)

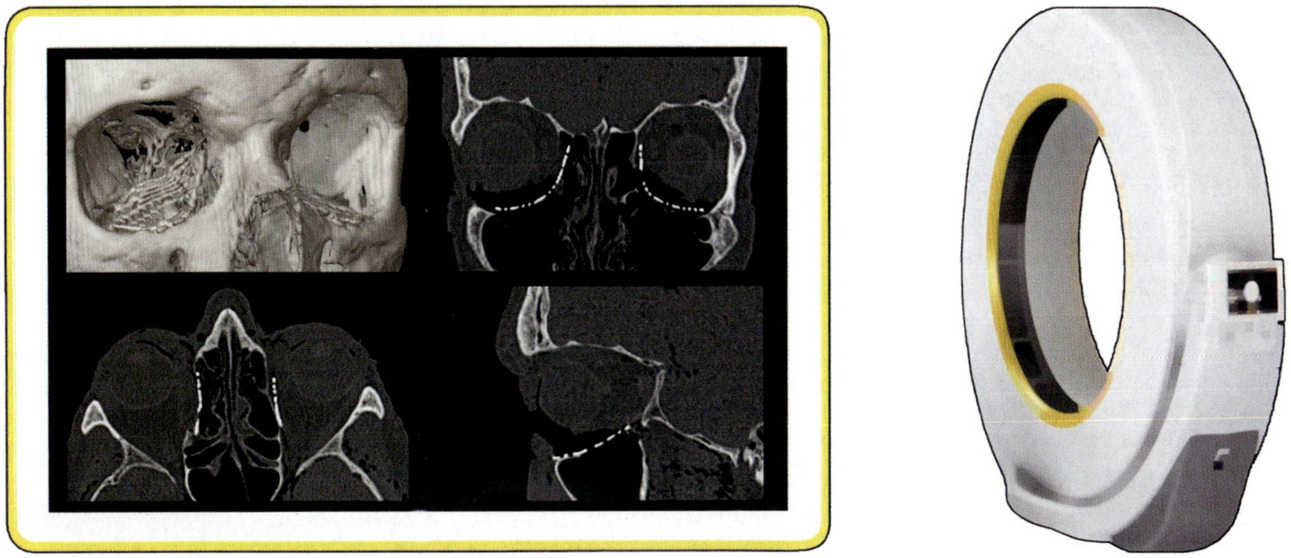

Fig. 5 Intraoperative scanning feedback. The result of intraoperative imaging is visualized on the screen (the necessary hardware is also shown). Based on these images, the surgeon could decide whether adjustment of the implant position was necessary. (Courtesy of Ruud Schreurs, MSc, Alfred G. Becking, MD, DMD, PhD, FEBOMS, Jesper Jansen, MD, DMD, PhD, and Leander Dubois, MD, DMD, PhD.)

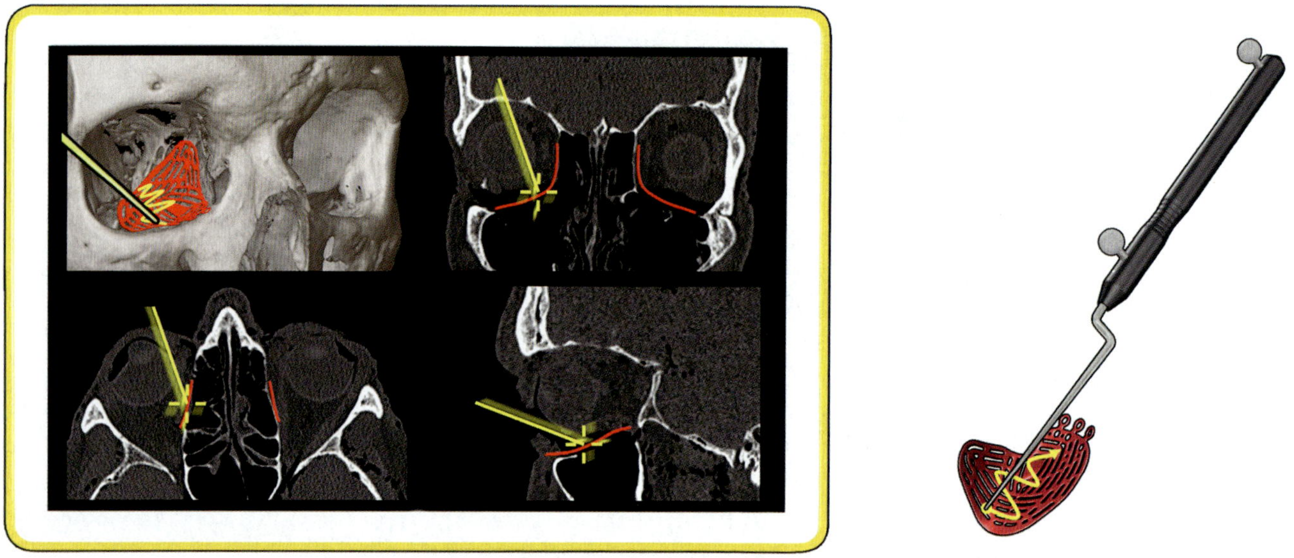

Fig. 6 Image-guided navigation, where information is collected through the use of a navigation pointer. The pointer is moved along the contour of the implant; the position of the pointer is shown in the multiplanar views, where it can be compared with the planned contour of the implant. (Courtesy of Ruud Schreurs, MSc, Alfred G. Becking, MD, DMD, PhD, FEBOMS, Jesper Jansen, MD, DMD, PhD, and Leander Dubois, MD, DMD, PhD.)

Reconstruction with virtual surgical planning (study 3)

In the third session, the surgeons had access to a 3D virtual computer environment and to virtual planning tools in iPlan Cranial, such as segmentation and mirroring. Information on the ideal position of the orbital implant, which had been planned with the help of a skilled and experienced technical physician, was available during reconstruction (Fig. 4). The surgeons were challenged to put the implant in the best position according to the virtual plan. The results of reconstruction with preoperative 3D virtual planning were compared with the baseline results (study 1).

Reconstruction with intraoperative imaging (study 4)

An intraoperative CT scan was made after reconstruction of the orbits in this study. A scanning protocol identical to the T0, T1, and T2 studies was used for intraoperative imaging. The implant position was verified by the surgeon on the information seen in Fig. 5 and, if required, the orbital implant position was corrected. The procedure and the scans were repeated until the surgeon was satisfied with the resulting implant position. The results were compared with baseline (study 1).

Reconstruction with intraoperative image-guided navigation (study 5)

All orbits were reconstructed with assistance of intraoperative image-guided navigation (Kolibri; Brainlab AG). The preoperative virtual surgical plan was linked to the intraoperative position of the cadaver head (registration).[15–19] The cadaver head was tracked using a skull reference marker array (Brainlab AG). After a stable position of the orbital implant was achieved intraoperatively, the navigation pointer was moved along the implant. The result was verified on the multiplanar views: the surgeon could compare the trajectory of the pointer with the contour of the planned position of the implant, which was shown as an overlay (Fig. 6). Results were compared with the baseline study (study 1).

Reconstruction with intraoperative marker-based navigation (study 6)

In this study, intraoperative navigation was again used, but feedback was obtained by indicating orientation markers in the implant design. Three markers were embedded in the preformed implant design, in a triangular fashion (Fig. 7).[11,20] The markers were indicated as landmarks in the virtual surgical planning, which allowed comparison between the current position of the marker (indicated with the navigation pointer) and the planned position. This feedback was both visual, to obtain information about the direction of displacement, and quantitative, on the amount of displacement (as seen in Fig. 8). The

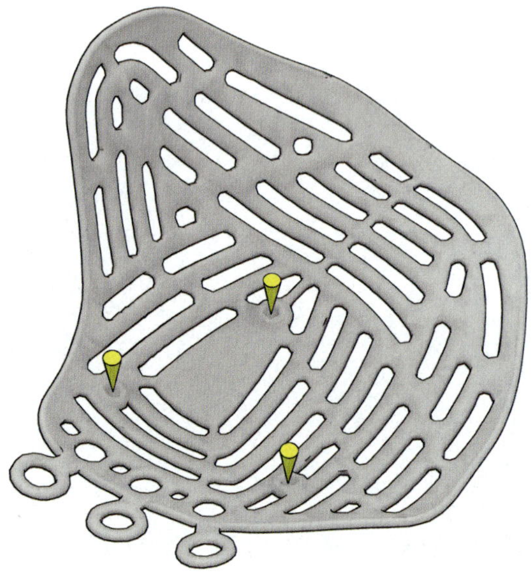

Fig. 7 Navigation markers embedded in the preformed implant (*arrowheads*). (Courtesy of Ruud Schreurs, MSc, Alfred G. Becking, MD, DMD, PhD, FEBOMS, Jesper Jansen, MD, DMD, PhD, and Leander Dubois, MD, DMD, PhD.)

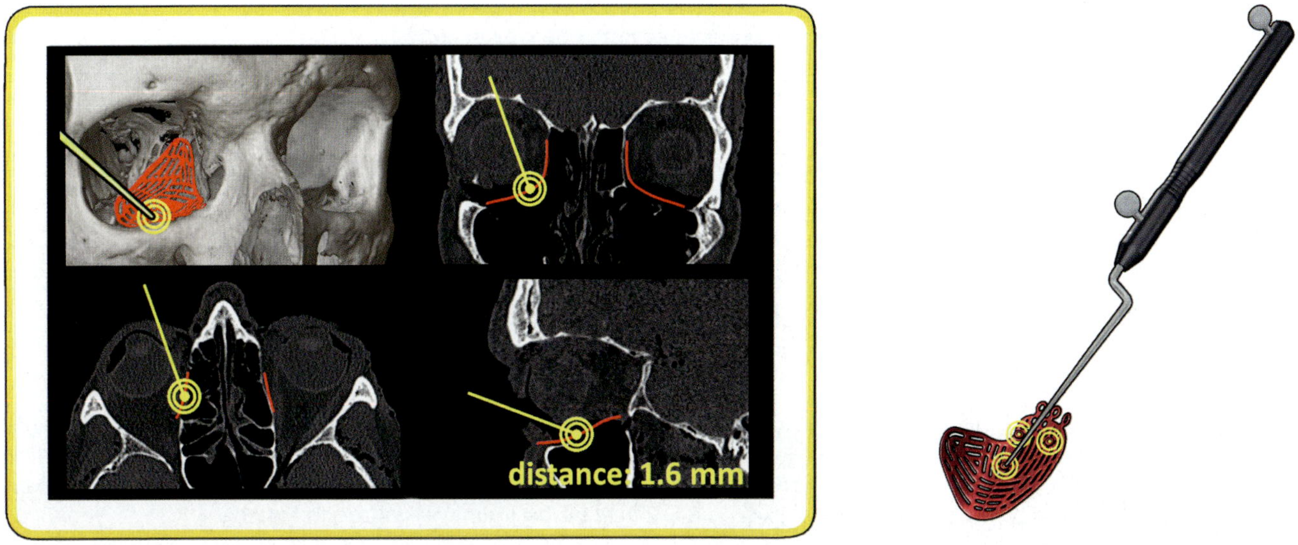

Fig. 8 Feedback obtained if the pointer is positioned at one of the marker points. In the multiplanar views, the position of the marker in relation to the landmark in the virtual surgical planning is compared for guidance. Quantitative feedback on the deviation between pointer position and planned marker position is also provided. (Courtesy of Ruud Schreurs, MSc, Alfred G. Becking, MD, DMD, PhD, FEBOMS, Jesper Jansen, MD, DMD, PhD, and Leander Dubois, MD, DMD, PhD.)

implant-guided navigation workflow results were compared with the results of the image-guided navigation workflow (study 5).

Reconstruction with intraoperative real-time navigation (study 7)

For this study, a real-time navigation workflow was developed and used. An instrument (Titanium Orbital Positioner) was designed that attached to the preformed orbital implant and was compatible with tracking by the navigation system. The cohesion between implant, instrument and navigation tracking allowed calculation of the implant position from the instrument's position, even during positioning of the implant. Real-time feedback on the current implant position in comparison to the planned position was provided, both visually and quantitatively, and the surgeon could be steered to the correct implant position under navigation guidance. The instrument attachment to the preformed implant and the feedback obtained during positioning are shown in Fig. 9. The reconstruction was compared with reconstruction with implant-oriented navigation (study 6).

Results

The results are all presented in later discussion in the same manner; statistical workflows, however, differed in some situations because of study design or scientific insights over the years. The outcome of the Orbital Implant Positioning Frame (shown in Fig. 1) parameters (roll, pitch, yaw, and translation) are provided in tables, and graphic representation of the mean obtained implant position with each technique (in relation to the planned position) is provided in the figures.

Conventional transconjunctival reconstruction (study 1)

The rotational and translational deviations of the acquired implant position in relation to the planned implant position are provided in Table 1. The mean and standard deviations of the positioning parameters show that there is minimal control in positioning of the orbital implant: the mean rotation around the z-axis (yaw) is larger than 15° and the mean translation is 5 mm. A maximum value of 47.6° is seen for the yaw. Precision, the consistency of positioning, is also low, as seen by the large standard deviations. Visual appraisal of the average acquired position of the implant (Fig. 10) illustrates the size of the quantitative deviations found. These results underline the need for intraoperative control during reconstruction.

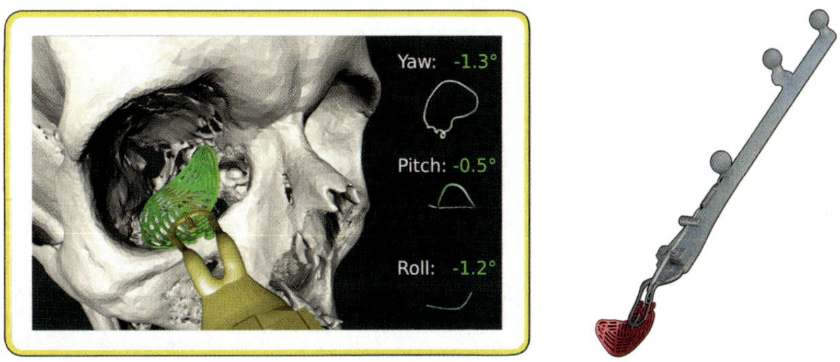

Fig. 9 Real-time navigation feedback and hardware. The designed instrument attached to the implant (and could be released after fixation). This made visualization in 3D possible (with the color of the implant changing according to the amount of deviation still present) as well as quantitative feedback on all positioning parameters. (Courtesy of Ruud Schreurs, MSc, Alfred G. Becking, MD, DMD, PhD, FEBOMS, Jesper Jansen, MD, DMD, PhD, and Leander Dubois, MD, DMD, PhD.)

Table 1 Rotational and translational deviation in conventional reconstruction (baseline)

	Conventional	
	Mean	SD
Roll (deg)	−9.8	9.1
Pitch (deg)	−1.3	3.1
Yaw (deg)	17.8	10.9
Translation (mm)	5.0	2.2

The mean and standard deviations (SD) of the rotations (roll, pitch, yaw) and translation are given.
Abbreviation: deg, degrees.

Reconstruction with transsinusoidal endoscopy (study 2)

The rationale behind endoscopic-assisted orbital reconstruction is that a bidirectional view is created for the surgeon: the implant's position may be visually assessed both transconjuctivally and, with the aid of an endoscope, transsinusoidally.[7] The resulting implant positions are quantified in Table 2 and visualized in Fig. 11. The results suggest that there is no significant improvement with the use of an endoscope compared with the baseline. Although there are some unrelated advantages regarding exhibition of the procedure for training surgeons,[21,22] accuracy and consistency of implant placement are again low.

Reconstruction with virtual surgical planning (study 3)

With virtual surgical planning available, the surgeon is able to check the information in the planning during the reconstruction of the orbit. In Table 3, the results are compared with the baseline study: roll, yaw, and translation are significantly more accurate with 3D virtual surgical planning. The standard deviations are smaller than in the baseline reconstructions as well, demonstrating improved precision. The addition of 3D virtual planning is considered to be superior to conventional reconstruction with multi-planar reconstruction information from a CT scan. Additional anatomic landmarks of the preoperative 3D planning, enhanced insight in the extent of the fracture, and the detailed knowledge of the ideal implant position help the surgeon to achieve a better reconstruction result (in terms of implant position).[1,23,24] The mean acquired implant position is visualized in Fig. 12.

Reconstruction with intraoperative imaging (study 4)

With intraoperative imaging, major deviations from the ideal position can be identified and may be altered intraoperatively, to avoid a second procedure and potential complications.[13,25,26] The position of the orbital implant improves significantly in terms of roll, yaw, and translation compared with the baseline study (Table 4), showing the advantageous effect of an intraoperative imaging during reconstruction. In Fig. 13, the improvement on implant positioning yielded by intraoperative imaging is shown. Significant improvement in yaw, the parameter with the largest deviation, is also recorded if the position after the first reconstructive attempt and the final CT scan are compared (Table 5), demonstrating the learning effect of intraoperative imaging and the guidance it provides.

Reconstruction with intraoperative image-guided navigation (study 5)

Image-guided navigation feedback may be generated immediately after the implant is first positioned. From comparison of the pointer's trajectory with the implant's contour in the

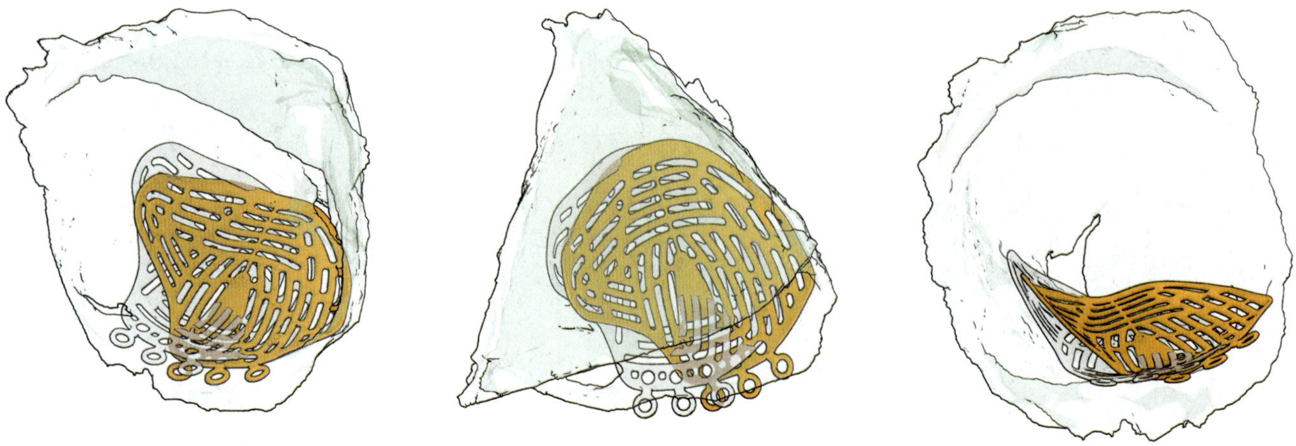

Fig. 10 Angulated, top, and frontal view of the mean acquired position of the orbital implant with conventional reconstruction (*orange*). The planned implant position is visualized in gray. A deviation in yaw can be best appraised in the top view, whereas roll is best seen in the frontal view. (Courtesy of Ruud Schreurs, MSc, Alfred G. Becking, MD, DMD, PhD, FEBOMS, Jesper Jansen, MD, DMD, PhD, and Leander Dubois, MD, DMD, PhD.)

Table 2 Quantification of endoscopic-assisted implant positioning, compared with conventional implant positioning

	Conventional		Endoscope		
	Mean	SD	Mean	SD	*P* Value
Roll (deg)	−9.8	9.1	−7.1	5.6	.19
Pitch (deg)	−1.3	3.1	−0.3	3.7	.24
Yaw (deg)	17.8	10.9	14.5	11.8	.14
Translation (mm)	5.0	2.2	4.2	2.1	.19

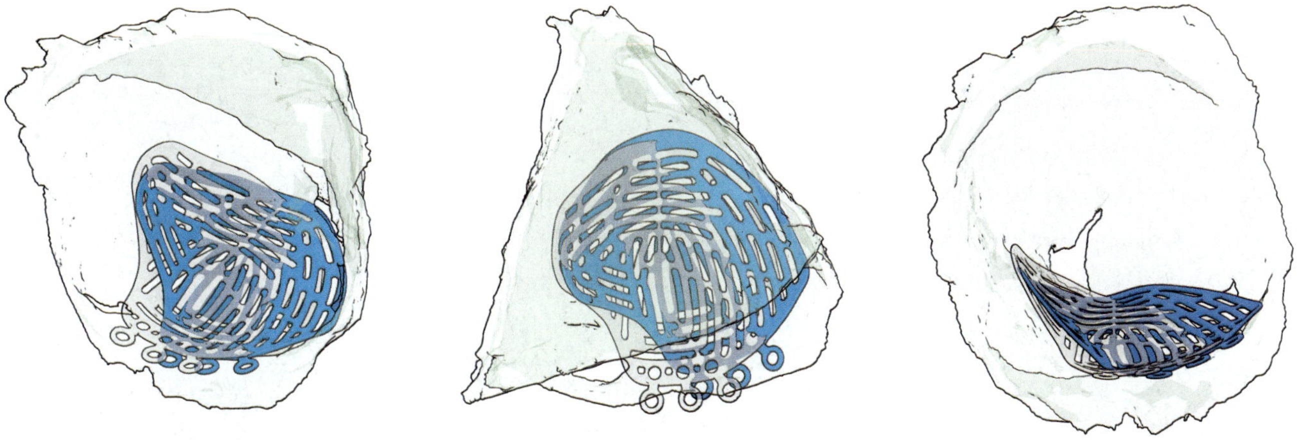

Fig. 11 Mean acquired position with endoscopic-assisted orbital reconstruction (blue) compared to the planned position (grey). (Courtesy of Ruud Schreurs, MSc, Alfred G. Becking, MD, DMD, PhD, FEBOMS, Jesper Jansen, MD, DMD, PhD, and Leander Dubois, MD, DMD, PhD.)

Table 3 Results of reconstruction with virtual planning versus results of conventional planning

	Conventional		Virtual Planning		
	Mean	SD	Mean	SD	*P* Value
Roll (deg)	−9.8	9.1	−4.5	3.5	.01
Pitch (deg)	−1.3	3.1	−1.1	2.2	.78
Yaw (deg)	17.8	10.9	5.2	6.8	<.01
Translation (mm)	5.0	2.2	2.6	1.7	<.01

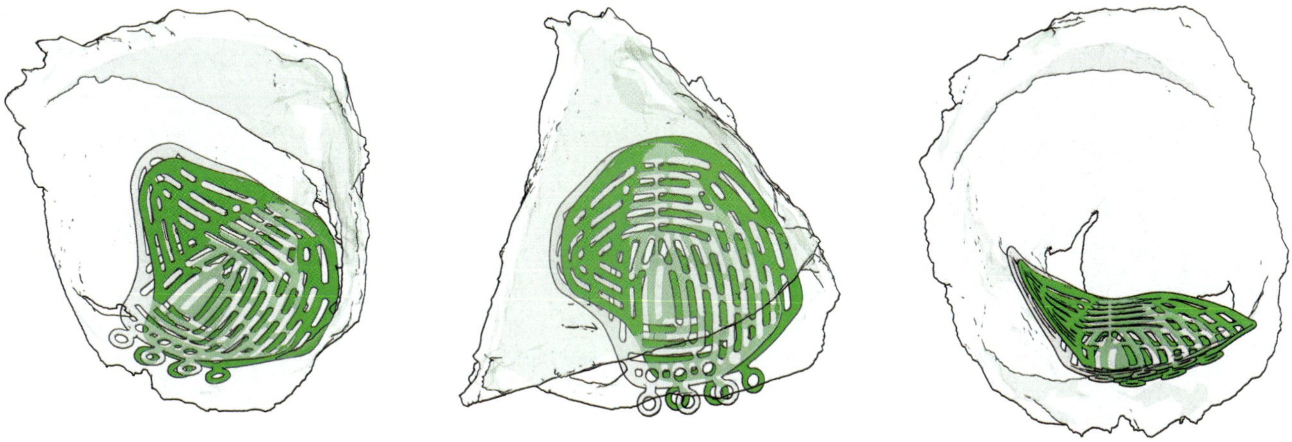

Fig. 12 Average position of the implant for reconstruction with preoperative virtual planning (*green*). The planned position is visualized in gray. Compared with Figs. 9 and 10, the average obtained position resembles the planned position more closely. (Courtesy of Ruud Schreurs, MSc, Alfred G. Becking, MD, DMD, PhD, FEBOMS, Jesper Jansen, MD, DMD, PhD, and Leander Dubois, MD, DMD, PhD.)

Table 4 Quantification of orbital implant position obtained with intraoperative imaging

	Conventional		Intraoperative Imaging		
	Mean	SD	Mean	SD	*P* Value
Roll (deg)	−9.8	9.1	−2.5	4.2	.01
Pitch (deg)	−1.3	3.1	−1.8	3.7	.37
Yaw (deg)	17.8	10.9	6.8	7.8	<.01
Translation (mm)	5.0	2.2	3.0	1.4	<.01

Compared with conventional reconstruction, significant improvements for all parameters but pitch are seen.

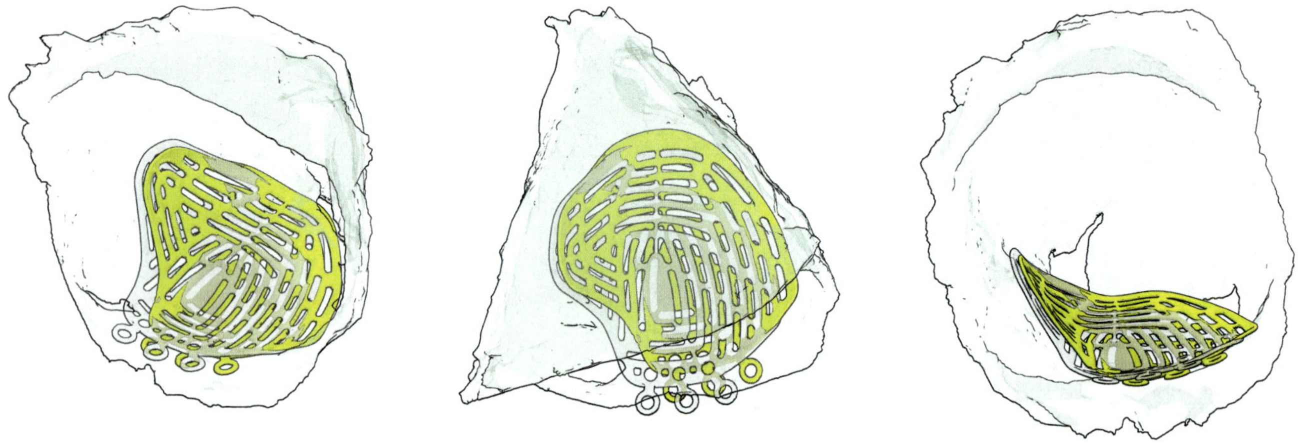

Fig. 13 Obtained implant position after reconstruction with intraoperative imaging (*yellow*). The mean of the final implant positions is visualized. (Courtesy of Ruud Schreurs, MSc, Alfred G. Becking, MD, DMD, PhD, FEBOMS, Jesper Jansen, MD, DMD, PhD, and Leander Dubois, MD, DMD, PhD.)

Table 5 Comparison of first result and final result in the cadaver group with adjustments after the first intraoperative image

	First Intraoperative CT		Final Intraoperative CT		
	Mean	SD	Mean	SD	*P* Value
Roll (deg)	−2.1	8.2	−1.5	3.6	.78
Pitch (deg)	−1.2	2.9	−1.9	4.5	.48
Yaw (deg)	10.2	13.2	5.6	10.1	.02
Translation (mm)	3.6	1.4	2.9	1.0	.16

Table 6 The effect of image-guided navigation on translation and rotation of the resulting implant position

	Conventional		Image-Guided Navigation		
	Mean	SD	Mean	SD	*P* Value
Roll (deg)	−9.8	9.1	−2.3	4.8	<.01
Pitch (deg)	−1.3	3.1	−1.1	2.2	.77
Yaw (deg)	17.8	10.9	8.8	8.1	<.01
Translation (mm)	5.0	2.2	3.3	1.6	<.01

The baseline results, conventional reconstruction, are used for comparison.

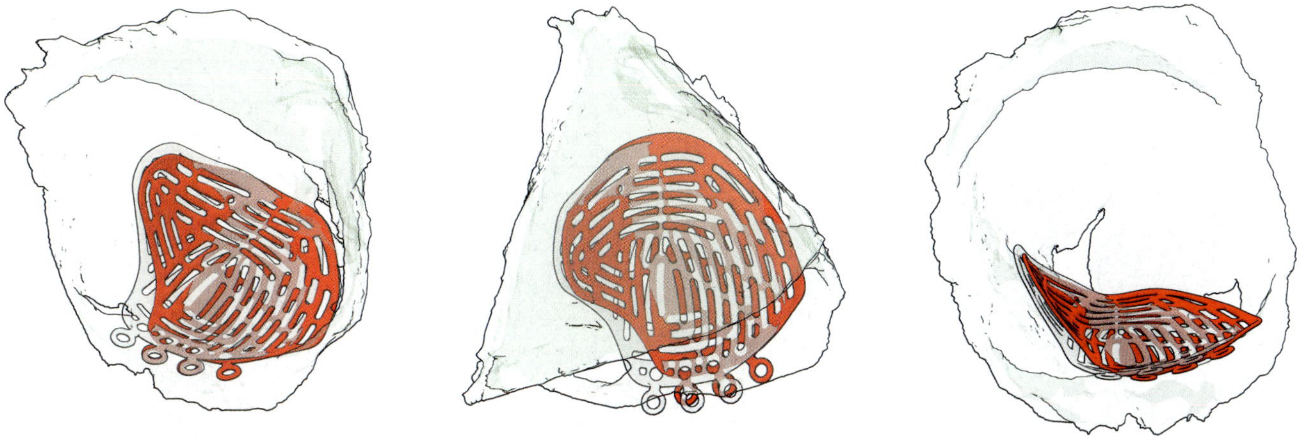

Fig. 14 Mean position of the implant after image-guided navigation reconstruction (*red*). The planned implant position is also visualized (*gray*). (Courtesy of Ruud Schreurs, MSc, Alfred G. Becking, MD, DMD, PhD, FEBOMS, Jesper Jansen, MD, DMD, PhD, and Leander Dubois, MD, DMD, PhD.)

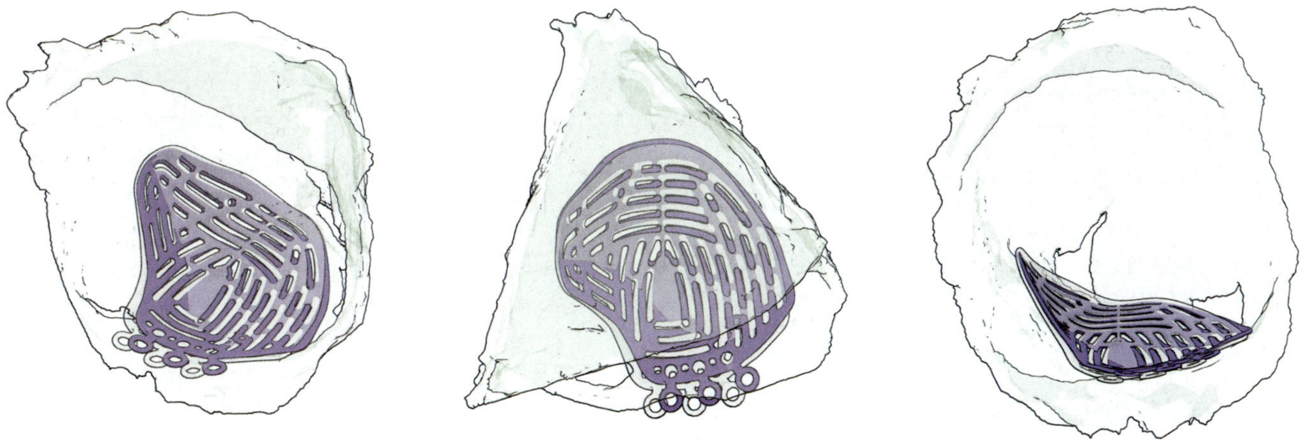

Fig. 15 Marker-based navigation result (*purple*). The mean position resembles the planned position (*gray*) closely. (Courtesy of Ruud Schreurs, MSc, Alfred G. Becking, MD, DMD, PhD, FEBOMS, Jesper Jansen, MD, DMD, PhD, and Leander Dubois, MD, DMD, PhD.)

Table 7 The effect of image-guided navigation on translation and rotation of the resulting implant position

	Image-Guided Navigation		Marker-Based Navigation		
	Mean	SD	Mean	SD	*P* Value
Roll (deg)	−2.3	4.8	−2.3	3.1	.16
Pitch (deg)	−1.1	2.2	−2.2	2.8	.52
Yaw (deg)	8.8	8.1	6.0	8.1	.02
Translation (mm)	3.3	1.6	1.4	0.7	<.01

The baseline results, conventional reconstruction, are used for comparison.

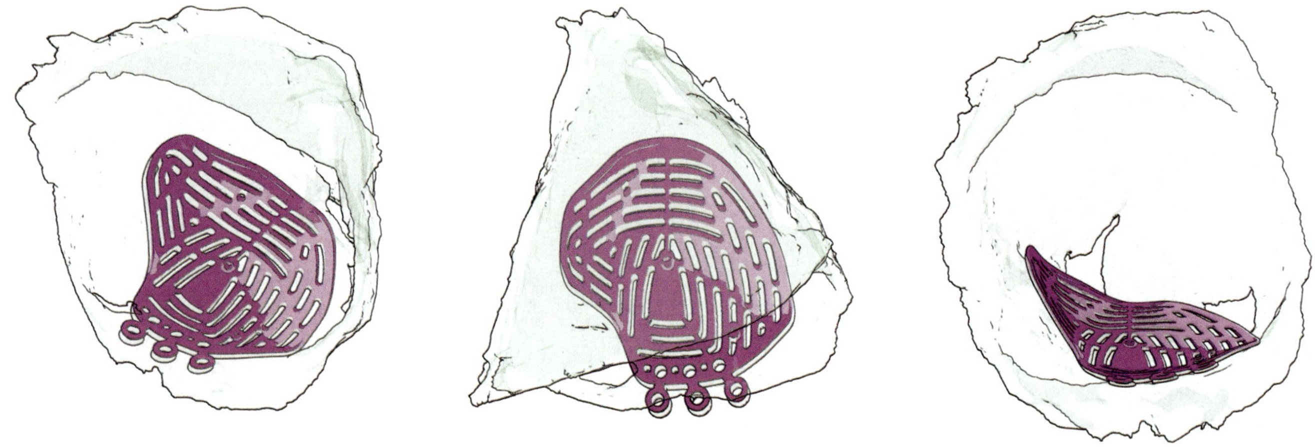

Fig. 16 Mean position of the implant obtained with the real-time navigation workflow. The result (*pink*) is virtually indistinguishable from the planned position (*gray*), indicating excellent accuracy. (Courtesy of Ruud Schreurs, MSc, Alfred G. Becking, MD, DMD, PhD, FEBOMS, Jesper Jansen, MD, DMD, PhD, and Leander Dubois, MD, DMD, PhD.)

Table 8 Linear mixed model estimates for the effect of technique on the outcome parameters

	Marker-Based Navigation	Real-Time Navigation	
	Model Estimate	Model Estimate	*P* Value
Roll (deg)	3.2	2.0	.03
Pitch (deg)	1.5	1.3	.53
Yaw (deg)	3.4	2.2	.01
Translation (mm)	1.8	1.3	<.01

The *P* values are generated from Likelihood Ratio tests between a model with and without navigation.

multiplanar views, the surgeon is able to evaluate the need for adjustment of the position of the implant.[1,2,18] After adjustments are made, their effect is again assessed directly afterward. This short feedback loop for control and improvement of implant position yields significant improvement in acquired implant position in comparison to the baseline reconstruction (Table 6). Roll, yaw, and translation are further improved through image-guided navigation. Fig. 14 demonstrates the mean position with image-guided navigation and the planned position of the implant.

Reconstruction with intraoperative marker-based navigation (study 6)

Although image-guided navigation provides direct feedback after positioning and leads to better outcome in terms of positioning, the feedback itself could be improved: moving of the probe along the implant means that the surgeon needs to evaluate the implant's position through interpretation of continuously shifting multiplanar views.[27] The thought behind marker-based navigation is that more static, and quantitative, feedback is obtained from the marker positions; the triangular fashion makes interpretation of the 3D position feasible. Marker-based navigation is compared with image-guided navigation (study 5) and proves to be significantly more accurate in positioning an orbital implant in translation and yaw (Fig. 15, Table 7). The precision is improved as well, as seen from the smaller standard deviations. With marker-based navigation, intraoperative handling thus becomes more intuitive.

Reconstruction with intraoperative real-time navigation (study 7)

The real-time navigation workflow leads to very accurate positioning of the orbital implant, with small deviations compared with the planned position (Fig. 16, Table 8). Compared with the marker-based approach, positioning improves in terms of translation, roll, and yaw. This improvement may be explained by the real-time nature of the feedback.[12] In image-guided or marker-based navigation, the surgeon can either obtain feedback or adjust the implant's position and needs to switch between these processes. In real-time navigation, adjustment of the implant position is possible under navigation guidance. Feedback is presented in a true 3D fashion. Next to an improvement in implant position, surgery time is reduced and appraisal of the feedback by the surgeon is higher.

Discussion

These studies have been designed and executed to assess the relevance of individual parts of modern technologic advancements for orbital reconstruction, instead of the grouped results of computer-assisted surgery (3D virtual planning, intraoperative imaging, and navigation). Significant progress in reliability and predictability has been achieved by introducing 3D virtual preoperative planning in which surgeons are thought to gain better insight in local anatomy, defect size, and complexity. This enhanced insight in turn generates helpful additional anatomic landmarks, leading to improvement in implant positioning.[1,23,24] The same is true for traditional intraoperative imaging with CT, which also demonstrates a significant improvement in implant positioning, and it is hoped, decreases the need for secondary procedures.[25,26]

Three methods of intraoperative navigation have been assessed in combination with 3D virtual planning. Image-guided navigation significantly improves implant positioning compared with traditional reconstruction; however, marker-based navigation increases implant positioning even further and brings the mean translation within the calibration error. Using the Advanced Concepts of Orbital Reconstruction research protocol, the more user-friendly real-time navigation proves to be the safest, fastest, and most accurate way to place an orbital implant into the ideal position. The instrument for orbital implant positioning has not been clinically introduced yet: it is a proof of concept and in the process of further development.

The goal to assess different techniques for discriminative outcomes of individual steps in orbital reconstruction seems to be achieved, even with the restrictions in the materials and methods: small series, few surgeons, and no clinical circumstances (human cadaver models). Studies 1 to 5 were designed to be one-on-one comparisons of the assessed techniques, but studies 6 and 7 had a different design. Care has been taken to make the outcomes comparable, for instance, through repeating the marker-based reconstruction for the cadaver group of study 7. Still, interpretation of these results and translation to a clinical setting warrant caution.

The focus of the studies in this article, and of many other studies, is on orbital implant positioning.[4,16,25,28,29] Outcome evaluation and presentation lead one to believe that implant positioning will be improved tremendously by using these novel technologies. Of course, the overarching goal for orbital reconstruction is not to improve orbital implant position, but to improve the quality of life for patients with orbital wall fractures. Surgery itself is an additional trauma to the orbit and its contents and should be well indicated and balanced with the anticipated outcomes of nonsurgical or less-invasive treatment options.[30,31] Surgery and reconstruction with orbital implants have a distinct place in treatment of orbital wall fractures. When indicated, orbital implant positioning should be performed as accurately and precisely as possible, to improve bulb position, ocular movements, orbital volumes, and esthetic outcome.[13,23,32,33]

Clinics care points

- Significant progress has been made in terms of reliability and accuracy of orbital reconstruction with the introduction of computer-assisted surgery techniques. A significant effect is seen for each individual technique and techniques can be combined to further optimize feedback during reconstruction.
- The effect of intraoperative navigation can be enhanced by providing more intuitive feedback on implant position. The more intuitive and user friendly the feedback is presented, the more accurate the implant is positioned.
- Translation of results from a preclinical setting to a clinical setting always warrants caution.
- The focus in these studies, and many other studies, is on implant position. However, the main goal in orbital reconstruction is not to improve surgical precision but to improve quality of life for the patient. Accurate implant positioning should be viewed as a means to achieve the goal, rather than a goal in itself.

Disclosure

In the submission process, in kind funding was declared. In all these studies, Brainlab provided the navigation equipment in kind, while KLS Martin provided the preformed orbital implants in kind. Additionally, for the real-time navigation, Brainlab provided the IGT link license in kind. KLS Martin provided the instrument in kind. This sub-project was supported by the S.O.R.G. Research Grant Award 2017.

References

1. Gellrich N-C, Schramm A, Hammer B, et al. Computer-assisted secondary reconstruction of unilateral posttraumatic orbital deformity. Plast Reconstr Surg 2002;110(6):1417–29.
2. Bly RA, Chang S-H, Cudejkova M, et al. Computer-guided orbital reconstruction to improve outcomes. JAMA Facial Plast Surg 2013; 15(2):113–20.
3. Rana M, Chui CHK, Wagner M, et al. Increasing the accuracy of orbital reconstruction with selective laser-melted patient-specific implants combined with intraoperative navigation. J Oral Maxillofac Surg 2015;73(6):1113–8.
4. Zimmerer RM, Ellis E, Aniceto GS, et al. A prospective multicenter study to compare the precision of posttraumatic internal orbital reconstruction with standard preformed and individualized orbital implants. J Craniomaxillofac Surg 2016;44(9):1485–97.
5. Chen C-T, Pan C-H, Chen C-H, et al. Clinical outcomes for minimally invasive primary and secondary orbital reconstruction using an advanced synergistic combination of navigation and endoscopy. J Plast Reconstr Aesthet Surg 2018;71(1):90–100.
6. De Cuyper B, Abeloos J, Swennen G, et al. Intraoperative navigation and cone beam computed tomography for restoring orbital dimensions: a single-center experience. Craniomaxillofac Trauma Reconstr 2020;13(2):84–92.
7. Dubois L, Jansen J, Schreurs R, et al. Predictability in orbital reconstruction: a human cadaver study. Part I: endoscopic-assisted orbital reconstruction. J Craniomaxillofac Surg 2015;43(10). https://doi.org/10.1016/j.jcms.2015.07.019.
8. Jansen J, Schreurs R, Dubois L, et al. The advantages of advanced computer-assisted diagnostics and three-dimensional preoperative planning on implant position in orbital reconstruction. J Craniomaxillofac Surg 2018. https://doi.org/10.1016/j.jcms.2018.02.010.
9. Jansen J, Schreurs R, Dubois L, et al. Intraoperative imaging in orbital reconstruction: how does it affect the position of the implant? Br J Oral Maxillofac Surg 2020;58(7):801–6.
10. Dubois L, Schreurs R, Jansen J, et al. Predictability in orbital reconstruction: a human cadaver study. Part II: navigation-assisted orbital reconstruction. J Craniomaxillofac Surg 2015;43(10). https://doi.org/10.1016/j.jcms.2015.07.020.
11. Dubois L, Essig H, Schreurs R, et al. Predictability in orbital reconstruction. A human cadaver study, part III: implant-oriented navigation for optimized reconstruction. J Craniomaxillofac Surg 2015;43(10):2050–6.

12. Schreurs R, Dubois L, Ho J, et al. Implant-oriented navigation in orbital reconstruction part II: preclinical cadaver study. Int J Oral Maxillofac Surg 2020;49(5):678–85.
13. Jaquiéry C, Aeppli C, Cornelius P, et al. Reconstruction of orbital wall defects: critical review of 72 patients. Int J Oral Maxillofac Surg 2007;36(3):193–9.
14. Schreurs R, Dubois L, Becking AG, et al. Quantitative assessment of orbital implant position-a proof of concept. PLoS One 2016;11(3). https://doi.org/10.1371/journal.pone.0150162.
15. Eggers G, Mühling J, Marmulla R. Image-to-patient registration techniques in head surgery. Int J Oral Maxillofac Surg 2006;35(12):1081–95.
16. Metzger MC, Hohlweg-Majert B, Schön R, et al. Verification of clinical precision after computer-aided reconstruction in craniomaxillofacial surgery. Oral Surg Oral Med Oral Pathol Oral Radiol Endod 2007;104(4):e1–10.
17. Widmann G, Stoffner R, Bale R. Errors and error management in image-guided craniomaxillofacial surgery. Oral Surg Oral Med Oral Pathol Oral Radiol Endod 2009;107(5):701–15.
18. Schramm A, Suarez-Cunqueiro MM, Rücker M, et al. Computer-assisted therapy in orbital and mid-facial reconstructions. Int J Med Robot Comput Assist Surg 2009;5(2):111–24.
19. Yu H, Shen SG, Wang X, et al. The indication and application of computer-assisted navigation in oral and maxillofacial surgery—Shanghai's experience based on 104 cases. J Craniomaxillofac Surg 2013;41(8):770–4.
20. Gander T, Essig H, Metzler P, et al. Patient specific implants (PSI) in reconstruction of orbital floor and wall fractures. J Craniomaxillofac Surg 2015;43(1):126–30.
21. Bevans SE, Moe KS. Advances in the reconstruction of orbital fractures. Facial Plast Surg Clin 2017;25(4):513–35.
22. Moe KS, Murr AH, Wester ST. Orbital fractures. Facial Plast Surg Clin 2018;26(2):237–51.
23. Schmelzeisen R, Gellrich NC, Schoen R, et al. Navigation-aided reconstruction of medial orbital wall and floor contour in craniomaxillofacial reconstruction. Injury 2004;35(10):955–62.
24. Mahoney NR, Peng MY, Merbs SL, et al. Virtual fitting, selection, and cutting of preformed anatomic orbital implants. Ophthal Plast Reconstr Surg 2017;33(3):196–201.
25. Stuck BA, Hülse R, Barth TJ. Intraoperative cone beam computed tomography in the management of facial fractures. Int J Oral Maxillofac Surg 2012;41(10):1171–5.
26. Wilde F, Schramm A. Intraoperative imaging in orbital and midface reconstruction. Facial Plast Surg 2014;30(05):545–53.
27. Schreurs R, Dubois L, Becking AG, et al. Implant-oriented navigation in orbital reconstruction. Part 1: technique and accuracy study. Int J Oral Maxillofac Surg 2018;47(3). https://doi.org/10.1016/j.ijom.2017.09.009.
28. Essig H, Dressel L, Rana M, et al. Precision of posttraumatic primary orbital reconstruction using individually bent titanium mesh with and without navigation: a retrospective study. Head Face Med 2013;9(1):1–7.
29. Rana M, Holtmann H, Kanatas AN, et al. Primary orbital reconstruction with selective laser melted core patient-specific implants: overview of 100 patients. Br J Oral Maxillofac Surg 2019;57(8):782–7.
30. Zimmerer RM, Gellrich N-C, von Bülow S, et al. Is there more to the clinical outcome in posttraumatic reconstruction of the inferior and medial orbital walls than accuracy of implant placement and implant surface contouring? A prospective multicenter study to identify predictors of clinical outcome. J Craniomaxillofac Surg 2018;46(4):578–87.
31. Jansen J, Dubois L, Maal TJJ, et al. A nonsurgical approach with repeated orthoptic evaluation is justified for most blow-out fractures. J Craniomaxillofac Surg 2020.
32. Cai EZ, Koh YP, Hing ECH, et al. Computer-assisted navigational surgery improves outcomes in orbital reconstructive surgery. J Craniofac Surg 2012;23(5):1567–73.
33. Schlittler F, Schmidli A, Wagner F, et al. What is the incidence of implant malpositioning and revision surgery after orbital repair? J Oral Maxillofac Surg 2018;76(1):146–53.